PRAISE FOR
THE OXYGEN REVOLUTION

"Dr. Harch is a tireless researcher, brilliant clinician, and true pioneer in hyperbaric oxygen therapy. In this book, he offers compelling reasons for the widespread adoption and utilization of this remarkable, yet overlooked therapy."
    —Julian Whitaker, M. D., founder of Whitaker Wellness Institute and editor of Health & Healing newsletter

"One of the most important and insightful medical books in 40 years. If you or your loved one has a neurological condition, you cannot afford to be without this book; it has the potential to restore your lost life."
    —Vance Trimble, Pulitzer Prize winner and author of *The Uncertain Miracle*

"The second edition of *The Oxygen Revolution* is an essential text to understanding and using hyperbaric oxygen in a wide variety of indications. It is written by one of the true pioneer clinicians in this field with a wealth of clinical experience. I have personally seen HBOT make a significant difference in the lives of many people and have before and after brain SPECT scans to prove it."
    —Daniel G. Amen, M. D., CEO and Medical Director of Amen Clinics, Inc. and author of *Change Your Brain, Change Your Life*

"An authoritative, well-written book on a subject we all need to know more about. Highly recommended for physicians and health care consumers alike."
    —Nathaniel Altman, author of *The Oxygen Prescription*

"This excellent book is truly about a revolution, a recognition of the need to shift the emphasis in medicine away from the false hope that drugs will cure when tissues lack oxygen. Most diseases and injuries reduce oxygen delivery to tissues, but oxygen has been downgraded to the status of a supplement and there is no understanding of the importance of pressure in determining its dosage. Now that biological science has defined the key role of oxygen in the regulation of our genes, a new era beckons in which oxygen will be given its rightful place as a cornerstone of treatment by physicians and surgeons. *The Oxygen Revolution* deserves to be widely read because it will open minds."

—Philip B. James, Professor of Hyperbaric Medicine, University of Dundee, Scotland

"Paul G. Harch, M. D., is a medical maverick in the tradition of Dr. Ignaz Semmelweis. Both had the resolute beliefs, confidence, and outcomes that the treatments they endorsed saved lives. Both were doubted, dismissed, and discounted by peers, colleagues, and critics. Semmelweis was later proven and declared a visionary and pioneer for his promotion of 'hand washing,' which saved, and continues to save, millions of lives from bacterial diseases. I suspect the expanded use of hyperbaric oxygen therapy will eventually earn its place in medicine's accepted armamentarium. History has demonstrated the value, role, and contribution of medical mavericks like Dr. Harch and the need for more of them. This book serves as a valuable compendium in delivering the hard science demanded but often overlooked by mainstream medicine in controversial treatment arenas. It should be incorporated into what I anticipate will be further debate and demands regarding the use of HBOT for (currently) unindicated neurological disorders. Dr. Harch and his colleagues should be applauded and admired for their efforts in expanding our understanding of the ever-changing landscapes in neuroscience. This book will change lives, lives that haven't been born yet."

—Rick Rader, M. D., President of the American Academy of Developmental Medicine and Dentistry

"One must be a courageous enthusiast to espouse an innovative therapy! Such a person is Paul Harch, M. D., dogged in his determination to prove that hyperbaric oxygen in appropriate dosage is valuable as a therapeutic intervention for many neurological disorders.

It is surprising that this is an argued point when it is common knowledge that oxygen in the air is as necessary as water! Of issue is whether oxygen under greater than atmospheric pressure can maintain diseased tissue and accelerate healing in wounds caused by blood vessel problems, multiple sclerosis, viruses, birth injuries, strokes, and dementia. By today's standards, use of hyperbaric oxygen therapy (HBOT) to treat some of these is experimental, but because they have never been subjected to randomized prospective trials their benefit cannot be known for certain. However, in the past, penicillin was never subjected to a prospective trial nor was the use of digitalis! Furthermore, who would have thought that botulinum toxin, one of the world's most potent toxins, would become a valuable therapeutic intervention? Consequently, I have an open mind regarding HBOT while advocating prospective randomized trials to prove its indications or lack thereof.

Dr. Harch has produced a lucidly written, interesting, and thought provoking book that I recommend not only for those with disease of the nervous system, but for others who want to be informed regarding hyperbaric oxygen therapy."
—James F. Toole, M. D., Teagle Professor of Neurology and Professor of Public Health Sciences, Wake Forest University School of Medicine

"*The Oxygen Revolution* is a fascinating book written by one of the great pioneers in the field of hyperbaric medicine. Dr. Harch shares his incredible knowledge and experience in a compelling book that is both comprehensive and accessible to the lay person. It opens tremendous horizons in the treatment of numerous conditions and will give true hope to millions of people with chronic diseases."
—Pierre Marois, M. D., F. R. C. P., Ste-Justine University Hospital

"Dr. Edward Teller, Nobel Prize winning physicist and father of the hydrogen bomb and a friend and patient of mine the last ten years of his life once said to me: 'Hyperbaric oxygen is just too simple for most doctors to understand; they have forgotten their basic gas laws of physics.'

In this book, Dr. Harch has explained this treatment so simply and fundamentally that anyone, even most doctors, can grasp the concept. I consider Dr. Harch one of my co-workers and believe that this book is a brilliant, enjoyably readable, yet in-depth explanation of hyperbaric oxygen therapy (HBOT).

I am very proud of his work and trust him to continue to further my most fervent dream, the acceptance of HBOT in brain injuries and the healing processes of the human organism at an intra-cellular level.

The concepts in this book should be taught in every medical school and hospital and known in every household."

—R. A. Neubauer, M. D., founder of the Ocean Hyperbaric Neurologic Center

"Finally, a reader-friendly description of the miracle effects of hyperbaric oxygen therapy used to treat a yet-to-be-determined myriad of medical conditions! This chronicle, written by the most brilliant true scientist in the hyperbaric field, reveals the medical science behind this simple, noninvasive, life-altering treatment. Through this book, *The Oxygen Revolution*, Dr. Paul Harch has successfully revealed the exciting potential of this underused healing phenomenon. A must read for anyone wanting information about hyperbaric oxygen therapy.

This book will single-handedly bring hyperbaric oxygen therapy (HBOT) into the limelight it deserves and will serve as a tool for parents of children with cerebral palsy, other brain injuries and autism to fight to get HBOT covered by Medicaid and insurance companies. No longer will parents have to second mortgage their homes, treat their children at the bottom of a swimming pool or travel hundreds of miles to access HBOT."

—Julie Gordon, Director of MUMS National Parent to Parent Network

THE OXYGEN REVOLUTION

THIRD EDITION

HYPERBARIC OXYGEN THERAPY:

Breakthrough Gene Therapy for
Traumatic Brain Injury & Other Disorders

THE
OXYGEN
REVOLUTION
THIRD EDITION

HYPERBARIC OXYGEN THERAPY:

Breakthrough Gene Therapy for
Traumatic Brain Injury & Other Disorders

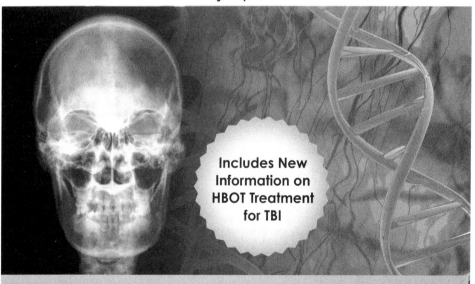

Includes New
Information on
HBOT Treatment
for TBI

PAUL G. HARCH, M.D., AND VIRGINIA MCCULLOUGH

Foreword by William A. Duncan, Ph.D.

Hatherleigh Press is committed to preserving and protecting the natural resources of the Earth. Environmentally responsible and sustainable practices are embraced within the company's mission statement.

Visit us at www.hatherleighpress.com and register online for free offers, discounts, special events, and more.

The Oxygen Revolution: Third Edition

Library of Congress Cataloging-in-Publication Data is available upon request.

ISBN: 978-1-57826-627-2

DISCLAIMER

The ideas and suggestions contained in this book are not intended as a substitute for consulting with a physician. All matters regarding your health require medical supervision. Names of medications are typically followed by TM or ® symbols, but these symbols are not stated in this book. Most of the patients who contributed their medical histories to this book have allowed their real names to be used. In the remainder of cases, the names of the patients have been changed.

Interior design by Jacinta Monniere, Jasmine Cardoza, Allison Furrer

Cover design by Adam Kesner, Deborah Miller

Printed in the United States

10 9 8 7 6 5 4 3 2

THIS BOOK IS DEDICATED TO:

The mothers of special needs children, who live quiet lives of hardship, immense sacrifice, often broken marriages, and loneliness in their pursuit of a better quality of life for their children; all the brain injured patients who can improve the quality of their lives with the information in this book; Dan Greathouse, who fortuitously changed my career with the privilege to treat him in 1991; and to my mother, who benefited from HBOT. She held our family together during many hard years as a single parent and encouraged me to apply to medical school when I was not so sure. She also believed in me as only a mother could. She said at the time of my birth that a "terrible mistake" had been made. (In 1954, mothers were heavily sedated during labor so her first introduction to me was after I'd made a trip to the nursery. When a red-haired boy was presented to a dark-haired Italian mother she just "knew" the hospital staff had mistaken identity. Over the years she has come to think otherwise.)

ACKNOWLEDGEMENTS

THE PUBLICATION OF THIS BOOK WOULD NOT HAVE been possible without the contribution of many people past and present. In my more youthful days I had the delusion that I could be successful, independent of the help of others: the controversion of "no man is an island." I've since learned otherwise and would like to mention just some of the people to whom I am indebted.

In the past several years, I have been introduced to a number of professional authors as possible collaborators, but the "fit" wasn't right until I was introduced to my coauthor Virginia McCullough by PR consultant and patient advocate, Julia Schopick. Thank you, Julia, and thank you, Virginia. From our initial agreement to a rough outline, through the many revisions and updates, to its present form, the writing of this book has been a smooth process, due not only to the comfortable working relationship that we have developed, but a common sense of purpose and perspective. Again, thank you, Virginia.

To Hatherleigh Press, thanks for taking a chance on us and our idea. I hope that together we can continue reaching those who need this information.

To my children, for their forbearance. The time taken to write this book, added to the other demands on my time, has collectively taken away from the time I would have liked to and could have spent with them. I hope they will understand in later years their component contribution to what I hope will be the impetus to revolutionize neurology with hyperbaric oxygen therapy.

To Phillip Tranchina, nuclear technologist *par excellance*! Had he not taken an interest in the SPECT brain imaging I was performing on the early patients in 1990–91 and personally overseen this project for the next 24 years, the beautiful images in this book, medical book chapters and other scientific publications, the leverage these images have provided would not have been possible.

To Jana Knight, an exceptional woman and hyperbaric technician who helped pioneer this world of hyperbaric neurology with me for 13 years. Her facility and relationship with countless brain injured children and her keen observation when I was not present helped make this all possible.

To Dr. William Duncan. Through his tireless efforts and extensive contacts within the government infrastructure I was able to launch a new medical society, the International Hyperbaric Medical Association, and gain access to critical government officials and agencies. He was crucial to the eventual approval of reimbursement of HBOT for diabetic foot wounds by Medicare. The American public owes him a debt of gratitude as well, especially in his latest heroic effort with the Patriot Clinics in Oklahoma. His and his wife Anita's sacrifice to deliver HBOT to our brain-injured servicemen and women is immeasurable.

To my late aunt, Gloria Russo who, through her generosity and moral support, helped keep our family together during a critical period in my childhood. If not for her timely intervention, it's likely that my life would have taken a different course. Thank you.

A thank you to Pat Ridge for expeditious transcription of the original manuscript.

And, most importantly, thanks to my wife, partner, and confidant, Juliette Lucarini—a beautiful woman in so many ways—for literally saving my life and the lives of my children in August 2005. Deepak Chopra says that we cannot ignore coincidences in our lives, and Juliette's appearance in my life was no coincidence; I know that she was God-sent, when she came into my life just before Hurricane Katrina. She saved my family and me as we traversed through the evacuation after the storm, relocation, salvage, FEMA trailer living, and the road show of working in multiple emergency departments in California, Louisiana, and Mississippi. It's difficult to believe that, just four months after the Hurricane, the first edition of this book was due. With Juliette at my side, I dictated the first draft of this book as we stayed in the California desert. Juliette: my family, this book, myself, and this body of work would not be here without you.

Lastly, a begrudging tip of my hat to Hurricane Katrina. While she wreaked so much havoc on the Southeast United States, residents of New Orleans, and me personally, my temporary unemployment and forced evacuation to a remote region of the California desert, specifically Lone Pine and Southern Inyo Hospital, afforded me the time to write this book.

It is now August 2015. Last night, we passed the tenth anniversary of Hurricane Katrina at a restaurant in New Orleans with friends who were similarly devastated by the Hurricane, the Gremillions. Their story is told in a book by Jennifer Gremillion, just released: *Life Storms*. At the time, they were in New Orleans for their inaugural book tour.

Reading her book prompted me to write this acknowledgement. It is no coincidence that I am rewriting this book exactly 10 years after I first started dictating it, while we were being evacuated from the site of Hurricane Katrina to California. All while meeting with friends *from* New Orleans *in* New Orleans, who had evacuated to California and are now living there. It is a time of great emotion and reflection; a time to realize that time itself is fleeting, that there is an urgency to be even bolder in Virginia's and my exhortation for people worldwide to seek, demand and obtain this life-saving, and quality-of-life-saving therapy—for themselves *and* their loved ones.

CONTENTS

INTRODUCTION   xvii

AUTHOR'S PREFACE   xxi

PART I   WHAT IS HYPERBARIC OXYGEN THERAPY?   1

          CHAPTER 1   WHY YOU SHOULD BE AWARE
                      OF HYPERBARIC OXYGEN THERAPY   3

          CHAPTER 2   OXYGEN DEPRIVATION AND THE
                      BODY'S INFLAMMATORY REACTION   29

          CHAPTER 3   THE CURRENT USES FOR HBOT   45

PART II   CONDITIONS THAT HYPERBARIC OXYGEN
          THERAPY CAN HELP   65

          CHAPTER 4   TRAUMATIC BRAIN INJURIES (TBI)
                      AND OTHER MEDICAL EMERGENCIES   67

          CHAPTER 5   BIRTH INJURIES AND CEREBRAL PALSY   99

          CHAPTER 6   STROKES   117

          CHAPTER 7   AUTISM   131

          CHAPTER 8   ALZHEIMER'S, PARKINSON'S, AND
                      OTHER NEUROLOGICAL DISEASES   141

CHAPTER 9   DIABETES AND CARDIAC DISEASE   161

CHAPTER 10   JOINT REPLACEMENT, ARTHRITIS,
             AND BONE REMODELING   169

CHAPTER 11   AIDS, ASTHMA, ALCOHOL ABUSE,
             AND OTHER USES FOR HBOT   181

CHAPTER 12   HBOT: AN ANTI-AGING TOOL   199

PART III   HOW YOU CAN TAKE ADVANTAGE OF HBOT   219

CHAPTER 13   THE TREATMENT EXPERIENCE
             AND COSTS   221

CHAPTER 14   ROADBLOCKS AND GATEWAYS
             TO THE FUTURE   239

CONCLUSION   WHEN IS HBOT RIGHT FOR ME OR MY
             LOVED ONE?   263

APPENDIX A   MAKING—AND CHANGING—HEALTH
             CARE POLICY   271

APPENDIX B   MORE ABOUT SPECT   277

GLOSSARY   279

RESOURCES   285

SPECIAL NEEDS RESOURCES   289

REFERENCES   291

INDEX   297

Introduction

WHY IS SOMEONE WITH A DOCTORATE IN political science and economics writing an introduction to a book about hyperbaric medicine, and specifically, one that includes using hyperbarics to treat brain injuries? In fact, this book explains that, contrary to popular belief, treating brain injury can be as routine as breathing, watching TV, and being able to fly in an airplane.

This medical treatment, hyperbaric oxygen treatment (HBOT), dramatically changed my life, the lives of my brother and my mother, along with other members of my family. The changes have been positive and permanent. Over the 15 years I've been involved with HBOT (and part of what I consider a true movement within medicine), I have seen hyperbaric medicine change the lives of thousands of individuals. Taking it one step further, seeing this treatment in action, I now believe we were bioengineered to use oxygen to heal and live.

For 10 years I had the privilege of serving the American people as one of just 34 congressional staff with direct oversight of the appropriated budget for the nation's healthcare infrastructure, including the National Institutes of Health (NIH), the Centers for Disease Control (CDC), the Agency for Healthcare Research and Quality (AHRQ), Medicare, the Food and Drug Administration (FDA), and so forth. In addition, I had considerable input into the welfare infrastructure, prisons, and education policy, and oversaw the budgets of over 80 federal agencies.

In the course of my work, I learned of hyperbaric oxygen therapy, an effective treatment for brain injuries (insults), which had been in use since 1937. At the time I learned about HBOT, it was already approved for three kinds of brain injury and three kinds of non-healing wounds. Nearly 80 years of world-wide research existed that confirmed what I witnessed in a number of people. Despite this record of effectiveness, HBOT was either not being used at all, or woefully underused.

Further, research conducted at the Department of Defense (DoD) and the Veterans Administration (VA) was looking at diagnostics, not treatment. Across the board, government agencies charged with healthcare had not moved beyond the myth that no treatment existed, or *could* exist to heal the brain. Hanging on to this stubborn belief prevented even looking at treatments that had the potential to work. The myth really prevented medical professionals—clinicians, researchers, and administrators alike—from adopting rational prevention and treatment strategies at the public policy level.

Sadly, I also discovered that at each critical point in the history of hyperbaric medicine, the decision to not recommend HBOT was never about its effectiveness or the science supporting it. It was always some other consideration.

However, at the public policy level, some of us working with HBOT and advocating for it set out to correct that problem, through the appropriations process. Dr. Harch and I gave DoD Medicine, the VA, the CDC, and the NIH the complete chronic brain injury protocol in 2001 that Drs. Harch, Neubauer, Van Meter, and Gottlieb had developed over the previous 23 years. (Acute protocols were already known.) Had the treatment been used starting at the time, we could have prevented the tragedy of over 1 million improperly treated young war veterans in our society (and countless millions of civilians). From the point of view of self-interest, the treatment would likely have saved billions in VA disability claims and medical benefits. HBOT found success in other areas. For example, using Dr. Harch's research and protocol, HBOT was approved for Medicare reimbursement for diabetic foot wound healing. The International Hyperbaric Medical Foundation (IHMF) created the National Brain Injury Rescue & Rehabilitation Project (NBIRRP) and as a result, hundreds of veterans and civilians have received HBOT. Government researchers received millions in research dollars and Dr. Harch, through my efforts with ex-Secretary of the Army, Martin Hoffmann, received $1.2 million to conduct his present TBI study.

But, not all the news is good. Suicide rates among veterans continue to rise, and have now reached 22 per day. On day-to-day practical terms, think of the billions in lost manpower from untreated injuries, and all because some in medicine refuse to recommend the treatment for chronic brain injuries because they have failed to conduct the so-called "definitive" study. In the end, the inability to do the necessary work to make this treatment an accepted healing tool has cheated both patients and tax payers.

It's often said that watching legislation be written and passed is akin to watching sausage being made. And so it is. Starting in 2008, the International Hyperbaric Medical Association (IHMA, sister organization to the IHMF)-endorsed bill, the TBI Treatment Act, passed in the U.S. House of Representatives, only to have the VA and others in military medicine block it in the Senate. Unfortunately, it became clear that the VA did not want HBOT to be paid for or become the standard through which their other therapies for TBI could be compared to. As a result, veterans were unable to go outside the VA system for reimbursable treatment.

After this failure at the federal level, the states have begun to rebel, since their budgets are being destroyed by untreated brain injury, especially in veterans. As a result, in 2013, Oklahoma led the way when the legislature passed the Oklahoma Veteran Recovery Plan. (The Oklahoma bill is discussed in this book.) It eventually passed in spite of efforts to prevent its passage. Under the Veterans Bureau Act of 1921, the state will be able to recover its costs of treating veterans with hyperbaric and other effective therapies for brain injury, PTSD, Agent Orange dementia, and other brain insults caused by federal government military service. Ten states are prepared to follow Oklahoma's example. This is tangible progress, and has occurred despite efforts to block it.

Finally, in 2014, I created Patriot Clinics, Inc., in Oklahoma, in order to start providing free treatment for our war veterans, my fellow service members (I served in the Army for eight years), who were being abandoned and harmed by the managed care system that focuses on treating symptoms and not the cause of the symptoms. We also treat others who need hyperbaric oxygen therapy, especially for those whose lives have been shattered by brain injury.

The Patriot Clinics have done 10,000 hyperbaric treatments in the past 21 months for nearly 300 patients, starting with a two-person multiplace chamber and growing to five treatment berths, and now adding another three at our new location. We expect to treat over 100 per day at our Oklahoma City facility, and eventually will have equipment to treat 300 per day. We have also combined other synergistic therapies with hyperbaric oxygen. This is just the beginning.

We have demonstrated to many state officials that our system should be adopted nationwide. We are partnered with many private clinics across Oklahoma who are prepared to join in getting veterans treated through this state partnership.

Clinics all across the nation are poised to join in the effort to deploy effective treatment for brain injury. At the International Hyperbaric Medical Foundation, we have launched a major nationwide charity effort to raise money to enable patients to be treated as close to their homes as possible. We are raising money for every qualified clinic willing to treat these men, women, and children. (For more information about this charity, check our resource list in the back of this book. You'll find our website address and I urge you to explore the information on our site. On a personal note, I urge every reader to act, and join our movement.)

Making this treatment routine, from acute treatment at ERs or urgent care centers, to treatment for chronic conditions, will cut mandatory and entitlement spending by many billions per year. It will restore lives, restore families, restore productivity, and reduce substance abuse, crime, and suicide. As we sit, 15 years into the 21st century, we are poised for an effective care revolution. Hyperbaric medicine shows the pathway to the kind of effective care I'm talking about. Its routine adoption is essential in order to achieve the kind of health care we want for our loved ones and for society.

By the time you finish this book, you'll understand the wide range of diseases that can be effectively treated with HBOT. One million men and women have battle casualties from our current military conflicts; but we can't forget victims of car accidents, those with sports injuries, and those injured in crimes, such as battered and abused women and children. Plus, we can address a range of work-related industrial injuries and those sustained by police officers and fire fighters. In other words, serious brain injuries treatable with HBOT can occur in countless situations we encounter in everyday life.

Put simply, current and future generations are depending on us to succeed. This book will show you why I feel so strongly about the possibilities of HBOT. With the publication of this new edition, I hope many more individuals will come to know the true miracle that a little oxygen can create in the lives of billions around the world who suffer from a range of diseases and disabilities. For those readers who themselves suffer, I assure you that there are few experiences in life as wonderful as feeling your brain switch on. For me, it all started with Dr. Harch restoring my health and the health of several people close to me. The impact it has had on us is profound and life-changing.

William A. Duncan, BA, MBA, PhD, HMT
President, Patriot Clinics, Inc.
President, International Hyperbaric Medical Association
Vice President (Development), International Hyperbaric Medical Foundation
Oklahoma City, Oklahoma
2015

AUTHOR'S PREFACE

JUST FOR A MINUTE, IMAGINE THAT I'M TELLING YOU a story about being locked in a stifling hot, sealed room, empty but for one chair. I explain that I had been in the room for hours, and the only window, though large, was painted shut. Every few minutes I tried to open that window, but it just wouldn't budge. Finally, I tell you that I'd given up and accepted my doom. "If someone hadn't rescued me," I say, "I'm certain I would have died for lack of oxygen."

You've been listening politely while I've told my story, but you're puzzled. Surely, a piece of information is missing. Finally, you scratch your head and ask the question that's been on your mind from the beginning: "Dr. Harch, why didn't you just pick up the chair, break the window, and let the air in?"

I slap my forehead with the heel of my hand. "Wow," I say, "why didn't I think of that?"

The first edition of this book was about breaking the window. With this new edition, we have broken the "big picture" window. In the 351 years since the advent of hyperbaric therapy in England (in 1664), no one has understood exactly what we are doing when we deliver a hyperbaric treatment. We know now. As I explain below (and have published previously in a medical journal), the ground-breaking news is that we are performing gene therapy. (You can read this important article online, as well as view the lecture I gave on this subject at HBOT 2014 in Albuquerque in August 2014 at the 9th International Symposium on Hyperbaric Medicine: Roadmap for the Future, at HBOT.com.)

Hyperbaric oxygen therapy (HBOT) is the "stupidly simple" answer to many health problems. Some of these conditions result from injury, some from disease. They can occur at any time of life, including during the birth process itself.

I originally wrote this book to help you understand the theory behind HBOT and to help you seek the treatment for yourself or your family should the need arise. My mission hasn't changed. In fact, it has become more urgent.

A rapidly increasing amount of clinical use and research validates the contents of the first edition of this book, so much so that I can't overemphasize your need to learn more about this overlooked and misunderstood treatment. It is a life- and quality-of-life saving treatment that you can't ignore—and one that you should demand when the situation calls for its use.

Patients routinely ask me why their doctors either know little about the treatment or have a dismissive attitude about it. At one time, I would have dismissed HBOT out of hand, too. I recall the day I first heard about hyperbaric oxygen therapy. I was in my third year of medical school at the Johns Hopkins University School of Medicine, and HBOT was mentioned in passing. Having never heard of it before, I asked my supervising resident doctor what it was. He didn't know a great deal about it himself, so he repeated what someone else had told him: "It's a type of oxygen therapy, it's performed in chambers, and it's worthless, unscientific, been thoroughly disproven, is charlatanism, snake oil sales, and fraud."

This incident occurred in 1978, and I quickly filed his answer in the same place I put all the other so-called cures or remedies that had been labeled snake oil. I also took his dismissive words as gospel, considering the source, the setting, and the school. In other words, I let someone else, in this case a doctor, do my thinking for me. It might come as a surprise to some readers that therapies such as acupuncture, chiropractic, and biofeedback were once relegated to the snake oil file of medicine, too. In fact, some doctors still have little faith in these therapies.

For a variety of reasons, most of which are rooted in ignorance and the "boom-bust" cycles of HBOT, the treatment has long had a cloud hanging over it. With the exception of a few applications, the treatment remains on the fringes of medicine—part of alternative or complementary medicine, much of which is subject to great suspicion. We'll explain the reasons for this in great detail as we go on.

Much has changed. I believe HBOT is now poised for acceptance into mainstream medicine. In fact, this is already occurring, for a number of reasons. Reports about the usefulness of the treatment for a variety of diseases have made their way into the media. For example, many heard about HBOT for the first time when the sole survivor of the Sago mine accident was transported from West Virginia to Pittsburgh, Pennsylvania, where a hyperbaric chamber was available. In addition, there has been a dramatic increase in the number of high-quality scientific studies on HBOT published in medical journals in the past 10 years.

It seems that hyperbaric oxygen therapy has made its way into public awareness through popular culture as well. As an example of the latter, the final episode of *Star Trek* features a scene in which a character was rushed to a hyperbaric chamber in an effort to save his life. A popular soap opera used a hyperbaric chamber as a "prop" in a hospital set, and even made it part of a story line. A few years before the *Oprah Winfrey Show* ended, frequent guest Dr. Mehmet Oz rolled out a hyperbaric chamber to demonstrate HBOT as one of the modern anti-aging tools. This trend will undoubtedly continue as HBOT enters the mainstream.

In addition, information about HBOT has been available for many years in a variety of sources, and patients seeking treatment for themselves and their loved ones have done their own research. Some patient advocacy organizations (discussed later in this book) have spread the word about the value of HBOT for specific conditions.

Unfortunately, however, a few badly designed studies have convinced some doctors that the treatment is worthless. Imagine hearing about a new, revolutionary pain medication. Some doctors show mild interest, but others are very skeptical because they believe they have all the necessary knowledge about controlling pain. Still, they agree to conduct a study of this new drug, but they give half the recommended dose and the patients in the study aren't helped. That study is a big step on the road to a bad reputation for this new drug. In medicine, that kind of reputation is difficult to overcome. Let's say another group of scientists also decides to study the new pain relief drug, but they triple the dose and some patients in their study become ill—some even report internal bleeding. Now reports go out that the treatment is not only worthless, it's dangerous, too!

Had a similar sequence of experimental under-dosing and overdosing been used at the outset of its application and development, aspirin would not be available to us today. Very low doses of aspirin are ineffective for pain relief and very high doses frequently cause stomach bleeding. Were it not for its long and established history, one of the most common medications on our planet could have ended up in the snake oil file—not because it's ineffective, but because it was misused. In the wrong hands, any treatment can become worthless.

The modern-day example of this misuse, mis-dosing, misunderstanding, and misperception of treatment lies in the unfortunate studies put out on the use of hyperbaric oxygen therapy in the treatment of persistent post-concussion syndrome of U.S. war veterans. As a result of widespread public and congressional pressure, as well as the precedent I set with treatment of U.S. veterans in 2008, a series of poorly-designed studies were conducted by the U.S. Department of Defense and individuals with very little experience treating chronic brain injury with HBOT. The result has been a confusing mixture of data. However, when examined, the data showcases the effectiveness of the doses that I, and others like me, have used to treat brain injury. Other data show an ineffectiveness of some doses, which have never before been used to treat brain injury; still more data suggest the possible harm of yet another dose. The issue of dosing will become clear as you move through the information in this book; however, the result of this research is the unequivocal proof that HBOT *is* effective in the treatment of traumatic brain injury of all severities and injuries of any age and in any person. *The evidence is now so compelling that every patient with a brain injury should seek this treatment as soon as possible after receiving a brain injury.*

Someday, medical history books are going to say that HBOT is an example of a treatment that came into acceptance not because doctors introduced it to patients, but because patients demanded access to the treatment from their doctors. This is going to start with traumatic brain injury. In my experience, patients and the lay public in general do not have difficulty understanding the vast benefits of the judicious use of oxygen therapy in situations in which oxygen deprivation has resulted in injury. For patients, "breaking the window" usually makes perfect sense. Based on countless conversations with patients and their families, once these individuals understand the specific and unique way we use oxygen therapeutically, they embrace its possibilities.

You will get the scientific foundation from this book, which will then help you seek HBOT on your own. I know for certain that once you absorb the information in this book, you will never let anyone, not even physicians, tell you that HBOT is without value.

This brings me to a final, critical point that I want you to burn into your memory. An unfortunate and damaging habit has permeated and dominated the medical profession for decades, and must now come to an end. Perhaps it is simply a specific example of a more ubiquitous human habit, but in the medical profession it has had devastating consequences and should no longer be tolerated. In a nutshell, the habit is: offering negative opinions, often in strident tones, without a factual basis for these statements. Others presume doctors have authority and knowledge of medical matters far beyond that of the lay public. And in some ways this is true—but in a commonsense way, it is *not*.

Because doctors are *exposed* to vast amounts of medical information, this has led to the presumption that we *possess* vast knowledge—indeed we are *expected* to have knowledge about all matters in medicine. So, when patients ask questions and seek opinions, doctors feel compelled to give answers. Many doctors find it difficult—nearly impossible—to answer a medical question by saying, "I don't know."

However, as you likely know from your own experience, *titles do not confer knowledge—they presume knowledge.* Just because someone has the title of "Doctor," or is Chairman of the Department at XYZ University School of Medicine, does not mean that that person has specific knowledge about everything in medicine. This is especially true when it comes to a subject about which so few doctors have ever received instruction, like hyperbaric medicine. Like all doctors or experts in any field, any doctor you consult should be required to demonstrate their supposed expertise; in fact, you should demand it.

In the case of hyperbaric oxygen therapy, and especially hyperbaric oxygen therapy for neurological conditions, many physicians almost compulsively give the answer that I was given in medical school. The problem, aside from it being totally false, is that this answer violates the Hippocratic Oath. Traditionally, physicians have tried to abide by the Hippocratic Oath (or at least some components of it). The single component of the oath that should be viewed as inviolate and to which all doctors must adhere is the promise to "do no harm." And the first step in doing no harm is *"saying no harm;"* if physicians don't have a sound factual basis on which to offer an opinion, they should say, "I don't know," or else defer to someone more knowledgeable. The consequences of a negative, ignorant opinion are devastating beyond comprehension. Patients will take that opinion as authoritative, which will in turn deny them, their family members, loved ones, or friends the possibility of life or an improved quality of life. And that is totally unacceptable.

I admonish you not to accept a physician's negative opinion about this therapy. As you will see, very few people in medicine are as informed about hyperbaric oxygen therapy as you will become after reading this book. Case in point: Dr. Sarah Parks is a seasoned cancer surgeon, now retired from Tulane University School of Medicine. She was one of my hyperbaric medicine doctors-in-training, and in 2011 she performed a survey of 120 U.S. medical schools and found that 75 percent of them had nothing in their curriculum about hyperbaric medicine. This means that current doctors-in-training (along with those from my generation) have never received formal instruction in the principles and practice of hyperbaric medicine. This, more than any other fact, should provide all the proof necessary to understand the need to do your own research. Ask questions, seek answers, read this book, and come to your own conclusions.

Life-Changing Discoveries

It's interesting that medical therapies are often advanced by famous individuals who are afflicted with certain diseases. For example, Mary Tyler Moore has been a tireless public advocate for juvenile diabetes. Both Michael J. Fox and Mohammed Ali have testified before Congress about Parkinson's disease. Former Attorney General, Janet Reno, has also gone public and discussed her experience with Parkinson's disease. Ronald Reagan's family has raised awareness about Alzheimer's disease, and while they were alive and able, Dana and Christopher Reeve educated others about spinal cord injuries. It's certainly true that "celebrated" cases stimulate both advances in medical application and additional research. This happens in part because the public begins to advocate for it, too. From time to time in this book, you will read about "non-famous" citizens who have joined together to help educate each about HBOT and find the treatment they need.

On a personal level, it's been interesting to come across a curious feature of hyperbaric medicine. The field has always been filled with physicians who have tried HBOT on patients and saw such dramatic—often phenomenal—results that the physician's career changed just as dramatically. I know this is true, because it happened to me. In the late 1980s and early 1990s, I used HBOT with divers who had resistant, untreatable, or delayed cases of brain decompression illness, and the results so impressed me that it altered the course of my career and by extension, the course of my life. I saw patients improve to such an extent that it couldn't be explained in any way other than to attribute it to a single cause, the HBOT they had received. Or, put another way, the effectiveness of the therapy was proved by treating individual cases, and no other treatment had brought about these results.

In the late 1980s and early 1990s, when I began to work with HBOT for neurological conditions, I saw the positive—even amazing—results firsthand. I saw divers whose lives had been completely shattered by chronic brain decompression illness recover and begin to live normally again. My early work challenged previous assumptions in diving medicine and it led to an expansion of the potential applications for HBOT, especially to brain injured children. What I had been told was impossible happened before my eyes. (You will read brief case histories of a few of these and other patients throughout this book.)

Using This Book

IMPORTANT NOTE: A critical feature of this book is the series of Internet links to videos, articles, newspaper pieces, patient testimonials, and so forth, all of which powerfully illustrate the healing power of hyperbaric oxygen therapy. These have been included to augment the information in this book and lead you to resources that will expand your knowledge of this important treatment.

To view these news articles and patient testimonials, go to www.HBOT.com and click on the Oxygen Revolution tab on the home page. This will take you to all of the videos, articles and other resources mentioned in this book.

I've arranged this book to be as informative and helpful as possible, with the goal of making you aware of all your treatment options for a wide range of diseases and conditions.

The medical profession claims that randomized, controlled experimental clinical studies are the foundation of medical care. However, the medical decisions made by every doctor for a patient are often dictated by a previous patient's response to a given treatment. Similarly, a patient's choice of treatment is often guided by the results a friend or family member experienced with a given treatment. We know these as individual testimonials, and when doctors publish them they're called case reports. Throughout this book, you will be encouraged to read articles and view videos documenting patient responses, before and after HBOT treatment. In all but one of these news articles (the Major Ben Richards' story is the exception), the piece was prompted by the patient, television or radio station, or some institution because of the life-changing effect HBOT had on the patient. In these cases, the patient or family was so moved by the response of the person to HBOT that they went to the media to announce the result.

One day, HBOT will be a universally recognizable term, with its uses widely known. However, since the numerous applications of the treatment are still relatively new and some are not yet accepted within conventional medical circles, I have arranged the information in this book to first provide a foundation on which the rest of the information builds.

In the following chapters, you'll find essential explanations of HBOT, the body's inflammatory reaction, and a discussion of the range of conditions for which HBOT is currently used. It's been my experience that when individuals comprehend the mechanisms of the treatment, they gain confidence in its usefulness. Any medical treatment can sound theoretical or abstract, but the provided case studies should help illustrate the way in which this treatment has changed lives.

I've arranged the information in such a way as to help you find the disease or condition of primary interest to you, and I've also addressed a range of medical emergencies, from cardiac arrest to serious accidents, such as near drowning and carbon monoxide poisoning. You will also find individual chapters that discuss the application of HBOT for a wide variety of diseases, including: traumatic brain injury, seizures, birth injuries, strokes or cerebrovascular accident (CVA), autism, a range of neurological diseases, from multiple sclerosis (MS) to Alzheimer's disease, diabetes and cardiac disease, joint replacement and arthritis, alcohol and drug detoxification, cancer, and a variety of other illnesses, from environmental disease to AIDS to chronic fatigue syndrome.

Unfortunately, for some conditions, such as Alzheimer's disease and MS, few good treatments are available and currently, most believe that the best they can hope for is to control symptoms and perhaps retard the progression of the disease. Although HBOT is not yet "approved" (which means "typically reimbursed") for use with these common neurological diseases, a considerable body of research (including my own) demonstrates that it is a safe and effective treatment option. For this reason, I believe that patients have a right to explore HBOT. (I also address the issue of "off-label" use of HBOT so that you will understand the context in which the term is used.) This book offers my vision for the future of

HBOT, including expanded research applications and its potential use in anti-aging medicine.

I assume that you're curious about the practical issues surrounding treatment, so later in this book you will find information about the experience of HBOT treatments, including descriptions and photos of hyperbaric chambers. Throughout the book, you will see SPECT brain scans that show the physiological changes brought about by HBOT. (In addition, you can see brain scans and patient video exams at HBOT.com.)

HBOT stands poised to take its rightful place in the world of healthcare, but in order to complete its journey to acceptance and entrance into mainstream medicine we will need a coalition of educated patients, physicians and researchers, and public and private policy makers. I hope we can use recently gathered research information to strengthen the current dialogue about this treatment, and my hope is based in part on the contribution of educated citizens like you.

Finally, a glossary that defines medical terms and presents the "language of HBOT" appears at the back of the book, along with a list of resources you may find helpful as you do your own research.

Without question, my work with brain-injured children has been incredibly rewarding, which is why I dedicated this book to the mothers whose determination to find help for their children has touched me so deeply. It isn't easy to put into words, but I have been privileged to witness the painful beauty of these mothers, who often do so much more than simply seek treatment for their individual children. These women are driven by the most basic biological and human instinct in that they each seek to improve the ability of their child to be self-sufficient. They know that once they are gone, their children's fates are likely to be determined in a harsh economic environment where only the strongest survive. The mothers whose children I treat have also faced the heartbreaking reality that their children will never be normal. Given the framework of reduced expectations they set their sights on simply improving the quality of life for their injured children. These women have formed support and exchange networks and have even raised their own research funds.

Over the last decade, I've treated children diagnosed with cerebral palsy, autism, certain learning disabilities, and genetic disorders. In addition, I know of a child diagnosed with fetal alcohol syndrome (FAS) who has also benefited from HBOT. One driving force behind this book is to educate parents, and parents-to-be, about HBOT. Far too many remain unaware that the treatment may benefit their children, even long after the event that caused the injury.

For the last 26 years or more, the driving force behind my professional life has been treating patients and conducting HBOT research. Some of my patients had been seen by multiple specialists, and were told that "nothing more could be done." They were also given a list of what I have come to refer to as "never-evers:" your child will never ever smile, drink from a cup, sit up, interact with you, walk, talk, know you, and so forth. These are predictions that can never be accurately made in the very early stages of an injury or disease, and one after another, many of these children exceed these predictions *before* they receive HBOT, only to go even farther *after* HBOT.

I've also lectured widely to my colleagues about the many applications of HBOT. In addition to my rewarding clinical practice, I've been especially gratified by speaking to audiences comprised of lay men and women, most of whom don't allow outdated information to prevent them from absorbing new ideas.

This book is a natural outgrowth of my work with patients, patient advocacy organizations, the lay public, and my colleagues. It's a far cry from my original intentions of practicing surgery. Mine has been a non-linear, unpredictable path. What I first thought was just happenstance, I now know was a calling. Countless patients come into Room #3 at my clinic, imbued with the drive from a higher power. I finally realize that I have been driven by the same. If not for God's hand in my life, I would have died in a life-changing auto accident 35 years ago, at the start of my surgical training. Unknowingly, it launched me onto my current path, one that has defined my purpose in life. I exist to advance this life-saving and quality-of-life-saving therapy, plain and simple.

I believe that it's no exaggeration to say that HBOT represents a healthcare revolution in the making. By the time you finish reading this book and you understand the vast number of conditions for which HBOT is a valuable treatment, I think you will agree. Then, together, we will "break the window."

Paul G. Harch, M. D
2015

PART I

WHAT IS HYPERBARIC OXYGEN THERAPY?

B Y THE TIME YOU FINISH THE CHAPTERS INCLUDED in Part I, you will have a working understanding of hyperbaric oxygen therapy, including an overview of its history. It often surprises newcomers to this information that innovative pioneers have been looking at ways to harness the power of oxygen since the late nineteenth century! However, HBOT pioneers exploring the possibilities of the therapy in the twentieth century worked at significant disadvantage. While they could see that the treatment had positive effects on a variety of diseases, they were unable to explain why HBOT worked; furthermore, they were unable to demonstrate physiological changes in the brain. Today, however, we understand why HBOT is effective and modern technology allows us to demonstrate our results using Single Photon Emission Computed Tomography (SPECT), the sophisticated imaging technology described in this book.

Chapter 2 is of particular importance, because an understanding of the body's inflammatory reaction is the key to comprehending the vast number of applications for HBOT. Primarily, you'll see why HBOT promotes wound healing throughout the body, from traumatic brain injuries to diabetic foot wounds. With this foundation of practical knowledge (plus the more recent information on HBOT's effects on the genes of inflammation), you will find the explanations of HBOT for individual conditions quite easy to understand. You'll also likely begin to ask why HBOT isn't applied more liberally to the vast majority of conditions dominated by inflammation!

CHAPTER I

WHY YOU SHOULD BE AWARE OF HYPERBARIC OXYGEN THERAPY

O XYGEN MAKES LIFE POSSIBLE. AS YOUNG CHILDREN, we all learned this when our first science lessons taught us about oxygen, the "element in air and water needed by every living thing." In our Western outlook, oxygen is more than just "one element among many." It is what we view as our "life force."

This fundamental understanding of oxygen is one of the reasons that patients and other lay people I encounter on a daily basis have no trouble with the concept of hyperbaric oxygen therapy (HBOT). They nod their heads, showing their willingness to expand their knowledge of this essential "life force "element. Since these individuals are open to the concept of using oxygen therapeutically, then generally, all they need to convince them of its value is more information. That's the purpose of this book. In order to consider HBOT for yourself or a family member, you need to educate yourself. You may even need to educate your doctor!

Harnessing the Power of Oxygen and Pressure!

In the most basic terms, we used to believe that HBOT consisted solely of the use of elevated pressures of oxygen to treat many conditions in which tissues have been damaged by varying degrees of oxygen deprivation. This sounds simple enough, but it's not true. Harnessing the power of oxygen is a more complex proposition, and the oxygen has a partner in HBOT. This oxygen-only understanding of hyperbaric oxygen therapy was naïve and partly responsible for the medical profession's long-standing misunderstanding of this therapy. It also points to another curiosity of science and medicine, which is that basic scientific research sometimes doesn't translate to clinical understanding and implementation.

The revelation of these two facts came to me in a most unusual way, and as you learn more about HBOT, the full meaning of this experience will be become clear to you. In the summer of 2008, Bill Duncan and I were preparing a congressional appropriation request for $10 million dollars to perform a research study using HBOT to treat our brain-injured veterans. In conjunction with this request, I submitted a question to the FDA to learn if I needed permission from them to perform the study. I was requesting permission to treat U.S war veterans from Iraq and Afghanistan with 1.5 atmospheres of hyperbaric oxygen (a dose of oxygen over seven times what we are breathing in room air, at a pressure 1.5 times our atmospheric pressure at sea level). Four years later, the answer I received from the FDA stunned me: I was told that it was simply unacceptable for me to study a single dose of HBOT. They viewed HBOT as a drug with two components: increased pressure and increased oxygen. They said I needed to study multiple doses of pressure, multiple doses of oxygen, and multiple doses of both (to conform to scientific rigor).

When I read their response, I immediately thought of all of the lay and commercial drug industry criticisms of the FDA. In my nearly 34 years of exposure to hyperbaric oxygen therapy since medical school, I had never heard of anyone mention that the effects of hyperbaric oxygen therapy were due to anything other than the exposure to increased pressure of oxygen. No physician had every talked about the pressure itself as an independent factor. At the same time, the FDA had no idea if increased pressure had any biological effect. One can think of increased pressure of a gas more easily when thinking of the equivalent increased pressure of water, or hydrostatic pressure. (To clarify, hydrostatic pressure is the weight of the fluid above any point in the depth of the fluid; in other words, the pressure exerted by the fluid above. So, the pressure of all of the seawater above you if you are 33 feet under water is 14.7 pounds/square inch of water. In the case of a gas it is the weight of the gas above whatever measuring point you choose. For example, our atmospheric pressure at sea level is also 14.7 pounds/square inch. That is the weight of all of the gas in out atmosphere from sea level up to outer space.) The FDA professionals were looking at HBOT with fresh eyes, and said that since you are putting people in a chamber where you turn up the pressure *and* give them increased oxygen, there are naturally two active components: increased pressure *and* increased oxygen.

How right they were.

So: when the going gets tough…the tough go to the library! I performed a literature search on the biological effects of increased hydrostatic pressure. I found 70 years of basic scientific research, beginning in the 1940s, that documented the effects of even very small amounts of increased atmospheric pressure on all organisms, ranging from algae to man. (You will read more about this in the chapter on arthritis, but as you likely know, arthritis patients often tell their doctors that they can sense approaching weather changes hundreds of miles before the weather reaches them—the origin of statements like, "I feel it in my bones." These expressions reflect exactly what these patients experience.) I could only shake my head; it seemed as if basic science researchers had never talked to clinical hyperbaric doctors, and vice versa.

The implication of these findings was that it helped unlock one of the two keys to understanding HBOT, its past, and its future. It also led to *redefining HBOT* physiologically for the first time in 351 years and publishing that definition in a medical journal, specifically, *Medical Gas Research: HBOT is the use of increased pressure and increased pressure of oxygen as drugs to treat basic disease processes and their diseases.* In other words, HBOT is a *combination drug* whose activity consists of the independent actions of increased pressure, the increased pressure of oxygen, and the combined effects of both.

What's more, the basic science research and clinical experience suggests that the *effects of HBOT can vary across a wide range of different doses of pressure and increased oxygen.* Once you understand this, you will understand the controversy surrounding HBOT in the previous 351 years along with the different results that doctors and patients have experienced throughout the roller coaster ride that is HBOT's history. This is especially true of the conflicting results now generated by the Department of Defense in their studies on HBOT in chronic concussion. The different results are due to the different doses of HBOT used, just like our previous example of aspirin.

The second key to understanding HBOT was discussed as a hypothetical in the previous edition of this book, but has now been confirmed in the past seven years. For decades, doctors and researchers have documented that a daily exposure to HBOT for patients with chronic non-healing wounds has resulted in healing of those wounds (diabetic foot wounds and radiation wounds are two of the most common examples). What we haven't known is what is happening with each HBOT—what is responsible for healing these wounds? What are the intervening steps after each HBOT that cause the amazing effects we see with this therapy?

Well, let's think it through. To heal a wound you need to grow new tissue: new blood vessels, new connective tissue, new bone, new skin, and in the case of a brain disorder, new brain tissue. To grow new tissue, you have to stimulate cells to divide and multiply. For cells to divide and multiply, the DNA of the cells must be stimulated in some fashion. In 1997, a researcher named Dr. Siddiqui suggested that HBOT was a DNA stimulant. The hyperbaric medicine field yawned. Over the next 12 years, researchers reported increases in individual proteins, hormones, and enzymes after hyperbaric treatment. While this was interesting, it still did not have an impact on the field.

By 2008, however, critical advances in mass DNA analysis techniques were developed that opened our eyes to a revelatory understanding of HBOT. In 2008, Dr. Godman and colleagues, basic science researchers all, found that a single hyperbaric treatment to the human cells that line all of our blood vessels turns on and turns off as many as *8,101 genes in the 24 hours following HBOT.* If the cells are given another treatment at 24 hours, even more genes are activated, and the cells begin to roll up and form small blood vessels.

So: not one gene, not two genes, or even the handful of genes that were implicated in the previous 12 years of research, but 8,101 genes—*8,101 genes!* Furthermore, the turned-on genes are those genes which code for growth and repair hormones and the anti-inflammatory genes; the turned-off genes are the pro-inflammatory genes and those that code for cell death.

Other research followed and found that *different pressures turn on different and overlapping sets of genes and different levels of oxygen turn on different and overlapping sets of genes. Oxygen was responsible mostly for turning on the genes and pressure for turning off the genes.*

Essentially, hyperbaric oxygen therapy is the oldest, most enduring, most effective, and most extensive gene therapy known to man. And it's totally organic. Each time a patient undergoes a hyperbaric treatment, the physician is playing a symphony with their genes using different pressures and different amounts of oxygen. The dissemination of this fact alone will prove to be one of the most important factors in the advance of HBOT. It will also help you to understand everything that follows in this book. (Again, I encourage you to watch the lecture on HBOT and Gene Therapy that I gave to the 9th International Symposium, available at HBOT.com. Pay attention to the Venn diagrams showing all of the overlapping and independent genes at different pressures and different doses.)

So, because of its profound implications, let's look at this again: when oxygen is under pressure, it acts like a drug, and has drug-like effects on the DNA and other components of each cell, bringing about permanent changes in the cell and surrounding tissue. The actual increase in pressure alone is doing the same thing. Over the decades of experimentation with HBOT, we've discovered that its "secret of success" is its cumulative effect, meaning that after 25–35 treatments, the body's tissues have been permanently changed.

At the same time, HBOT also has a host of other effects. In particular, and perhaps most important, is that a variety of studies have shown HBOT seems to recruit stem cells to wounded areas. In using HBOT, genes are stimulated to produce growth and repair hormones simultaneously with stem cells acting as a stimulus to tissue regeneration. This is what makes HBOT such a versatile treatment.

In the treatment of acute conditions, HBOT also affects the patient's DNA. Evidence points to its ability to reverse injury to the DNA or overcome a type of freeze that is put on the DNA from various insults. (I use the term "insult" throughout this book when referring to a variety of harmful injuries and events.) It's been my experience that when people understand the treatment in terms of using oxygen as a drug, they quickly open their minds to the idea that the treatment has far-reaching implications.

For many people, the next logical question is: "What conditions can be helped by using hyperbaric oxygen therapy? "The short answer is that HBOT is useful for conditions caused or aggravated by reduced oxygen levels in the tissues, and other forms of injury as well. As you can see, this covers enormous ground.

If we look at only brain injury or "insult," as it is called in medicine, tens of millions of individuals in the United States alone are affected by one or more of the following:

- Birth injury, e. g., cerebral palsy and hypoxic-ischemic encephalopathy that can be caused by oxygen deprivation during or shortly after birth.
- Other pediatric neurological conditions such as autism.

- The long-term effects of head trauma.
- The lingering effects of stroke.
- Degenerative neurological diseases, such as multiple sclerosis.
- Parkinson's disease, Alzheimer's disease, and non-Alzheimer's senility.
- Accidents that result in oxygen deprivation, including common emergency situations such as near drowning, near hanging, carbon monoxide poisoning, cardiac arrests, and exposure to neurotoxins.
- Alcohol and drug detoxification and the treatment of the brain injury resulting from these and other substances, including pharmaceutical drugs.
- Cancer.

It's no exaggeration to say that hyperbaric oxygen therapy should be universally available, both as an emergency treatment and as standard therapy for diseases that develop as we age. Just as we need oxygen from our earliest stages of development until we take our final breath, we may benefit from HBOT at any point in our lifetime that we encounter situations in which tissues anywhere in the body are deprived of adequate oxygen. I realize the great implications of that statement, because indeed, this therapy may have a profoundly positive effect on the course of the diseases we associate with aging. Accidents and diseases can occur at any stage of life as well, thus making HBOT a potentially valuable therapy over a lifetime.

You or a loved one may be intimately acquainted with one of the devastating conditions that result from oxygen deprivation, and as you will see, HBOT may be useful long after the injury has occurred or the disease has developed. Furthermore, we will be able to use HBOT to prevent the secondary effects of oxygen deprivation in certain situations, such as near drowning or carbon monoxide poisoning. The ideal way to do this is to treat with HBOT at the earliest possible opportunity—at the scene of the accident.

This concept of "earliest possible intervention" was attempted in England in the 1960s for carbon monoxide poisoning. My partner, Dr. Keith Van Meter, revived this idea at a special Stroke/HBOT conference in 1997. He suggested that we equip ambulances in New Orleans with HBOT chambers so that stroke patients could be treated at the scene. Then, in 2005, a doctor at the institution where that stroke conference was held submitted a grant to the NIH (National

Institutes of Health) on the same issue. Since that time, he has received funding to advance this project, but it will likely take at least another decade or two before ambulances throughout the country are equipped with an HBOT chamber.

No human being can be kept safe from the range of risks that are part of normal living, including serious injuries sustained in accidents. However, just imagine how different the aftermath of these events could be if we had immediate use of a treatment that could prevent a substantial amount of the long-term tissue damage and the range of disabilities that result when the brain is deprived of oxygen.

HBOT also has an important role in wound healing. In 2003, the U.S. Medicare program approved HBOT reimbursement for the treatment of foot wounds in diabetics. Medicare approval represents an important step in acceptance of HBOT into mainstream medical treatment. To those working in the field, however, this acceptance is quite late in the game, because decades ago it was shown that HBOT promotes wound healing, including burns and skin grafts.

Why Haven't I Heard More About This Treatment?

Patients often look puzzled when they hear about HBOT. They scratch their heads and ask me why they haven't heard about it before and why it isn't available in a facility near their homes. Well, many of us who use hyperbaric oxygen therapy scratch our heads, too, and wonder why such a safe and effective treatment continues to have a difficult time finding its rightful role in the treatment of numerous diseases and conditions. In one of the first lectures I heard on hyperbaric medicine in 1986, I saw a picture of the classic radiation wound that hyperbaric physicians had been treating for 20 years. I immediately wondered why HBOT couldn't and wouldn't work for similar wounds, such as a stroke. The short answer is that it does; the long answer has been entombed in the history, politics, and culture of medicine.

I sometimes attach the label "revolutionary" to HBOT, and while that's true, it implies that medical science only recently discovered this specialized use of oxygen for therapeutic purposes. In fact, HBOT has been used for many decades in diving medicine to treat decompression illness (caused by air bubbles that enter the bloodstream and form in tissues). At various times in the twentieth century, it was used to treat other conditions, too.

In the 1930s, the U.S. Navy began its investigation into using HBOT to treat decompression illness in divers. Unfortunately, applications and protocols for HBOT became stuck in the realm of diving and within a small branch of medicine controlled by experts within the U.S. Navy. Applications outside the field of diving medicine were dismissed both within the military and lay medical communities as impossible, end of story. Sadly, research into other areas was largely discouraged or even ridiculed.

Despite the lack of support for further investigation, some pioneering physicians (both in the United States and abroad) took information learned in diving medicine and used it to expand the use of hyperbaric oxygen therapy. Little by little, however, HBOT has made its way into the wider medical arena, and the lay public has been introduced to it as well.

In February 2000, Larry King interviewed Nick Nolte, who at that time was using a variety of treatments and nutritional supplements. King had Dr. Andrew Weil "live" on the air from a distant site to comment on the therapies as they came up. At one point, Dr. Weil remarked that HBOT is useful in the treatment of stroke and other conditions and he would use HBOT himself. When therapies are introduced to the public consciousness, they sometimes are linked with certain "eccentricities," which was the case with Nick Nolte and others, such as the late Michael Jackson. Dr. Weil's presence during the King interview served to clarify and, if you will, lend "gravitas" to the discussion, because of Dr. Weil's prominent role in educating the public about health concerns.

But even with Dr. Weil's presence, the Nick Nolte interview did not have a major impact on the field of hyperbaric medicine. Neither have any modern day scientific advances or testimonials. The reason lies in a curious fact, outside the realm of science. In the first edition of this book, we decided to avoid this controversy. But in the 10 years since its publication we have been besieged by patients, newspaper reporters, radio interviewers and physicians who continue to ask why this therapy has not been accepted "if, as you say, it works so well." The answer resides in the "belief system" of medicine—what can legitimately be termed "the culture of medicine." Once something is "believed" in medicine, it is extremely difficult (if not impossible) to reverse that belief, even in the presence of a mountain of evidence to the contrary. This is the story of hyperbaric medicine, particularly in the modern era, and is due to a combination of factors.

Hyperbaric medicine was introduced clinically in the United States through both the U.S. Navy's application of HBOT in cases of diving accidents and a famous experiment in the Netherlands in the late 1950s involving severe infections, surgery, and carbon monoxide poisoning (discussed in the following pages). Initially, doctors couldn't see a connection between the diving application and the other applications. However, as initial interest and use spread in the United States, doctors began to report astounding success with a variety of conditions. Some of these successes were with untreatable diagnoses that were seemingly unrelated to one another, e.g., balding, cancer, impotence, longevity, acne, and so forth. As patients and doctors stood up and proclaimed their successes, the remainder of the medical profession demanded an explanation. Due to the immaturity of the field, the science was not understood. In the face of criticism, an inability to connect the diving medicine experience with the Dutch data, and an inability to reconcile the "sensational claims" with the science as understood, hyperbaric medicine was at a severe disadvantage.

Simultaneously, one of my mentors, Dr. Richard Neubauer (who died only a few years ago), began to apply HBOT to chronic neurological diseases, along with other physicians. Believe, me, this caused no small furor. First and foremost, Dr. Neubauer was not a neurologist; within the neurology specialty, it had been taught (and considered settled) that nothing could be done for a neurological disorder except to allow the passage of time. The brain was thought to be distinctly different from all of the other organs in our body, with the unusual characteristic of being impervious to medical intervention or outside interference in its own self-determined slow repair process. Dr. Neubauer's claims were deemed heretical by the neurology community and he was widely scorned, yet no one could refute the science of what he was saying. The objections were emotional and non-scientific—they violated the "belief system" of neurology.

This antagonism from the neurology community was surprisingly aided and abetted by none other than the hyperbaric medicine community itself. The hyperbaric medicine community was fighting for credibility and had only one neurologist within its ranks, a Navy diving neurologist. To take on the neurology specialty *and* fight a century-old belief that the brain could not be repaired by human intervention, all while trying to gain a toehold in the field of medicine, was a daunting task.

The bigger problem, however, had nothing to do with the science. It had to do with money: specifically, reimbursement for HBOT. The hyperbaric medicine community was fighting for reimbursement at a fairly generous rate from Medicare and insurance companies in their hospital-based hyperbaric departments. Dr. Neubauer was charging one-fifth (or less) for the same treatment in his clinic in South Florida. Not only was Dr. Neubauer's treatment challenging the scientific foundations of medicine, it was thought to be threatening the financial underpinning of this fledgling specialty. In the process, Dr. Neubauer became the object of resentment and outright hatred by an influential element of the hyperbaric medicine community.

The final straw was the hyperbaric medicine community's inability to understand and define its own therapy. As explained above, HBOT was felt to be a phenomenon resulting from exposing patients to increased amounts of oxygen above sea level pressure. Eventually, a definition emerged that said the treatment "...can be viewed as the new application of an old established technology to help resolve certain recalcitrant, expensive, or otherwise hopeless medical problems...pressurization should be at 1.4 atmospheres or higher."

So what's wrong with this definition? First, it has no definitive "is" in it. Second, which "certain recalcitrant, expensive, and otherwise hopeless medical conditions" are we talking about? Virtually every chronic medical condition is untreatable, and thus "recalcitrant, expensive, and otherwise hopeless." Many acute conditions would also fall into this category. Third, this treatment is defined by the diseases it treats. In other words, it is not a physiologic definition. Lastly, why does the pressure have to be 1.4 atmospheres or higher? Does this mean that 1.399 atmospheres is *not* HBOT?

The key problem with the definition was that the "certain recalcitrant, expensive, or otherwise hopeless medical conditions" was actually a disjointed list of diagnoses. You will see in a later chapter that this list of diseases seemed to bear no relation to one another, e.g. diving disease, bone infections, burns, and so forth. When the medical profession was presented with this definition and the list of diagnoses, it led to further confusion about HBOT.

The convergence of all of these elements provided the perfect storm for the rejection of hyperbaric medicine by the medical community. The fact that the hyperbaric medicine community itself did not support neurological applications was a particularly stinging condemnation. It is what led to the widespread belief that HBOT was "worthless, unscientific, has been thoroughly disproven, is charlatanism, snake oil sales, and fraud," as I was taught in medical school.

Without exception, this was assumed to be true for applications to neurological diseases. As these false perceptions became part of the belief system in medicine, the hyperbaric medicine community itself rallied around the mis-definition of the therapy and its selected core list of diagnoses. By doing so, they joined the rejection of any application to chronic neurological disease, mostly on personal and financial grounds.

Once the rejection of hyperbaric medicine was thoroughly ingrained into the belief system of medicine, it became very difficult to change it, for a range of reasons. First, huge amounts of reputation capital, as I'll refer to it, were expended in the fight. In other words, countless prominent, credible, and purportedly informed physicians denounced the therapy, decade after decade. Human nature itself plays a role here as well, because once this reputation capital was spent, it became virtually impossible for those doctors to admit they had made a mistake.

In the medical profession, admitting a mistake has an additional element beyond human nature. As I mentioned previously, doctors are expected to know about *all matters* in medicine. We're expected to give answers and even feel *compelled* to provide answers. To admit that you gave incorrect information to a patient is extremely difficult for doctors, not just because of the human nature issue, but also because of ego involvement (and in today's world, fear of malpractice litigation).

But an additional reason exists that dwarfs all of the rest: if you have denounced a therapy that not only has the potential but also the *probability* of saving or improving lives, how can you reverse the harm done by your uninformed opinion, given to countless patients who have been denied their life or improved quality of life because of your words? In short, you can't; no apology, no amount of words can reverse this harm. This is particularly relevant with the application of HBOT to acute severe traumatic brain injury (TBI), and now to our valiant war veterans with persistent post-concussion syndrome who are committing suicide in heartbreaking and record-breaking numbers.

The difficulty that physicians have in reversing existing belief systems has been well documented in other scientific disciplines, most notably by the famous theoretical physicist Max Planck. When Dr. Planck was developing the new science and math of quantum theory, he became dismayed over the scientific community's resistance to his proofs. In frustration, he noted that new ideas must outlive their detractors to succeed with the newer generation. This has been paraphrased as, "Science advances one funeral at a time." The problem is that you and your injured loved ones cannot wait for the advancement of HBOT by the attrition of its detractors. You have to act now.

Which brings us to a very important point in this book: nowadays, medical consumers have more influence than ever before. As a consumer, however, you must be aware that a treatment exists before you can talk with your healthcare providers about it. You also need hard information if you decide to take matters into your own hands and seek a treatment you believe in. Of course, you should be skeptical, too, and ask for information and scientific evidence before accepting any medical recommendation. Over the last decade or so, HBOT has emerged as an extremely versatile therapy, backed by solid science, whose full range of applications continues to develop. In that sense, HBOT is a revolutionary development in medicine and is poised to come into its own.

How Can One Treatment Do So Much?

Admittedly, it is difficult for some to take seriously any claim that a treatment can effectively treat both skin wounds and brain injuries. But in a way, that's a bit like doubting that water, a compound of two elements, oxygen and hydrogen, can be used to generate electricity, float ocean liners, or be an essential part of sustaining the life of every cell in the body. No human being questions the need for water or oxygen to maintain life. But for many inside the medical field, it's been a huge leap to take the knowledge about the use of therapeutic oxygen gleaned from one field—diving medicine—and apply it across the range of conditions and diseases to which humans and other animals are vulnerable. In a sense, this is where the "revolution" comes to fruition. It's as much a revolution of understanding as it is of treatment. The understanding is that we are simply using pressure and oxygen, two entities to which all living organisms are sensitive, to manipulate gene expression and suppression in order to prompt the body to heal itself.

We have learned that low levels of oxygen and pressure affect all the body's cells in much the same way. By logical extension, the therapeutic introduction of oxygen and pressure has a similar positive effect on the DNA and structural components of the cells in the brain, spinal cord, bones, and skin. In addition, an excellent scientific reason exists to explain why HBOT has such wide applicability. HBOT specifically treats the common secondary injury processes that cause the majority of damage in all of the acute and chronic conditions named in the list above.

The simple fact is that nearly every injury process, whether its cause is trauma, toxins, loss of blood flow, low oxygen, and so forth, causes a secondary injury, which is the same regardless of the cause. Each injury, regardless of cause, is like plugging in the DVD of inflammation at the outset of the injury. That DVD plays from start to finish, years down the road, the same way each and every time. This secondary injury, the inflammatory reaction (explained in Chapter 2) generates the majority of the injury that leads to disability. HBOT treats the acute inflammatory process and long-term end products of the body's inflammatory reaction.

Once you come to this simple realization, it is easy to see how HBOT could have such profound far-reaching applications to seemingly unrelated conditions. It is also easy to see why it could have such applicability to chronic wounds anywhere in the body.

As reasonable as the above explanation sounds, it challenges what has been, until recently, the bedrock belief in neurology—that we really can't do much about brain injuries, and that the brain recovers, to whatever degree possible, on its own. Therefore, treatments focus on rehabilitation and adjusting to the injury. We see this in stroke rehabilitation and in the treatment of children with birth injuries.

This older belief about the brain includes the idea that the inactive or "dead" brain cells cannot be changed, so the best we can do is work around the injury. In fact, most neurologists believe that there is no such thing as inactive brain cells that exist longer than a few hours. If that were true, why do we repeatedly see newspaper articles and TV stories about people who awaken after years in a coma? If all of the brain cells responsible for their "awakeness" died, they would never be able to awaken. At the same time, technological advances have brought us sophisticated imaging tests, including SPECT imaging (see Chapter 3). We're beginning to understand that, in some cases, damaged brain cells and the surrounding tissue can live for extended periods of time and "wake up," at least to some degree. This new information then opens the door to treatments that may have been dismissed in the past.

The Treatment is **Not a Cure-All for Human Ills**

Just as it's important to grasp the vast potential of HBOT, it is equally important not to view the treatment as a cure-all, a panacea for all human illness. Historically, when a treatment is billed as a miracle cure for just about everything, from the serious to the minor, its days are usually numbered. The history of HBOT is littered with periods of sensationalism that ultimately detracted from the serious purpose of its early pioneers. So, while I point out that HBOT has potential applications to a very large and diverse range of maladies in medicine based on HBOT's effects on the basic components of the diseases I want to be a bit cautious about making panoramic recommendations. In many cases, it makes excellent sense to apply HBOT, but in other situations we may want to wait for additional information and research.

Before we understood why HBOT worked, the treatment took on the look and feel of "voodoo." For example, to perform the treatment, patients enter a chamber, into which oxygen is introduced. In the past, that alone added a certain mystery to the treatment. Some claim that it is this "ritual" of going in the hyperbaric chamber that produces its effect. Not only does it involve a chamber that looks imposing, it also delivers the treatment without causing discomfort or pain, which adds to the skepticism about its efficacy. Furthermore, HBOT is delivered in the same way regardless of the condition under treatment—only the specific dose of oxygen changes.

In addition, HBOT is most certainly a "whole person" treatment because the oxygen and pressure are introduced to every cell in the body. In a sense, it is a type of holistic therapy. Since it is a whole body treatment, all damaged areas of the body are simultaneously exposed to its therapeutic effects. Inadvertently, while patients are receiving treatment for their radiation or diabetic foot wound, other sites of chronic injury or the patient's systemic illness can also benefit, such as a patient's diabetes or brain injury. It is not uncommon in such situations to have the patient report an overall improvement in their sense of well-being. So, while the whole patient, mind and body, is not the initial target of the hyperbaric oxygen, sometimes the indirect effect of treatment benefits the entire person. In fact, most individuals report increased well-being, regardless of the condition treated.

Some people believe that a treatment without significant side effects is too good to be true. In this case, the good news *is* true. *Hyperbaric oxygen is one of the lowest risk medical treatments available today.* One measure of the risk (or lack thereof) is the minimal rate ascribed by malpractice insurance companies to HBOT, which falls into one of their lowest ranking categories. This is particularly true for chronic conditions. Using HBOT for acute, life-threatening conditions, those in which the patient is deathly ill and on a breathing machine in the chamber, there is certainly risk. But even in these severe situations, the treatment is better than the disease.

In early experiments with HBOT, sensational claims were made about things like renewed sexual vigor. Now that we understand that HBOT causes new blood vessel growth (angiogenesis), has effects on the tone of blood vessels and blood flow, and wounds in the brain, we can explain why the treatment has systemic effects and seemingly unrelated side effects, even the positive effect on one's libido or erectile function.

Not a Case of Either-Or

As useful as HBOT is, it will not necessarily replace other treatments for the specific condition being addressed. In many cases, we can view it as an additional treatment that adds healing power to existing therapies and makes them more effective. For example, while the treatment may be of great benefit to victims of stroke, even years after the event, it does not replace rehabilitation therapies. HBOT may help improve circulation for those with diabetes and promote healing of skin wounds that afflict many with the disease, but it does not replace insulin or the importance of diet and exercise. In other cases, it may become the first choice of treatment, such as in near-drowning, cardiac arrest, or other conditions where there has been absence of oxygen or interruption of blood supply.

This "*both-and*" approach, as opposed to "*either-or*," is important. Too many patients are discouraged from seeking non-traditional therapies because their health providers are afraid they will stop their current treatments. However, in most cases, HBOT is not a therapy given in isolation. In an ideal situation, primary physicians and hyperbaric specialists should be able to work together with their patients to bring about the best outcomes using all therapies at their disposal. Diabetic foot wounds represent a perfect example. Patients need

HBOT, but they also need to control their glucose, prevent infection, wear special protective footwear, and use other supportive therapies.

A Brief Look Back

What we call hyperbaric oxygen therapy, or HBOT, has its roots in seventeenth century medicine[1], when its predecessor was referred to as "hyperbaric air therapy," which is simply compressed air, or increased pressures of ambient air. When patients breathe compressed air, all components of the air are compressed, including oxygen. So, patients receive increased oxygen through the lungs, which eventually reaches all the tissues in the body. An Englishman named N. Henshaw built a chamber in 1664 he called a domicilium, to which he attached two large bellows that he operated to increase or decrease the pressure in the room in relation to atmospheric pressure.

In modern parlance, Henshaw's air therapy was the equivalent of a "wellness tool." Had modern technology been available to him, he might have created infomercials that played on late night TV. It would have been promoted as a method to help maintain good health and prevent disease. In particular, he thought it could prevent lung diseases. (Unfortunately, Henshaw's first name has been lost to us, and we aren't sure if he was a physician or a clergyman—he may even have been both.) In view of the fact that Henshaw's theories never caught on with the English medical establishment, I have come to think of Henshaw's domicilium as the beginning of the boom-bust cycle that has characterized HBOT.

Almost two centuries later, the idea of compressed air resurfaced in France. Called "air baths," this treatment ended up in spas throughout France and Europe. At the time, air baths were considered akin to the water spas already used to treat a wide range of medical conditions and promote overall health. Long before we had tools or techniques to measure or "prove" the effects of compressed air, the French physician, V. T. Junod, theorized that the compressed air increased blood flow to the brain and all other organs. He was correct, and today we know that the repetitive application of hyperbaric oxygen results in new blood vessel growth.

In the late 1800s, experiments with pressurized air included performing surgery. A body of research accumulated over time. Still, because researchers couldn't say why the treatment worked, it never became part of mainstream medicine in the U.S. or in Europe. It remained a kind of healthcare fad up until the 1950s, when physicians in the Netherlands performed a famous experiment on pigs showing that the pigs could live in a hyperbaric chamber without blood. In this experiment the doctors removed all of the pigs' blood and replaced it with salt water while the pigs were under pressure with pure oxygen. This rekindled the use of HBOT for surgery and spawned the application to pediatric heart surgery for blue babies.

Another likely reason for down cycles of hyperbarics in its early development is related to the fact that no one could explain how or why the treatment worked, as explained previously. Of course, medical experts often say that the reasons a particular medical procedure are effective are "not well understood." One need look no further than the FDA and the current Physicians' Desk Reference, the compendium of FDA approved drugs available to physicians to prescribe. Nearly half of these drugs have no known mechanism of action. Yet that fact doesn't prevent the FDA from allowing them to be marketed and used in the U.S. for any condition for which a physician feels it might be effective. In the middle of the twentieth century, a Dutch physician, Nicolaas G. Meijne, said he thought hyperbaric treatment had definite value, but since he couldn't understand how the very small amount of increased oxygen brought by compressing air could account for it, he concluded that the benefits were probably due to the treatment's psychological effects.

It's also possible that hyperbaric air treatment fell into disuse because it may have been applied indiscriminately and the results exaggerated. During the early years of hyperbaric development, one clinician was quoted as saying, "The confidence this treatment deserves might be lost by overemphasizing its value." This echoes the thoughts of many of us who use and support HBOT, but who do not want it touted as a cure-all!

One of the best known chapters in the history of HBOT occurred in the United States during the infamous epidemic of Spanish flu in 1918. Dr. Orval Cunningham, who practiced in Kansas City, Missouri, noticed higher death rates from the flu among those who lived at higher elevations than for those living at sea level. Cunningham reasoned that the rarified air—that is, the decreased oxygen concentration in the air at altitude—explained the phenomenon. The lungs are one of the main organs attacked by influenza viruses, so this line of reasoning is certainly logical.

Cunningham extended his thinking beyond influenza, and while on a trip to Colorado he considered that those living at higher elevations had greater incidence of certain diseases, including neuritis, a condition affecting peripheral nerves. There are many types of neuritis, including sciatica and diabetic neuropathy. He also observed that these and other conditions usually improved when patients moved to lower altitudes. Cunningham linked the improvement to the increased oxygen in the air at sea level. He then extended this thinking to believe that a further increase in pressure above sea level would provide even more oxygen to treat diseases.

After Cunningham successfully treated flu patients by first saving the life of a dying young man, he received referrals from all over Kansas City and eventually the entire country. As he continued using the treatment, he found that the hyperbaric air was particularly effective for lung diseases, just as earlier pioneers had observed. What is so amazing is that at the heart of Cunningham's results lay the answer to our realization that HBOT is a gene therapy, with effects that last far beyond the treatment. Cunningham was delivering just one hour of compressed air a day to his dying flu victims. Reason would argue that the increase in oxygen during that single hour should only reverse the low oxygen levels in the flu victims for that limited time they were in the chamber. However, some additional effect had to be working the rest of the day (what we now understand to be gene therapy) that sustained the patients and allowed them to slowly recover.

Given what we know today, we understand why treating lung conditions with hyperbaric (HB) air makes so much sense; it is the first organ to see the increased amounts of oxygen in HB air. As oxygen diffuses across this lining to the blood vessels in the lungs there is a 30–35 percent drop in oxygen concentration in the blood. As a result, all of the rest of the tissues in the body see far less oxygen than the lungs. In the 1970s, Russian physicians successfully used low pressures of hyperbaric oxygen therapy to treat chronic lung disease and reported this at the 7th International Congress on Hyperbaric Medicine.

As you can imagine, word of Cunningham's "mysterious" and "revolutionary" treatment traveled quickly, although Cunningham never advertised his treatment; in fact, he believed it was unethical for a physician to advertise. But, much like what happens today, people heard about him anyway, and those who had the means made their way to his clinic for treatment, later telling others about their amazing results.

Cunningham also treated a few famous individuals, including Miriam Rand, who was married to James Rand, Jr., the president of Remington-Rand Corporation. Mrs. Rand developed severe high blood pressure in her thirties. She went to Cunningham for help, and was brought out of what was called "hypertensive crisis" a number of times. Another industrialist, Henry Timkin, brought Cunningham to Cleveland, Ohio, after Cunningham saved Mr. Timkin when he was dying of renal failure. In gratitude, in 1925 Timkin spent $1 million to build the famous five-story steel ball hyperbaric hospital in Cleveland.

Putting any tendency for "hype" aside, Cunningham's results provide powerful scientific testimony and can't be written off as merely anecdotal. However, Cunningham's success and discoveries didn't conform to what was accepted at the time, so he became an easy target. Personal jealousies were played out in the arena of medical societies and organizations just as they have in more modern times. In the end, Cunningham's pioneering work and writings were discredited by those more powerful within the medical community.

This whole story represents a very ugly chapter in medicine, and Cunningham did not live long enough to be vindicated. Equally damaging, these initiatives against Cunningham led to yet another HBOT boom going bust. But in spite of what happened to Cunningham, interest in HBOT never completely faded away. Where relevant, I have noted research that led to advances or further investigation into the expanded uses for HBOT mentioned in this book.

The Field of Diving Medicine

Despite its odd history, hyperbaric oxygen therapy flourished in the field of diving medicine as an effective treatment for decompression sickness (commonly known as "the bends"), which is one of the hazards involved in SCUBA diving. It results from exposure to increased pressures of the gases divers breathe at varying depths. (The word SCUBA comes from the term "self-contained underwater breathing apparatus.") The breathing gases in SCUBA diving are usually air or oxygen-enriched air called Nitrox. In commercial, military, and science diving, divers can breathe mixtures of helium and oxygen—called heliox—or other exotic mixtures of gases such as hydrogen, neon, argon, and so forth. The different mixtures of gases are used to fine-tune the needs of the diver on special dives, such as very deep prolonged dives where the diver needs to control nervous system sedation, or excitement, or control body temperature.

From the second divers go underwater they are exposed to the increased pressure of the water above them. With every inch of increasing depth the water pressure increases; the deeper they go, the greater the pressure above them. The SCUBA tank on the diver's back contains compressed air at very high pressure, the equivalent seawater pressure of about 7,000 feet underwater or 200 atmospheres. With each breath the regulator at the diver's mouth lets the very high pressurized air out of the tank to the diver's lungs and adjusts it to the exact pressure the diver's body is at underwater. So, the diver breathes pressurized air equivalent to the depth he is in the water. If not for the regulator, the diver's lungs would be exposed to the 7,000 feet of pressure in the tank, which would rupture the diver's lungs, sending air into his heart, blood vessels, and brain.

So, when divers descend roughly 33 feet, the water pressure is twice surface pressure (the pressure of air at the surface of the water), and at 99 feet, it's four times surface pressure. At 33 feet divers breathe gas at twice surface pressure and at 99 feet, four times surface pressure. At every depth on the way to and from 33 feet or 99 feet divers breathe air at the pressure for that depth when they take a breath. The regulator on their SCUBA tank allows them to do this.

To appreciate the effects of seawater depth and pressure on the air we breathe we can look at how pressure decreases the volume of air in our lungs when we hold our breath and dive deep. Figure 1 on page 23 from the National Oceanographic and Atmospheric Administration's Diving Manual[2] shows a diver's lung volume when the diver takes a breath, holds it, and dives deep. This occurs in snorkeling and free-diving, such as performed by the Japanese pearl divers and competition breathhold divers, or anyone who dives to the bottom of a pool. Since the amount of air in the lungs is fixed due to the breathhold, the increasing effect of pressure is to compress the air (and lungs) as the diver dives deeper. This is known as Boyle's Law (one of the Universal Gas Laws) which says that a fixed volume of a gas changes inversely with the pressure on it. So, at 2 atmospheres (33 feet below sea level) the diver's lungs are one-half of their volume. At 4 atmospheres (99 feet) the lung volume is one-fourth, and the air in the lungs is under four times the pressure on the surface. You can perform this same exercise by inflating a balloon and diving with it to the bottom of a pool. You will see a change in size of the balloon. (See Figure 1.)

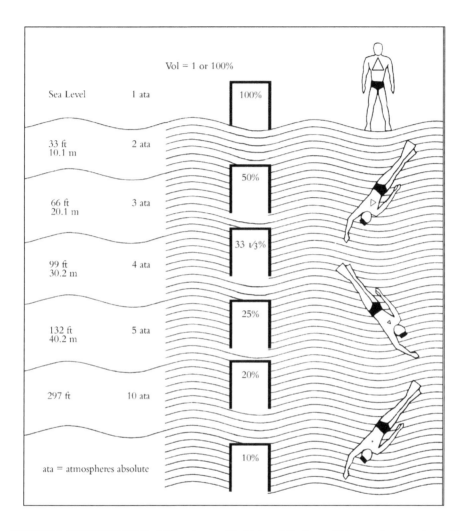

FIGURE 1. BOYLE'S LAW. Boyle's Law is one of the Universal Gas Laws which states that any volume of gas in a closed space will change its volume as the pressure on the gas is increased or decreased. If the pressure is increased, the volume is reduced and if the pressure is decreased, the volume will increase. This law applies to all closed spaces of gas, such as the air in your lungs when you hold your breath and go underwater. In the diagram the man on the surface jumps into the water and holds his breath. His lung volume is 100 percent. For each 33 feet he descends the volume of air in his lungs decreases. At 33 feet, the depth that snorkelers can achieve, the volume of air in his lungs is 50 percent. At 297 feet underwater, a "shallow" depth for competition breathhold divers (the record is 831 feet), the lungs and compressed air would have shrunk to 10 percent of the volume on the surface (the littlest triangle). In SCUBA diving the diver would be breathing air from his SCUBA tanks all the way down as he dives. At 297 feet he would have 100 percent lung volume as on the surface, but he would have 10 times as much air (10 little triangles) in his lungs as on the surface, at 10 times the pressure.

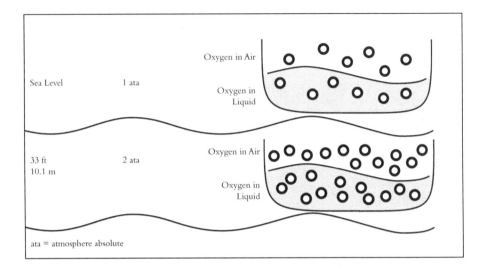

Sea Level   1 ata   Oxygen in Air

Oxygen in Liquid

33 ft   2 ata   Oxygen in Air
10.1 m

Oxygen in Liquid

ata = atmosphere absolute

FIGURE 2. HENRY'S LAW. Henry's Law is also one of the Universal Gas Laws which states that the amount of a gas that is dissolved in any liquid changes with the pressure of the gas. So if the pressure of the gas increases, more of the gas is dissolved in the liquid and if the pressure of the gas decreases, more of the gas comes out of the liquid. This is true for all gases. The diagram shows two glasses of liquid that interface with a gas (air) at two different pressures, sea level (1 atmosphere) and 2 atmospheres of pressure (equal to the pressure at 33 feet underwater). The amount of gas at 2 atmospheres is twice the amount of gas at 1 atmosphere and so the amount dissolved in the liquid at 2 atmospheres is twice the amount in the liquid at 1 atmosphere. In SCUBA diving it is the nitrogen in the air (79 percent of air) that we worry about the most. As the diver dives deeper more and more nitrogen passes through the lungs into the blood, where it is delivered to all the tissues in the body. When the diver returns to surface, the ascent must be slow enough to prevent this nitrogen from erupting as bubbles in the tissues and causing decompression illness (the bends). In hyperbaric oxygen therapy it is the oxygen dissolved in the blood that is so important. At 1.5 atmospheres of pure oxygen, for instance, we have seven times the oxygen dissolved in our blood that we have breathing air at sea level. It is the dissolved oxygen that is primarily responsible for the healing effects of HBOT.

In actual SCUBA or commercial diving, our lungs don't get compressed because we are freely breathing from a SCUBA tank or a hose connected to compressed air/gas supplies on the surface, from a boat or barge. But, we're still getting compressed air to breathe. The compressed air is delivered to us through the mouthpiece connected to the SCUBA tank or the hose to the surface, and the pressure is regulated by the mouthpiece/regulator, as described above, to give us the pressure of gas at the exact depth at which the diver is positioned under water.

When any gas is in contact with any liquid surface, some of the gas dissolves in the liquid. It is one of the Universal Gas Laws called "Henry's Law." (See Figure 2.) When we take a breath, the air we breathe and the oxygen in it comes into contact with the inside lining of our lungs. Just barely under that lining of cells are the blood vessels that absorb a certain amount of all the gases in the air, especially the oxygen and nitrogen.

As divers go underwater, the increased pressure of air or gas breathed at every depth of the dive causes increased amounts of oxygen and nitrogen to be dissolved in their blood. The blood takes this nitrogen and oxygen to all parts of the body where they are absorbed. The oxygen poses no problem, and we metabolize it; but the nitrogen and helium give us a problem. That dissolved nitrogen or helium has to be gradually released back into the blood and breathed off from our lungs as we come up from a dive and while we are on the surface. If the diver follows the diving tables or his dive computer and ascends slowly enough to dissipate all of the dissolved nitrogen, everything is okay. If the diver stays at depth too long or ascends too quickly, the nitrogen then forms bubbles (pockets of gas) in the blood and other tissues; this is what causes decompression sickness. Symptoms, which usually appear within 24 hours following a dive, include itching, joint pain, visual problems, numbness and tingling, dizziness and difficulty maintaining balance, weakness in the legs, confusion, and sometimes chest pain, chest tightness, or shortness of breath.

Nowadays, we treat decompression sickness with HBOT. The raised pressure of HBOT compresses the bubbles in the tissues, thus allowing them to dissolve and become reabsorbed. In addition, the increased oxygen replaces the nitrogen and heals the damage to tissue done by the bubbles. As the bubbles are slowly dissolved and reabsorbed, the symptoms usually disappear, and no permanent harm is done.

The idea of recompressing divers with decompression sickness originated around 1900. During its early development, hyperbaric air was all that was used in diving accidents. Then, in the late 1930s and 1940s, Dr. Edgar End, located in Milwaukee, Wisconsin, and two Navy physicians, Behnke and Shaw, began to recompress divers using oxygen instead of air. These doctors documented reduced treatment times and better results, which ultimately led to the oxygen treatment tables the U.S. Navy released in 1967. These tables (an example of which is shown in Figure 3) are still used today.

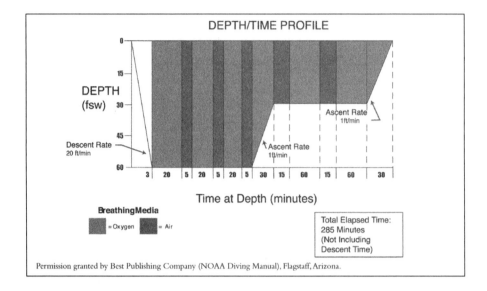

DEPTH/TIME PROFILE

Permission granted by Best Publishing Company (NOAA Diving Manual), Flagstaff, Arizona.

FIGURE 3. OXYGEN TREATMENT TABLE. This figure depicts the most common treatment table used for treating decompression illness, U.S. Navy Treatment Table VI. On the vertical line is the depth of pressure that the injured diver is subjected to during the treatment in a hyperbaric chamber. The chamber and diver start on the surface at 0 feet of seawater equivalent pressure (1 atmosphere at sea level) and then are pressurized with air down to 60 feet of seawater equivalent pressure (2.8 atmospheres). There is no water in the chamber. On the horizontal line is time. The first pressurization to 60 feet from surface occurs in 3 minutes. The treatment proceeds with different breathing gases (the different shaded columns) for different periods of time. After the third 5-minute air breathing period the chamber pressure and diver are decompressed to 30 feet of seawater equivalent air pressure while breathing oxygen and then continue with air and oxygen treatment periods. The air periods are given as "air breaks" to give the patient time off from oxygen to prevent oxygen toxicity. After 150 minutes at 30 feet, the chamber and diver are decompressed back to surface while breathing oxygen. The total treatment time is 285 minutes, or 4 hours and 45 minutes.

While most people in the United States associate hyperbaric oxygen with decompression sickness, researchers in other countries have studied its many other uses. We saw another brief HBOT boom in the 1960s and 1970s because of research that suggested wider application. Then, we also learned that HBOT can be effectively used at varying pressures, or put another way, at different doses of oxygen and pressure. This has been both a breakthrough and a source of controversy. (Again, I will be citing this research throughout this book, when relevant to today's applications of HBOT.)

As you will see, we now understand why HBOT is effective for a much longer list of conditions than once believed. Because we understand that HBOT is a drug with particular effects, HBOT is no longer shrouded in mystery and we can remove barriers to continued research and treatment.

Let Others Define Their "Miracles"

I hope the material included in this chapter gives you a general understanding of HBOT and the range of conditions for which it can be successfully used. I've had the opportunity to treat individuals of all ages, some of whom are members of the same families. (You will read about a few of these patients throughout this book.) I have seen men and women who were once severely disabled complete hyperbaric oxygen therapy and return to a normal life. These men and women speak of miracles, and rightly so. An autistic child that becomes more responsive, perhaps even carrying on complex conversations, is a miracle, too. However, we need to be careful, not only about using the word "miracle," but about defining it. After years of practicing medicine, I prefer to let others define their own miracles.

It is sad but true that no treatment, HBOT included, can guarantee complete recovery from some of the most devastating injuries and diseases. In some cases, we have to match our expectations to realistic possibilities. However, in addition to documenting the objective changes in the brain brought about by the treatment, I have heard the human stories of gratitude for seemingly small improvements in quality of life, which is—surprisingly—a component of health care that may not get the respect it deserves.

If your father suffers a stroke and you watch him live in a world of mental confusion, perhaps unable to feed himself, to you a miracle may be increased alertness and improved motor skills that enable him to eat independently. Or, the miracle might be your father's renewed interest in who wins the World Series. Viewed against the predictions that no therapy can improve your father, or that therapy has long since stopped improving him two to three years after the stroke, these improvements would actually seem to be miraculous to him, to you and to your family.

When I think about miracles, I recall the young mother whose child had been delivered by a physician impaired by alcohol and, as a result, the boy was horribly damaged for life. Through a series of events, the woman and her son ended up in my office. After having traveled from another state and without all the usual pre-visit screening procedures that establish the realistic hopes about what we can do for a child, I was extremely anxious when I walked into the room to see this young mother and her irritable son. So, my first questions to this mother had to be: "Why are you here? What are your expectations?"

She sensed my apprehension about false hope and quickly said, "Oh, Dr. Harch, I don't really have any expectations for my son. All I want for him is to be able to sit up one day, hold a cup, and enjoy a Happy Meal."

I had to turn away, because I was reduced to tears—I still have trouble keeping it together, so to speak, when I tell the story. Of course, I agreed to treat the boy. (I tell his story later in the book, but he far exceeded his mother's limited expectations—*and* those of his doctors).

So, while HBOT truly is a revolutionary treatment and can lead to vast improvements in numerous conditions, the degree of recovery or "miracle" depends on many factors. In the coming chapters, you will read about diseases and conditions for which HBOT offers hope, and miracles, too. But I leave it to you to define what that means for yourself or your loved one.

CHAPTER 2

OXYGEN DEPRIVATION AND THE BODY'S INFLAMMATORY REACTION

IMAGINE A MACHINE THAT CONTROLS A SYSTEM designed to perform hundreds of jobs; a machine which, while it's doing its work, must be able to withstand all manner of "abuse," including bouts with natural forces—wind, hail, sleet, lightning, floods, and so forth. And this complex machine must be tamper-proof, too, so that it can keep functioning even when curious kids or careless adults fool around with it.

One group of design engineers decides the machine must have more than one way to react to these various "insults." They attempt to develop a machine that has a specific damage control response to lightning, and a different one for freezing cold or scorching heat, and still another for a blunt force injury. As you can imagine, the software needed to regulate the machine's response to these possible conditions would be impossibly complex.

Another group of engineers goes back to the drawing board, so to speak, and designs a system that responds in a like manner to any assault, from being dropped off a truck to being dumped in a swimming pool, or having a child pound on it. No matter what happened to threaten its various functions, or even its life, the machine could immediately respond in one way to try to minimize the damage.

Our bodies are like the machine the innovative second group of engineers designed. We have within us the software needed to control a system made to absorb anything thrown at us. So, if we're exposed to cold, or fall off a ladder, drink too much, suffer blunt force trauma, experience stoppage of blood flow, or are exposed to lower than normal oxygen levels, our bodies respond in one specific way. In addition, the response to this vast array of everyday occurrences is the same whether the event affects the entire body, any of our organs, or the arms or legs.

This single response is called the inflammatory reaction. As you can see from the topics listed in the Table of Contents and the list in Chapter 1, this book covers many seemingly unrelated processes, including low or absent oxygen or blood flow. These include, of course, "everyday" events. Each incident may or not be major or dramatic, but lightning strikes and near-drowning accidents, ankle sprains or minor cuts, cardiac arrests or unexpected complications during birth, are everyday occurrences. In each case, our bodies activate the inflammatory reaction, and our understanding of this reaction allows us to explain why HBOT is so useful across such a wide spectrum of conditions and medical emergencies.

The inflammatory reaction is both fast and dramatic. It's also somewhat odd in that it has both beneficial and seemingly detrimental aspects. Imagine watching a fire start and then someone quickly dumps gasoline on it and a violent conflagration results. Barely an instant later, the same person brings in water and chemicals and puts the fire out. This is exactly what happens with the inflammatory reaction. After the initial injury the body brings all its "tools," including toxic chemicals and digestive enzymes, to bear on the site of injury, and causes a conflagration. If hyperbaric oxygen is delivered soon enough, it is like the person subsequently dumps water and chemicals on the conflagration to put the fire out. If no one intervenes with HBOT, the inflammatory reaction slowly cleans up the mess. So, in response to harm, the body causes more harm, and then, inevitably, in the clean-up process, heals by causing a "scar" to form. If the wound does not completely heal to scar formation, and rather becomes a non-healing wound, HBOT can often also treat this chronic wound.

It is important to note that the body can tolerate low oxygen levels fairly well, but it cannot tolerate low blood flow. This is important because the blood contains not only oxygen, but all the necessary nutrients the cells need to survive. Further, the body's threshold for low oxygen injury is lowered, that is, it occurs more "efficiently," when blood flow is low. What this means in practical terms is that an injury is more pronounced when blood flow is low. For example, an everyday gash on the skin of an otherwise healthy person usually heals in a given and expected amount of time because the blood flow remains adequate. But, if the same healthy person has a crush injury, such as a dog bite, which causes destruction to the blood supply, then it may be more difficult for the wound to heal. When a person with systemic wound healing problem, such as diabetes, experiences the same type of dog bite then healing becomes more complicated because of the many problems associated with diabetes that further compromise the wound.

I mention these seemingly small wounds because they are so common, and most of the time we don't pay much attention to them. But a change in health status, such as developing diabetes, can alter the person's response to the inflammatory reaction after a wounding incident.

The Cascade of Events

When oxygen levels are low, the inside lining of the blood vessels in the area low on oxygen are put on "high alert," particularly the smallest vessels at the tissue level of individual cells. In addition, a specific type of white blood cell is activated. They are called PMN (polymorphonuclear neutrophil) and they react early in acute injury, within minutes to hours.

Once blood flow and oxygenation is reestablished, the activated white blood cells stick to the inside lining (endothelial cells) of the tiny blood vessels, much like Velcro clings to carpet. The endothelial cells also activate when the blood flow is restored and begin to interact with white blood cells; hence, the inflammatory reaction.

The blood vessels are the same size or slightly larger than these white blood cells, a situation that then allows those white cells to act as a plug—or clot—in the vessel, especially if many of the white blood cells clump together. We end up with millions and millions of tiny clots in the vessels, and once the white blood cells stick, they discharge toxic chemicals and enzymes. A whole series of chemical reactions begins—the inflammatory reaction.

The chemical reactions are caused by the release of various chemicals and enzymes. They are like little "Pac-men" stored in tiny pouches inside the white blood cells. Or you could think of them as confetti stuffed into a little bag. When the white blood cells stick to the inside lining, the cells break open and release their "Pac-men," which then eat up tissues activated by the low blood flow, low oxygen event. They also dissolve the tissue and destroy it before they eat it up. Another way to think of it is to picture these Pac-men as Viking warriors. In the first phase of the inflammatory reaction, they destroy what's in their path; in the second phase, they gobble up what they've plundered in a "clean up" effort.

When clotting and other inflammatory processes in the blood are activated, you see blood clots forming at the site of an injury. In addition, in response to other chemicals contained in these pouches, the localized blood vessels dilate (stretch beyond normal size). Meanwhile, some of the white blood cells that are stuck to the blood vessel walls begin to reshape or deform themselves, which allows them to squeeze through the porous openings and out through the extremely thin (a cell thickness) walls of the blood vessels. (These white cells can be likened to mice gaining access to a house by reshaping themselves and pushing through tiny cracks in a wall.) This process is called diapedesis, meaning to "leap out," and leads to a more intense inflammatory reaction out in the tissues.

At some point in a traumatic event, blood and oxygen flow return. Think of a procedure that involves a tourniquet-like effect, meaning that blood flow is temporarily halted. As an example, imagine a surgeon creating a bloodless area on an arm or leg in order to perform a surgical procedure. Once the surgery is over, the blood is allowed to flow back to the area. But if this arm or leg has had zero blood supply or oxygen for some period of time, one to two hours or more, then the body responds dramatically to the restored blood and oxygen flow.

The secondary injury that results after interrupted blood flow is restored is called reperfusion injury. It is largely composed of the inflammatory reaction. The inflammatory reaction also can occur in the absence of an interruption of blood supply. If you are punched in the arm or suffer electric shock, you may sustain tissue injury, but the blood supply remains about the same initially. So, for example, the term reperfusion injury is used when we talk about resuscitation from cardiac arrest or after dissolving a blood clot in an artery.

In the process of re-supplying oxygen, the white blood cells create oxygen free radicals. A free radical is an unstable, reactive atom formed by an unpaired electron. The body can form free radicals from a variety of elements, but because they are unstable, they will immediately bind to anything, including protein and DNA. However, their primary target is fat. Fats (lipids) exist in every cell membrane, and of course in the fatty tissues of the body.

Oxidation occurs when oxygen free radicals combine with other chemicals and alter normal tissue—we say that they "digest" this tissue.

This process also results in "per-oxidation," of which the most common known type is lipid per oxidation. The brain is at least 60 percent fat; the greatest amount occurs in the covering of the brain cells. But all cells in the body have a covering composed of mostly fatty material.

As you will see, the specific consequence of the inflammatory response varies within the body. Individual chapters of this book describe how tissue damage occurs and how reintroducing oxygen in the form of HBOT may allow varying degrees of healing and improvement.

HBOT and Acute Injuries

Some subtle differences exist in acute injuries brought about by myriad causes, but almost immediately the inflammatory response is set in motion and this secondary reaction then causes the majority of the damage to our bodies and the net result is roughly all the same.

In simple terms, think about what happens to your arm if you're given a tetanus shot or a vaccine. The swelling and redness on your arm is a visible sign of the inflammatory reaction, as is the swelling and bruising around your ankle when you sprain or fracture it.

In childhood we become familiar with visible signs of injury and the changes that take place as these wounds heal. We take these signs for granted, even accepting that the pain serves a useful purpose. A sprained ankle hurts enough to keep us from putting weight on the injured leg and damaging it even more. In most cases, these familiar minor injuries don't worry us. We call them nuisances, manageable "side effects" of normal life.

And although we don't see it, the inflammatory reaction also occurs in the brain, the heart, and other organs when any of the previously mentioned injuries occur. It is also part of the injury process that occurs in a stroke.

What we now realize is that high pressure oxygen delivered within two to three hours after the injury, whether it's a stroke or other trauma, significantly quenches the secondary destructive inflammatory reaction. Hence, the major damage resulting from the injury is prevented or minimized. Actually, we also believe that HBOT delivered before or during the event may also minimize the damage done by the inflammatory reaction.

During the inflammatory reaction, oxygen free radicals are eating up and inflaming tissue, which leads to swelling, compression of blood vessels, less blood flow and less oxygen, a proverbial vicious cycle: tissue injury begets more tissue injury, which begets…and so on. This is why quenching the damage using a high dose of pressurized oxygen is so revolutionary.

The Oxygen Paradox

You might question the wisdom (and many have) of adding oxygen to a situation in which oxygen free radicals are pouring in. Isn't that like throwing more gasoline on a fire the body has already ignited? In other words, wouldn't this worsen the inflammatory reaction? This phenomenon is called the "oxygen paradox," and it is a matter of dosage and timing. Oxygen can act like gasoline if you get too much oxygen too late or even a mild increase early on, but a short, high pressure dose delivered at the time of the injury appears to stop this ongoing inflammatory reaction.

For years now, hyperbaric physicians have had to explain this to their colleagues in other specialties. We tell them to ignore the concern about inflaming the inflammatory reaction and concentrate on the clinical results. Ultimately, that's all that is important. Look at it this way: If HBOT was making the inflammatory reaction worse by increasing the free radicals, patients would become worse. But, in fact, they are better off as a result of treatment.

Like many things in medicine, this clinical result only told us there was a lot we didn't know. However, research has provided the evidence to explain this oxygen paradox: HBOT was quenching the inflammatory reaction. The scientific evidence for this is now overwhelming. In 2001, I gave a scientific presentation at the European Federation of Neurological Societies Meeting held in Copenhagen, Denmark. I asked if we could consider HBOT a generic drug for treating the acute inflammatory reaction after loss of blood flow to the brain. I assembled a variety of studies and found that regardless of the species of animal, the organ system involved, or the type of insult, hyperbaric oxygen had a remarkably positive effect in quenching the inflammatory reaction if delivered shortly after the damaging event. Today, there are nearly 100 studies reinforcing the same finding.

The most dramatic example of this was provided in 1983 by Ray Parrish (his real name), a commercial diver. Ray was diving in the Mississippi River, behind the famous Audubon Zoo in New Orleans, trying to salvage a sunken tugboat.

The diving company used an airlift, which is a diesel engine-powered vacuum cleaner that can suction mud off the bottom of the Mississippi River and throw it 50–100 feet in the air off the top of a barge. Ray was sucked up into the two-foot wide vacuum tube and eventually suffered a cardiac arrest in addition to decompression sickness. Finally hauled to the surface, he had laid on the barge for twenty-five minutes after his arrest before finally being put in a hyperbaric chamber. He was pressurized to 165 feet of water pressure and accidentally given 6 atmospheres of pure oxygen.

An uninjured or "normal" person given this dose of oxygen will suffer a grand mal seizure within five minutes, which is what happened to the "tender" diver who accompanied Ray into the chamber to do CPR and accidentally breathed the oxygen that was leaking from Ray's mask. Ray, on the other hand, came back to life and began to care for the seizing tender!

It shocked everyone when he came to life. Dr. Van Meter entered the chamber and oversaw the rest of his treatment. Ray left the chamber intact and went on to marry, have children, become a custom furniture carpenter in California, and see his case published in a textbook. In January 2010, Dr. Van Meter brought him to New Orleans to give him a medical checkup. A surgeon (Dr. Sabatier) and I also evaluated him and found him to be intact and normal, with a high IQ and a remarkably intact brain blood flow scan. (Ray was featured in a short news piece on New Orleans television, available for viewing at HBOT.com.)

Ray's dramatic case spawned a series of HBOT resuscitation experiments (first using guinea pigs, and then swine) at 6 atmospheres. Dr. Van Meter resuscitated pigs after 25 minutes of cardiac arrest, just like Ray. The scientific article on this experiment was published in *Resuscitation* in 2007. In modern medicine, if you can't apply CPR, drugs, and electric shocks to a cardiac arrested patient within about 12–15 minutes, 100 percent of the patients die. This 100 percent figure hasn't changed in 50 years with all of modern science and research. So, the potential for this HBOT application to humans is staggering.

Getting back to the point, Dr. Van Meter also found that the single resuscitation HBOT treatment stopped cold the inflammatory reaction in the brain. As mentioned above, it quenched the oxygen free radical reaction and reperfusion injury. It was a dramatic clinical example of the potential of HBOT.

Another Look at Diving Medicine

To date, diving medicine has served as the "training ground" for HBOT. However, in the late 1980s and the early 1990s, I realized that the divers our group treated in our hospital hyperbaric medicine department on the Louisiana Gulf Coast didn't respond to the first hyperbaric oxygen treatment in exactly the same way as the divers treated by U.S. Navy doctors. I could look at their reports and compare the results and immediately see the disparity. The reasons for this began to provide insight into other unanswered questions.

By Navy regulations, a hyperbaric chamber must be on site for every diving operation, so if a diver with the bends immediately reports his symptoms, he's usually within a chamber within one or two hours of the injury. In military diving, that first treatment, administered within an hour or two of the accident, cures the problem in over 90 percent of cases.

The commercial diving industry functions somewhat differently, however. A diver may not report symptoms—or may simply choose to ignore them— because a possible diagnosis of decompression sickness may lead to losing his job. In addition, in both commercial and sport SCUBA diving many divers aren't well enough aware of the symptoms to recognize decompression sickness, so they may seek medical attention after a significant amount of time has passed.

I was puzzled by the incongruity between the reported military experience and my own and my colleagues' experiences with treating our commercial and sport divers. In an attempt to answer these lingering questions about decompression sickness that affects the brain, the bubbles going through the brain blood vessels, I found animal research showing that bubbles directly injected into blood vessels of the brain for the most part pass through the brain in minutes. Only the largest ones get stuck. Researchers then took animals whose white blood cells had been chemically killed or removed and performed the same set of experiments. When they injected air into the blood vessels in the brain of these animals without white blood cells, the animals suffered almost no permanent injury.

That research has important implications for HBOT. When military doctors treat brain decompression illness within the first hour or two of a diving accident they are actually treating the white blood cell inflammatory reaction and not so much the bubbles. Yet, all this time, they hadn't understood what they were treating, which was the source of my ongoing curiosity and frustration. No one could tell me what we were actually doing when we treated divers. And, no one could explain the variation in results because no one could definitively explain what we were treating in the first place!

For me, this realization opened up a whole new world of possibilities for hyperbaric oxygen therapy. Now, the "Emperor Had No Clothes" in diving medicine and decompression sickness of the brain. It may seem odd to you that for so many years HBOT was approved only for diving medicine because the experts "believed" we were "treating bubbles;" yet all along in brain decompression illness we had been primarily treating something else—and we now had the evidence to show it (remember what I said previously about belief systems in medicine). Moreover, this evidence also clarified some of the past "amazing claims" about HBOT, which had been discredited because explanations were lacking.

This breakthrough further crystallized for me in 1990 and 1991, when I treated two amazing diving cases with HBOT months after their injuries (described later in this book). Then, in 1993, two different researchers showed that hyperbaric oxygen could inhibit the white blood cells that were involved in the inflammatory reaction. That research matched my treatment results, and revealed a huge piece of the HBOT puzzle that had been missing before.

Extremely important conclusions about HBOT logically followed:

1. During all of the years of using hyperbaric oxygen to treat brain decompression sickness we were, in fact, primarily treating this inflammatory reaction and not nitrogen bubbles. I published this argument in the 45th UHMS Workshop: Treatment of Decompression Illness, 1996[1].

2. Armed with this information, hyperbaric oxygen can now treat a whole slew of conditions affecting our bodies that have to do with loss of adequate oxygen and blood flow and involve the white blood cells and inflammatory reaction. This becomes especially clear in cases of acute injury: resuscitating patients from cardiac arrest (as my partner has done in pigs and humans), and further, resuscitating babies injured at birth, near-drowning victims, near-hanging victims, carbon monoxide poisoned individuals, and anyone experiencing severe low blood flow, low oxygen, and so forth.

Discovering what HBOT is actually treating when used in brain decompression illness opened the doors wider than we ever believed possible. For example, we can potentially use it to treat patients undergoing organ transplants, since the inflammatory reaction is part of the organ rejection phenomenon. If the white blood cells can be inhibited, thus preventing the inflammatory reaction when the organ is harvested as well as when it's transplanted, we may be able to prevent early organ rejections—that would change the nature of organ transplant medicine. HBOT is also safer than the anti-rejection drugs available today and because of other effects of HBOT, it may help rejuvenate these transplant patients who have been in a chronic state of ill health. Based on what I have seen after treating four chronic pulmonary transplant patients, HBOT may also have a role in chronic organ rejection.

Acute vs. Chronic Conditions

Hyperbaric medicine protocols have been dominated by using exclusively higher pressures of oxygen to treat all conditions, protocols which originated within the U.S. Navy HBOT practices. This habit and "belief" still dominates in hyperbaric medicine today, as you will see in the studies on persistent post-concussion syndrome. Briefly, the Navy's experience found that divers could be recompressed using an oxygen pressure of approximately 3 atmospheres, which is near the maximum pressure tolerated by humans. Then, military physicians experimented with slightly lower pressure to treat wounds that resisted healing. At the same time, animal and human experiments successfully used HBOT at the 3-atmosphere level for carbon monoxide poisoning.

Through experimentation, we learned that higher pressures are ideal when treating acute neurological conditions, especially within an hour or two of the accident. But, the same pressure is inappropriate when treating a brain injury that is no longer in an acute stage; that is, a longer period of time has passed between the brain injury and treatment.

When Navy doctors used 2.8–3 atmospheres of oxygen to treat divers, at least in the case of decompression illness, it is likely that they were actually treating more than the gas bubbles in the tissues, even though they were unaware of it. The presumption that we were continuing to treat residual bubbles in these divers with daily hyperbaric treatments confused me, and led to the realization that we could treat brain injuries longer and longer after the initial injury.

My reasoning went something like this: HBOT treats the bubbles responsible for the symptoms and physical exam findings in decompression illness. If we were treating bubbles on the first treatment, why weren't the patients completely healed after the first treatment? If the bubbles weren't completely gone from the brain after the first treatment, then they most certainly should be gone after the second treatment. However, many of the patients that we were treating were not healed after the first, second, or fifth treatment, yet they continued to improve with each treatment. In many cases, we were treating them hours to days after their accident, or after they had received their first hyperbaric treatment elsewhere.

I had read that bubbles are spontaneously absorbed after a period of time, and I coupled this with the fact that the bubbles were supposed to be compressed and absorbed after the first or second treatment. However, I realized that in almost all of these delayed or retreatment cases of brain decompression illness, we *weren't* treating the bubbles—we weren't treating what the U.S. Navy was treating all these years. Rather, we were treating the damage caused by the length of time the bubbles were in place *before* they were reabsorbed and/or the damage left after the bubbles passed through the tissue. If we weren't treating the same pathology, maybe the treatment needed to change. In other words, we needed a different dose of HBOT.

In 1992, I began to show the cases with brain decompression illness that I had treated months and even years after the diver's last dive. I pointed out that in the acute cases treated by the U.S. Navy the bubbles passed through the brain within a few minutes of the diving accident. I suggested that in these acute cases we were likely treating the inflammatory reaction that happens after bubbles pass through the brain.

Regardless, the results achieved by the Navy doctors lead directly to the following critical principle: more oxygen is more effective for these early conditions.

However, we have seen that this principle does not apply when treating neurological diagnoses in which treatment is delayed following the initial injury. In those cases, the higher pressures did not generate the same lasting results, and beyond that, it was possible that they had a toxic effect. These observations led to another critical principle: less oxygen may be more; in other words, lower pressures may be more effective in delayed cases, those in which the wound or condition has become chronic. (Again, this argument was presented in the 45th UHMS Workshop mentioned previously).

Different Stages, Different Targets

The key to understanding this principle is that this drug, hyperbaric oxygen therapy, has different targets at different stages in the disease process. In decompression illness, the early targets are bubbles and the inflammatory reaction. Later, the HBOT targets are blood vessel damage, low oxygen and blood flow damage to cells, and other effects.

These two guiding principles—let's call them the "principles of pressure"— represent a significant breakthrough in medicine, and ultimately allow us to understand why this unique treatment has such broad and deep potential applications. So, keep in mind that "more is more" applies to greater pressures of oxygen (up to 3 atmospheres absolute, and even higher in resuscitation) used in acute neurological events or situations affecting other organ systems, too. By using these higher pressures we can almost completely inhibit the body's inflammatory reaction that occurs after any insult to the body involving low oxygen and blood flow.

The "less is more" principle applies when considering the best way to use hyperbaric medicine to treat chronic brain injuries. In other words, as we progress from the acute situation to the more chronic one, the injury is no longer responsive to high pressures of oxygen, and in fact, this is when toxicity can result. So, days and weeks—and now we believe, even years—after an injury, the lower pressures appear more effective. German researchers showed this in the 1970s in the treatment of acute severe traumatic brain injury and acute severe stroke.

This information has not been routinely used in the United States, however. Unfortunately, because hyperbaric medicine in the United States has been dominated by military physicians who were trained (and train others) in diving medicine and use higher pressures of oxygen, other applications have been delayed. Nearly all of the early research in the 1960s and 1970s was performed with high pressure oxygen. So, regardless of the condition, or whether it was acute or chronic, relatively high pressures and long durations of exposure to HBOT were the norm. But now we know that "one size certainly doesn't fit all." In fact, this uniform application of high pressures likely was responsible for some of the uneven results seen with research.

Why Chronic Wounds are Different

When an injury, or the damage done by the inflammatory reaction following an injury, leads to chronic wounding, other disease processes are at work. For example, the reason many wounds are chronic is that the blood supply is compromised, and when this type of damage occurs, the cells in the area surrounding the wound don't have enough oxygen to carry on their reparative and normal function. (In other words, there are degrees of cell damage involved in an injury to various tissues.)

The initial low oxygen and low blood flow common to many chronic wounds seems to "freeze" or "stun" many of the cells in the tissues surrounding the injured area. Back in the 1920s, Dr. Cunningham treated syphilis, which affects nerve cells. He theorized that these cells could exist in an injured state for many years, and that they could be regenerated with HBOT. He believed this was why patients improved with HBOT. Many decades later, Dr. Richard Neubauer used the descriptive term "idling neuron" in his theory about the ability of injured brain cells to wake up or come back to life, so to speak.

In other words, it appears we have evidence that stunned or injured cells are prevented from performing their normal function, but they have not died. They exist in a neutral or "idling" state. Although this theory first applied to the brain, it has also been documented in heart attack and other organ injuries. In other words, heart cells may be stunned or injured, but, like brain cells, may be coaxed to get back to work and act like normal cells.

Nearly all chronic wounds in the heart, brain, or the skin or bones are characterized by low blood and oxygen supply. As I said earlier, we can think of HBOT as one of the premiere therapies that treats the "whole person," because the entire body is exposed to the increase in oxygen in the HBOT chamber. This means that, immediately upon starting HBOT, the increased oxygen can overcome the apparent DNA injury in the stunned or idling cells, and then the cells start to function more normally again.

This takes place with repetitive daily exposure to hyperbaric oxygen, which also stimulates new blood vessel growth in the old, chronic wounds. We have seen this in tissues damaged by radiation, compromised skin grafts and flaps, and burns, among other injuries.

Seizure disorders provide perhaps the best examples of chronic wounds resulting from the inflammatory reaction, the low blood flow/low oxygen tissue pathology in chronic wounds, and HBOT's beneficial effects on chronic wounds and pathology. Scars form on the brain as a result of trauma, infection, or low blood flow/oxygenation (e.g., near drowning or cardiac arrest). Scars anywhere in the body are usually characterized by low blood flow and oxygenation, and brain scars are no exception. In fact, we see this on SPECT brain blood flow scans (described in Chapter 3) when a patient is in between seizures. The areas of seizure foci are generally areas of low blood flow.

A similar example occurs in heart muscle after a heart attack. Scarred areas of low blood flow and oxygenation cause irritability of the heart cells. These cells suddenly "fire-off," which causes spontaneous electrical discharges, which can in turn progress to runaway heart rhythms and sudden death. In the brain, these irritable areas similarly "fire-off" and lead to electrical discharges that can spread throughout the brain to cause generalized seizures.

In 1993, I had the opportunity to treat a number of children after their near-drowning incidents, one of whom we'll call Mikey, who had a seizure disorder. As I treated Mikey, he showed a reduction in his seizures. Over the years, as I continued to treat children with near drowning and other brain disorders who also had seizures, I found the same result: namely, a reduction in the number, frequency, and often severity of seizures.

In the late 1990s, I came across literature from Brazil where Dr. J. Machado noted that cerebral palsy children treated with HBOT had a marked, permanent reduction in seizures. Similarly, researchers in China reported in 1995 and later that children with epilepsy had a reduction in seizures. In most cases, the dose of HBOT was generally lower than what had been typically used for chronic wounds elsewhere in the body.

In addition, over the past four years, my research has shown that HBOT can reverse some of the damage in chronic traumatic brain injury in animals. This research had never been done before with animals with any type of chronic brain injury. In that experiment, which used rats, we showed that with HBOT we improved the blood supply to the damaged area and that the damaged area began to function again, as demonstrated by improved measurements of spatial memory/learning. (In humans we saw the clinical improvements and measured it with various types of testing, especially SPECT, as explained in Chapter 3. The testing showed improved blood flow, but did not prove that we grew new blood vessels.)

So, after repeated exposure to HBOT, an old wound located anywhere in the body grows new blood vessels and the cells begin to function again. Growth hormones are developed, tissue grows, and the wounds heal. This is the basis for the dramatic claims made in hyperbaric medicine.

Once you understand the inflammatory response and the potential role of HBOT in minimizing its damage, it's easy to see how hyperbaric oxygen therapy could have such a wide application across so many fields of medicine. You can also understand my excitement for this field and its future for you and your loved ones.

CHAPTER 3
THE CURRENT USES FOR HBOT

BEFORE WE DISCUSS THE RAPIDLY EXPANDING USES of HBOT, we must remember how much we've learned from the original applications, especially diving medicine. Even in that field, we found out that we still had much to learn. One particular case, a diving tragedy, taught me a great deal.

In March 1990, I treated a 46-year-old man—we'll call him Tom—who had been injured in a diving accident seven months before. He had been a diver for 23 years for one of the major diving companies in the world. Because he was both competent and skilled, he had been put on the most difficult diving operations and his performance had always been exemplary. However, in September 1989, the company decided to start using a radical decompression method that hadn't been in use since the 1940s.

Tom's company started applying oxygen to divers decompressing from deep helium dives in the Gulf of Mexico. These dives were to depths over 300 feet. When the divers ascended to 60 feet of water, they were instructed to begin breathing pure oxygen. This amount of oxygen had not been used for commercial decompression before, and Tom developed oxygen toxicity. It manifested itself as they got him on deck in a chamber and re-exposed him to oxygen at the same pressure. He had a seizure, and while he was in the midst of the seizure they decompressed him further. His lungs expanded to the breaking point. Tom ended up having an internal air embolism—the small air sacs in the lung ruptured, sending air into the blood vessels, which took it to his heart and eventually to his brain. This caused damage to the brain similar to tiny strokes. It took Tom 20–30 minutes to finally wake up in the chamber.

My senior partner, Dr. Keith Van Meter, who had been called about this case, recommended a very slow therapeutic decompression that brought Tom to surface pressure over a period of about 20 hours. Once removed from the chamber, he was observed for 12 hours before being brought to New Orleans. Dr. Van Meter examined him there, conducting a meticulous neurological exam in the middle of the night in the emergency department. He found Tom to be intact; he did, however, want to perform some additional tests.

Unfortunately, the diving company took over the course of Tom's care, and a neurologist who had very little experience with diving medicine took on the case. This would have consequences for Tom: one of the tests the neurologist performed came back mildly abnormal, and his physical exam was abnormal. But Tom protested that he was fine, and the neurologist decided to comply with his request to return to work. Only two weeks later, 30 days after the initial seizure, using the same oxygen toxic protocol, he experienced a severe case of decompression sickness involving the brain, spinal cord, and bone. He had a headache, confusion, and pain and numbness in one of his legs. After his an air embolism in the chamber 30 days before, his brain and body had not yet healed enough to be challenged by the rigors of diving so soon. This is somewhat like the second concussion syndrome, in which an athlete who has a concussion returns to play and experiences another concussion soon after. We see devastating consequences when the effects of the second concussion are added to the effects of the incompletely healed first concussion. Tom was now severely injured. He was treated offshore with a single HBOT treatment, after which he showed partial improvement. He was then brought ashore for more treatments, but as a result of a series of miscommunications, he didn't receive those necessary follow-up treatments, and instead went home.

The next day, I was asked to track down Tom. I finally talked to his wife, who said he was sitting at the kitchen table, basically in a stupor; his decompression sickness had progressed. Although she'd encouraged him to see a doctor, he lacked the ability to act. By the time I finally saw this injured diver in the hyperbaric unit, he showed serious neurological impairment.

We treated Tom over the next month and saw some improvement, but when he reached a clinical plateau using the standard higher pressure protocol, we stopped treatment. At this point he was formally declared demented—that is, he had a severe impairment of intellectual and cognitive faculties. I have considerable experience with commercial divers and brain decompression illness, and along with that I've seen their employers declare them malingerers and fakers. Before long, these divers see their worker's compensation cut off.

Sadly, I have seen many of these divers go on to tragic deaths, and falling short of that, they end up with a variety of problems, from broken families to alcoholism or fatal car accidents, drug addiction, and so forth. Tom was no different. He ended up bankrupt, his family crumbled into disarray. Irritability and short-temperedness are hallmarks of organic brain injury, and Tom found himself in disputes that he mismanaged and made worse.

Brain decompression illness is difficult to diagnose. Before we had imaging technology to show brain blood flow, we found ourselves in a perpetual state of "it's your word against mine" between the company and the diver (and the company and the treating doctor, too). Almost invariably, the experts called in were former U.S. military diving doctors. They gained their experience with decompression illness in the Navy, where divers' immediate symptoms were rapidly treated and cured in the great majority of cases. With a residual injury, the most that would happen is medical discharge from the military, since lawsuits are impossible against the U.S. military.

In the commercial diving industry, however, when someone is injured and unable to work, and their worker's compensation is discontinued, a lawsuit naturally results. This is when the company's witnesses usually deny that an injury is present, because they aren't familiar with these injuries; but the treating doctors following the case can see a permanently brain-damaged individual.

Tom was so disgusted with his company's response after so many years of his service that he decided to take matters into his own hands, which meant loading two pistols, calling his brother and telling him he intended to shoot everyone in the company's offshore diving operations. In his brain-injured state, he thought he could even the score and avoid being caught. Fortunately, his brother managed to reach the attorneys on his case and together they got to him and managed to disarm him before he carried out his threats. They also put him in a car and brought him to me.

They wanted me to "do something with him." It was seven months after his accident, and at the time, there was nothing we knew to do, especially since he had already been treated. It was thought he'd reached maximum medical improvement. Frankly, everyone involved was desperate. Somehow, though, they managed to persuade me to look for other options.

The Important Twist that Illuminates HBOT

I decided to speak with Dr. Van Meter, an international expert in diving medicine, regarding Tom's condition. He reiterated that there was no treatment for this condition, but he recommended that I call a hyperbaric oxygen specialist, Dr. Richard Neubauer, in southern Florida. I found it amazing that after 10 or so years of hyperbaric medicine, living and practicing in Florida, Dr. Neubauer had never treated a diver. But in the previous 10+ years he had primarily treated individuals recovering from stroke and patients with multiple sclerosis. He then suggested that I try what he'd done for those two diagnoses, which was a shallow (lower pressure), short treatment. Since I had nothing to lose, I decided to give it a try.

Dr. Neubauer recommended that I give Tom 200 low pressure treatments. I listened to Dr. Neubauer's rationale for recommending so many treatments, and after further discussion we settled on trying 40 treatments. We proceeded, and Tom began to respond. His constant dizziness decreased, his behavior became more appropriate, his balance was better, and he began to talk and think at a higher level. At the end of 40 treatments he seemed noticeably better, and medical evaluation verified his improvement as well. So, I decided to try another block of 40 treatments.

During the seventy-ninth treatment, Tom had an extreme anxiety reaction in the chamber. He had been complaining that he was having increasing dizziness in the past few days and that he wasn't sure the treatments were giving him any further benefit. That day, he demanded that treatment end early. We took him out of the chamber and he literally ran out of our facility in tears. It appeared that he had likely reached his limits and may have even had a mild degree of oxygen toxicity, which fortunately was quickly reversed.

Ultimately, this man and his wife suffered enormously from the mishandling of his medical case. However, this diver decided to credit HBOT for his improvements, and maintained his gains and did well afterward. After a complex series of negotiations, he ended up being compensated for the career-ending injury. And, what we learned from treating Tom helped expand the use of HBOT.

Another Diver's Story Leads to Greater Knowledge

In September 1991, I had occasion to see another man: Dan Greathouse, a junior high school math and English teacher, a pianist, and principal of the nighttime GED school. He was also a recovering alcoholic, sober for nearly three years. He had recently taken up SCUBA diving, but on his final "checkout" dive in Lake Powell he suffered an air embolism and decompression sickness. Over the course of a week he became severely disabled. His doctor, Dr. Jeff Beall, is an old and good friend of mine. He realized the gravity of Dan's situation, but since he had no knowledge of or experience with diving medicine, he called me.

Dan's story takes many twists and turns, and involves communication from one state to another. I tried to get HBOT for him in Albuquerque, but insurance issues stood in the way, and when he was finally treated one month after his diving accident, he was given only standard diving medical treatment, which failed.

Through a series of events, Dan saw a neurologist who diagnosed him with balance problems resulting from damage to the cerebellum, the area of the brain that controls coordination, among other things. Later, he was given neuropsychological testing and found to have an IQ of 101—significantly lower than his normal IQ, which had helped him become his college's valedictorian. He also had an abnormal electroencephalogram (EEG).

Dan was told that his problems (cognition, gait, balance, coordination, speech, and so forth) were not organic, and were not caused by a diving accident; rather, they were due to emotional difficulties and his prior alcoholism.

This was a ludicrous conclusion, and didn't match the test data, especially the EEG results. What followed is a dramatic series of events and tragedies that took him to psychiatric hospitals, jail cells, and state hospitals. (In the next chapter I provide further information about the tragedy of brain injuries.) Eventually, I made arrangements for Dan to come to New Orleans. In fact, I had the judge prematurely release him from the psychiatric hospital. When we first saw him, he could barely walk straight and couldn't communicate effectively— clearly emotional problems were not at the root of his illness. However, over the next two weeks of tests and examinations by many doctors, he deteriorated dramatically, and experienced near-psychotic depression (I had taken him off his antidepressants for specialized testing).

All the test results and consultations were consistent with my diagnosis of brain decompression illness, but the clincher was the SPECT brain scan (see Dan's scans on page 1 of the photo insert.) All of the damage from the diving accident was visible in florid color. A SPECT done after one HBOT showed such blood flow improvement that I knew for certain that Dan was a candidate for HBOT.

We began HBOT, and indeed Dan improved dramatically. His balance corrected, his speech became fluid, his short-term memory returned, and his piano abilities resurfaced. As he said, "The music's back in my head." Repeat SPECT brain scans also documented this improvement. By the time he returned to New Mexico, his EEG had normalized— and when he had repeat neuropsychological testing his IQ measured at 123. Despite everything that happened to Dan, he returned to New Mexico and put his life back together—he even obtained two master's degrees in educational psychology and brain injury. He went on to test educationally handicapped children for the state of New Mexico for the next 15 years. After retiring, he continued as a specialist, testing brain-injured patients in a West Texas Hospital (where he remains employed today). We stay in touch, and in 2010 he completed his book, *Doc, I Want my Brain Back* (helped by my coauthor, Virginia McCullough), in which Dan tells his important— and frightening—story. What happened to Dan could happen to anyone. Dan's account of what it was like to be brain-damaged and have no one but his parents believe in him touched me deeply.

Dan's story is a powerful one, and he is a fully functional successful man. His case had tremendous meaning for me, because I knew that I had come on to something that was only the tip of the iceberg for neurorehabilitation. (You can see the video of a speech he gave to veterans in 2014, in which he tells his story in order to support the use of HBOT for veterans with TBI and PTSD, at HBOT.com.)

The Breakthrough Study

The above two cases had a great impact on my subsequent practice and the present day prescription for HBOT in chronic neurological conditions. After treating Tom, Dan, and a host of other divers and chronic trauma and stroke patients, I decided to begin research evaluating the ability of brain blood flow imaging to predict who would respond to hyperbaric oxygen therapy and who would not. Together with Dr. Sheldon Gottlieb, a colleague of Dr. Neubauer and the director of our research department, and Dr. Van Meter, we designed the trial to see if the SPECT imaging could be a quick and dirty test to screen patients for this type of therapy.

We decided to do a baseline SPECT brain blood flow scan, a single hyperbaric treatment the following day, and then repeat the SPECT brain scan immediately afterwards. (This test was originally used by Dr. Neubauer in 1990 in a patient 14 years after stroke). The patients would then go on to receive a block of 40 hyperbaric treatments. At the end of 40 treatments we'd repeat the brain scans and all other neurological testing that we had done prior to beginning hyperbaric oxygen therapy, including a video physical exam. Then, after I assessed the patients, they, their families, and I would reach a decision for continuing or discontinuing therapy. If therapy was continued, we would treat the patient with additional 40-treatment blocks of hyperbaric oxygen therapy, reevaluating at each interval. As long as the patients kept improving with each block of treatment we would continue the HBOT.

This research became known as the "Perfusion/Metabolism Encephalopathy Study," which we officially began at the JoEllen Smith Medical Center in New Orleans in 1994. Over the course of the next five and a half years, we evaluated nearly 200 patients including children and adults with nearly 50 different neurological conditions, including cerebral palsy, autism, traumatic brain injury, seizure disorders, near drowning, chronic effects of carbon monoxide poisoning, stroke, and so forth. What I found was that at 40 HBOT treatments, patients were noticeably better but not dramatically so. By the time 80 treatments had elapsed, however, patients further improved to the extent that all therapists, doctors, and examiners could document the improvement.

This study became the basis for the 80-treatment protocol frequently quoted on the Internet and now routinely used throughout the United States for hyperbaric oxygen in chronic neurological conditions. As it turns out, I investigated beyond this 80-treatmetn standard in a variety of patients, and what I found was that many patients did not tolerate continued 40-treatment blocks in the time period we were studying. Some would benefit, but many became fatigued, emotionally unsettled and "down" (dysphoria); some even showed some regression.

But once I became more attuned to the nuances of dosing HBOT, I found that this 80-treatment protocol is not set in stone. Frequently, patients will come to a plateau after less than 40, or between 40 and 80 treatments. It all depends on the dose of HBOT used, the peculiarities of the patient's diagnosis, his or her genetics, and other individual medical issues. Once I realized that I was dosing a tricky drug (oxygen and pressure) which was specific to each patient, I began to reflect on my past patients. While the great majority of them demonstrated benefit with the fixed, lower dose of HBOT I was using, many came to a plateau at some point and began to demonstrate side effects. Often the signs were subtle, but when HBOT was continued, the patients deteriorated.

The arguments regarding dosing HBOT came to a head in 2001, when Dr. Neubauer asked me to give a lecture on "The Dosage of Hyperbaric Oxygen in Chronic Brain Injury" at the 2nd International Symposium on Hyperbaric Oxygenation for Cerebral Palsy and the Brain Injured Child. Prior to this lecture, it was accepted dogma in hyperbaric medicine that you could not generate oxygen sensitivity or overdosing effects at the low doses we were using to treat chronic brain injury. This was well known to be the case at the *higher* pressures we typically used for diabetic foot wounds, carbon monoxide poisoning and decompression sickness.

I reviewed my previous 12 years of experience and presented 33 cases. Half of them were mine, patients that I had treated mostly under the previously mentioned Perfusion Metabolism Encephalopathy Study. Some were my very first diving cases, such as Tom and Dan. The other half was composed of cases from all over the world, those reported by patients and families who were inquiring as to why they had a negative outcome, when Dr. Neubauer and I were publishing positive results. What I showed was that, even at lower doses of HBOT, you could administer *too much* HBOT. Many of the doctors in the audience were furious with my presentation (including Dr. Neubauer), but the data was solid.

To this day, my wife, who is a seasoned hyperbaric technician/nurse, and my office/practice manager, receives phone calls every week or two from patients who were incorrectly dosed with HBOT or who developed side effects. While this number pales in comparison to the numbers who improve, it points to a very important concept. HBOT has similarities to all other drugs: the effect of the drug is the result of using the right dose, for the right disease, at the right time in the disease process, for the right patient. The hyperbaric physician has to interview, examine, monitor, and treat the patient, and adjust the dose as needed.

Treatment Blocks

As a result of the Perfusion/Metabolism Encephalopathies Study, HBOT is described in terms of 40-treatment blocks for chronic neurological conditions. This number was derived from the conversation above that I had with Dr. Neubauer about Tom, the commercial diver. Dr. Neubauer had recommended 200 treatments. For that patient at that time this number of treatments was impossible. What I wanted to do was give the diver the minimum number necessary to see a permanent, measurable improvement. Dr. Neubauer's answer was that I should try 40. When I asked, "Why 40?" he said that over the years, 40 treatments had seemed to be a pretty good number. While this sounds flippant and superficial, it was far from those things. In fact, Dr. Neubauer was summing up his 10–15 years of experience in hyperbaric medicine treating multiple sclerosis and stroke, and added in the other factors. For example, some people could only stay for a few treatments, and some stayed two weeks, and still others had treatment cut short for other reasons. He noted that if patients had about 40 treatments, then he and others could see the difference in the patients and the improvements showed some permanence.

As a result of this information, the experience with Tom and Dan Greathouse, and the subsequent Perfusion/Metabolism Encephalopathies Study, I developed a protocol that continues to dominate most hyperbaric treatment for chronic neurological diseases. I also investigated beyond the 80-treatment protocol (two blocks of 40 treatments) in a variety of patients and found that many patients didn't tolerate continued 40-treatment blocks at the low pressures and durations I was using (1.5–1.75 ATA/60 to 90 minutes/HBOT). While some showed benefit, many became fatigued or dysphoric, that is, they felt unhappy or disturbed in some way. Some patients also showed some regression.

Some patients have had the full 200 treatments that Dr. Neubauer recommended as optimal, and *have* shown marked neurological improvements. Unfortunately, these represent a limited number of cases, which then limits our ability to draw conclusions based on this number of treatments.

Interestingly, these 40-treatment blocks have precedence in hyperbaric medicine. If we look at HBOT for chronic wounding, specifically in radiation injury and diabetic foot wounds, we find that the minimum number of treatments for radiation injury is 40. In a 1995 review of many wound healing centers in Texas, the average number of hyperbaric treatments required to heal extremity wounds in diabetics and others was a little over 40 treatments.

This mounting evidence points to a constancy for the numbers of hyperbaric treatments in chronic wounding necessary to achieve permanent results. When I performed the animal experiments in 1995 on chronic traumatic brain injury, all four of my lab technicians independently remarked in the treatment book, unbeknownst to each other, that the rats receiving hyperbaric oxygen showed a noticeable change in behavior at approximately 25 treatments. Other research has determined that 25 treatments is roughly the point at which new blood vessel growth has occurred among patients treated for chronic radiation wounds. The overall conclusion is that, in cases of chronic wounding, 40 HBOTs in a concentrated block of treatments is necessary to achieve permanent improvement whether the wound is in the leg, arm, jaw, brain, or other tissue.

The Familiar Uses of HBOT

Beyond diving medicine, HBOT is now used to treat such things as carbon monoxide poisoning, which is why it came into public awareness when the Sago mine survivor was transported to another state to receive it. (I discuss this specific use in Chapter 4, which also provides information about acute brain injuries.) In addition, now that Medicare has approved HBOT for diabetic foot wound healing, it has become an accepted use. However, as you no doubt know, the issue of approved treatments for any given condition is complex, and does not necessarily correlate with the research showing its usefulness for that disease. (See Chapter 14 for a discussion of HBOT's off-label use.) As you can see from Table I, the current list of "typically reimbursed" uses may seem a bit odd because it mentions such a limited number of seemingly unrelated conditions. I have provided some brief explanation of some causes of these conditions.

As you will soon see, the conditions are not so unrelated; in fact, they are related by common underlying disease processes. HBOT treats these disease processes; however, it begs the question of what *other* diseases have these underlying processes. Fortunately, physicians in other countries have answered this question. As I mentioned before, this has been part of the problem in the acceptance of hyperbaric medicine—no one could "connect the dots." Knowing what you know about oxygen deprivation and the inflammatory reaction, you can now connect the dots and see why the list of treatable diagnoses is much greater in foreign countries than domestically: 20 diagnoses in Japan, 65 in China (with 18 investigative diagnoses), and 71 in Russia. Thankfully, these countries have led the way.

Table I:
Hyperbaric Oxygen Therapy Approved Indications

Condition	Description and Cause
Air or Gas Embolism	Air in the arteries caused by diving (internal rupture of the lung) or any invasive medical procedure that punctures an artery or the lung.
Carbon Monoxide and Carbon Monoxide Poisoning Complicated by Cyanide Poisoning	Inhaling carbon monoxide from any fossil fuel burning source. This includes gasoline, diesel, propane, natural gas, charcoal briquettes, and so on. Can also have carbon monoxide poisoning by inhaling methylene chloride, a common ingredient in floor and paint stripping agents. Methylene chloride is metabolized in the body to carbon monoxide. Cyanide is a chemical that metabolically poisons the energy generating machinery of every cell in the body. Oxygen displaces cyanide.
Clostridial Myonecrosis (Gas Gangrene)	Usually resulting from dirty wounds such as war wounds, wounds caused by animal hooves, punctures from rusty metal, and so forth. This is a rapidly progressive infection of muscle and is fatal unless antibiotics, aggressive surgery, amputations, and HBOT are used.
Crush Injuries and Skeletal Muscle Compartment Syndromes	Usually caused by heavy equipment and farm injuries to the extremities that involve crushing and loss of blood flow. With the swelling from the crush wound, blood flow is further compromised and the muscle compartments become gangrenous.

Decompression Sickness	"The bends." This is due to gas separation and bubbles that form in tissue or are released into the blood stream. Most of "the bends" is neurological, but it can affect any tissue in the body.
Central Retinal Artery Occlusion (CRAO)	CRAO is essentially a stroke of the eye where a clot forms in the main artery supplying blood to the eye. It is a cause of sudden blindness.
Enhancement of Healing in Selected Problem Wounds	Diabetic foot wounds and wounds from damage or disease to arteries and veins in the legs. The wounds that benefit best from HBOT are those where the blood supply has been damaged, there is swelling, or infection, or the body's immune system does not work properly, such as in diabetes.
Severe Anemia	Acute severe blood loss and the inability or lack of permission to transfuse with blood. This may occur with religious prohibitions, but it may have applications to battle casualties and severe trauma.
Intracranial Abscess	Abscesses of the brain tissue and the covering of the brain. Common in AIDS patients and in "Third World" countries.
Necrotizing Soft Tissue Infections	Commonly known as the "flesh eating bacteria," usually rapidly progressive severe infections caused by a mixture of bacteria that need oxygen and those that don't need oxygen to grow.
Osteomyelitis (Refractory)	Chronic bone infections that have resisted standard treatment. These are most common in the lower leg after motorcycle accidents and other severe trauma where the fracture was open.
Delayed Radiation Injury (Soft Tissue and Bony Necrosis)	Injury to both soft tissue and bone that usually results in wounds that lack blood supply due to radiation damage to the blood vessels.

Compromised Skin Grafts and Flaps	Grafts and flaps of tissue with compromised blood supply. Most common in breast reconstruction surgery.
Thermal Burns	Burns due to fire or heat.
Idiopathic Sudden Sensorineural Hearing Loss	Sudden loss of hearing in one or both ears.

Source: 2015 Undersea and Hyperbaric Medical Society[1]

The Significance of SPECT Imaging

Before you go farther into this book and address the issue of most importance to you, please take a look at the glossary in the back of the book, which represents the "language of hyperbaric oxygen." Using this glossary will help you to get the most out of this book. But, because you will encounter information about SPECT imaging in virtually all the chapters ahead, I want to take a moment to help you to understand its importance beyond a glossary definition.

Briefly, SPECT is an acronym for Single Photon Emission Computed Tomography. It is essentially CT or CAT scanning applied to nuclear medicine. Instead of shooting x-rays through patients, patients are injected with a small amount of a radioactive drug. Five percent of the drug is taken up in the brain and then emits a type of x-ray that is captured by a sophisticated camera that revolves around the patient's head.

SPECT is different from anatomic imaging, such as CAT (computerized axial tomography) and MRI (magnetic resonance imaging), which give us a roadmap-like picture of the brain that shows the different types of tissue. SPECT and its close cousin PET (positron-emission tomography) go a step further, allowing us to see blood flow and metabolism of brain tissue similar to seeing the movement of cars, trucks, and people on the roads as they go about their business. (Today's advanced forms of MRI can also do this.)

PET, by the way, is a more sophisticated and expensive type of functional brain imaging. It was developed after SPECT and validated with SPECT. Traditionally, it has had better resolution than SPECT, and using different radiopharmaceuticals has been able to measure blood flow, metabolism, and neurotransmitter receptors on neurons. On the other hand, SPECT has been exclusively a blood flow measuring technique that measures metabolism only indirectly. Recently, however, SPECT resolution has improved and is now nearly the equivalent of PET; in addition, receptor tracers have become available.

The development of SPECT is remarkable for many reasons, not the least of which is that we can document changes in the brain. We now have "before and after" imaging that demonstrates permanent changes in function brought about by HBOT. (I have included some before and after images where appropriate, so you can see this for yourself.) Needless to say, SPECT is both a valuable research and clinical tool. Despite all of the new whiz-bang imaging modalities, I have not found a single imaging technology that matches the simplicity, availability, and demonstration power of SPECT with HBOT.

How SPECT Imaging is Used

The ideal sequence of SPECT brain imaging is a baseline SPECT brain before any hyperbaric treatment, a repeat SPECT brain after the first hyperbaric oxygen treatment (within hours of the end of the treatment), and then another after a course of hyperbaric oxygen therapy. (This is the same sequence we used for over five and a half years on the Perfusion/Metabolism Encephalopathies Study.) If the second scan shows improvement as well as the final one, it overwhelms any argument of a placebo effect or spontaneous improvement, especially when the patient is a child, or so brain injured that he or she has no idea of the purpose of the scans and treatment. If we can demonstrate that the brain improves with one treatment and then it subsequently improves with a series of treatments, it's a very strong argument that the HBOT is responsible for any improvement observed in the imaging and the patient's condition. This is the paradigm of the SPECT imaging we published in the first HBOT veterans study in 2011. Although there was no treatment control group in the study, the imaging makes the argument of effectiveness of HBOT irrefutable. (You can view this study yourself at HBOT.com.)

Beyond serving as evidence to leverage against disbelievers and third-party payers for reimbursement of HBOT, SPECT brain imaging is useful to satisfy a patient's curiosity. Parents also demand information about their children's brain function; this is true for adults, too. It is only natural that brain injured individuals want to see a picture of what is wrong with their brain, and often the picture has the power to bring home, so to speak, the reality of one's medical condition. It also has the added benefit of arguing for a brain-injured patient to stop smoking or drinking, abusing drugs, working in a toxic environment, or risking repetitive head injuries in order to preserve what brain function is left and maximize long-term abilities.

It's been my experience that patients and their family members break down and cry in front of the scanner as they see a picture of the injured brain. They are finally able to visualize the damage that was done in an accident or by some other means. Equally impressive is the patients' elation when they see a repeat image after HBOT that shows improvement in brain blood flow that verifies the improvement in their clinical condition.

SPECT has the added benefit of demonstrating the improvements of hyperbaric oxygen to the current primary doctors and to anyone treating the patient in the future. I'm sure many doctors have referred other patients for HBOT based on what they see in these scans, combined with clinical improvements. The decision to obtain SPECT must be made prior to the first HBOT. Even one treatment can permanently change the brain. I often hear parents and others regret that they did not obtain a SPECT before starting treatment, especially if their child or other loved one has had dramatic improvement. In these situations, patients and families want to take this proof to their primary doctor or others, but because they don't have a pre-treatment scan, they don't have a baseline. For this reason, I encourage patients to at least obtain the baseline SPECT before any treatment or make very sure you do not want this scan before proceeding with HBOT. The decision on subsequent SPECTs can be obtained after they see the results of the first scan.

We found this imaging predictive of those who would respond to repetitive HBOT. However, since we now have so many cases with such a variety of neuropathology, we don't necessarily need SPECT unless it is an unusual diagnosis, the families or patients want additional evidence to demonstrate the effectiveness of hyperbaric oxygen therapy, they want to see if additional HBOT may have an added benefit, or they want to see the injury and "dysfunction" in the brain. Actually, the last reason listed may be the most important. When a patient can actually see a picture that displays the injury, the experience can have a profound effect, and lead to greater insight about the disability involved. I continue to be amazed at the number of patients with brain disorders I've seen in the past 30 years who have never had a blood flow scan of their brain. These powerful images show dysfunction not visible on CT or MRI. The lack of such scans has led to a phenomenal number of mistaken psychiatric diagnoses. You saw this in Dan Greathouse's case, but his story is only one instance of a tragic trend.

The image of the injury is also powerful when it is coupled with SPECT brain scans after treatment to show improvement. Scans of some of the cases described in this book appear in the photo insert. In addition, if you go to www.hyperbaricmedicalassociation.org (or www.harchhyperbarics.com) and click on the government testimonies link, you will see the brain SPECTs of the 22 patients I showed to the congressional sub-committees. They provide indelible images that, once seen, are not soon forgotten. This effect is not lost on agencies and companies that reimburse medical services. When the images are combined with caregivers' reports, they become another powerful proof for the beneficial effect of HBOT. This, too, may help patients obtain reimbursement. They are also not lost on legal teams. The ability to see brain injury and its improvement after HBOT has "made the case" for countless patients whose brain injury was disputed. This was what happened with our divers, allowing first the English physicians and then us to the see the injury, which before SPECT had never been visualized in 90 years of diving medicine.

Can You Determine the Likelihood of Response to HBOT?

The ability of a patient to respond to hyperbaric oxygen therapy is proportional to the size, volume, and location of ischemic penumbral tissue (described in Chapter 6) in relation to the rest of the normal brain. (Ischemic penumbral tissue is the low blood flow tissue that surrounds dead tissue, is not functioning, but is not yet dead). So, there may be a limit to the amount of stimulation and growth of brain tissue that hyperbaric oxygen therapy can generate through up-regulation of hormones, gene expression, and so forth (explained in Chapters 1, 6, 8, and 12). As patients lose greater and greater amounts of brain tissue, it is harder to recover function in the brain, which means that with larger amounts of lost tissue, the response to hyperbaric oxygen is less.

I have seen this most clearly in near-drowning patients (I've treated nearly 40 of these individuals). Near-drowning is the most devastating injury of all that I've been involved with, and I have seen only modest responses to hyperbaric oxygen among these individuals when treated years after the event (if treated immediately, the story is different). This is also true of those who have suffered massive brain injury, patients with advanced multiple sclerosis, and patients with significant brain atrophy.

The clinical diagnosis of dementia is correlated with the loss of about 50 grams of brain tissue. (The average human brain has between 1,100–1,300 grams of brain tissue; for men it is closer to 1,300 and for women, 1,100. By the time the patient is in a wheelchair or bedbound, completely disoriented, and nearly unresponsive, it's difficult to bring back meaningful function. Again, some amazing cases have been reported, but by and large, with greater amounts of lost brain tissue the response to HBOT is less, and requires a much greater number of treatments. Because of this, I often ask the families of patients who appear to fall into this category for a recent magnetic resonance imaging (MRI) of the brain. If I see massive loss of brain tissue, I make a very, very conservative estimate on return of function.

As discussed above, the change in pattern and appearance of the SPECT scan after a single HBOT can also help predict response. To illustrate, I have calculated the following predictive percentages: I have two SPECT scans placed side by side on a computer screen and I don't know if the baseline pre-HBOT scan is on the left or the right. If, after one HBOT, I correctly identify the "after" HBOT scan as the better scan, then I can predict a roughly 90 percent chance that the patient will experience improvement with repetitive HBOT. When I have picked the post-HBOT scan as worse or as showing no change, then roughly 50 percent of these patients will still see improvement with HBOT, and the other half will have no detectable clinical change if 40 HBOTs are delivered. This is one of the reasons for doing SPECT brain imaging in conjunction with HBOT.

Measuring Response

Ever since I began to use HBOT with patients who'd suffered neurological injury, I have performed video examinations. Some of these videos were sent home with patients to view with their families. They could then draw their own conclusions about the patient's improved condition—or the absence of gains.

When treatment begins, I have the patient and/or the patients' families generate a "problem list," which we then review at the end of treatment. The list has the advantage of letting the patient and family prioritize what they feel are the most important deficits that they can review at the end of a block of HBOT. In addition, I usually recommend that the patient and family keep a diary in which they can make entries of improvements or deteriorations in any function as they progress through treatment. For example, perhaps a patient was unable to use language normally, but then shows measurable improvement in that area after a block of HBOT. Sleep patterns may change, or motor skills might improve. Family members might note these improvements, or a patient might make this observation on his or her own.

So, we have a combination of recorded family and patient responses, video exams, and imaging, along with other before and after testing. Then we couple this with reports from independent caregivers, such as physical therapists, occupational therapists, and others on the medical team. With all of this information at hand, I usually see a consensus forming about the degree of improvement or the lack thereof.

Ultimately, the final answer rests with the patient and his or her family. If they decide that the gain or improvement has not been worth the hyperbaric treatment at any point, we stop. If they have seen benefit, we may continue with another block of treatment. Earlier, I discussed the widespread protocol of 80 treatments in use in the United States. This was reached not because hyperbaric doctors decided on it, but rather, it was driven by patients and their results as I investigated 40 HBOT blocks in successive patients.

Note: If you peruse YouTube, you will find four before-and-after videos of patients I have treated over the years. All four of them were treated either the day of the injury, or within 2–4 months of injury. (You can also find links to all of these videos on HBOT.com). These patients are:

- Chad Rovira, day of severe traumatic brain injury
- Curt Allen, four months after severe traumatic brain injury
- Vickie Harrison, reflex sympathetic pain syndrome or complex regional pain syndrome, over 2 months after injury to her foot
- Chloe Carlucci, blindness, four months after herpes encephalitis

While the great majority of these chronic patients have experienced notable changes (captured on video), the changes that occur when I can deliver HBOT in the first 4–5 months after injury are nothing short of dramatic. In this early period, the loss of brain tissue is incomplete. HBOT can truncate the injury process and stimulate repair; it "turns around" the injury and accelerates the path of recovery. The results speak for themselves.

Single vs. Multiple Therapies

Again, I want to emphasize that most conditions require multiple therapies, not just a single approach. In fact, I recommend visualizing a final care plan as a mosaic. This isn't such a revolutionary idea; after all, we treat bacterial pneumonia, for example, with antibiotics, a cough remedy, and chest percussion, along with bed rest and fluids. And, while we may say that the antibiotics are the primary treatment, they may not do their job well without the other components.

The need for different therapies may reflect the manner in which medical conditions develop. For example, many conditions result from a combination of insults, such as low blood flow, inflammation, toxins, trauma, psychosocial factors, and so forth. In order to reverse the process, we have to address the way the causes affect many different organ systems.

The perfect example of this phenomenon is Chad Rovira (further discussed in Chapter 4). He made immediate progress with HBOT, but then had combined therapy at an in-patient neurorehab facility while he continued to receive HBOT. With the combination of treatment, he made dramatic progress. However, once the HBOT was withdrawn he made almost no further improvement with inpatient neurorehab alone. But when we again combined the treatments, he made further leaps in progress.

The same scenario was true for a 17-year-old with traumatic brain injury, Curt Allen, Jr., also described in Chapter 4, who languished in the same neurorehab facility to which Chad had been transferred. It wasn't until we added HBOT that Curt made his dramatic gains, but we simultaneously continued his outpatient neurorehab. In each of these cases, and many more like them, I combined HBOT with existing therapy so patients could achieve the maximum recovery possible. *This* is individualized care, and is the essence of effective neurorehabilitation.

The key to this concept of multi-modality care, however, and the most important point I want you to take away, is this: *HBOT is different from almost all of the other therapies we have. It is a biological repair therapy, a foundation therapy upon which most other therapies can be added.*

As opposed to the multitude of stimulative, adaptive, symptom-masking or modifying therapies, HBOT actually *repairs* damage and generates new tissue growth. It does this through its widespread effect on a very large number of genes, and through the use of two ubiquitous agents that are involved with all life on this planet, oxygen and pressure. I predict that, because of the fundamental nature of HBOT, it is unlikely that we will ever discover a treatment that has so many biological effects and wide-ranging applications.

PART II

CONDITIONS THAT HYPERBARIC OXYGEN THERAPY CAN HELP

YOU MAY HAVE CHOSEN THIS BOOK BECAUSE YOU saw a condition listed in the Table of Contents that is of concern to you or a loved one. Now that you have a basic understanding of HBOT itself, you will see the ways in which it can be used to treat certain conditions. You may also gain an understanding about the condition that most drew you to learn about this treatment.

I hope you will pass on the information in these chapters to others. Educated patients are in the best position to obtain treatment in a timely way. I also know that we can expand the accepted uses of HBOT once readers like you bring what you've learned to your own doctors.

I am going to start with what I consider to be the paramount treatable diagnosis for HBOT, and we'll be devoting considerable time to this topic. It is one of the most important topics and ideas for you to retain when you are finished reading this book. Most of the information is directed to treating chronic traumatic brain injury (TBI), but I discuss the overwhelming evidence for treating acute TBI in Chapter 14: Roadblocks and Gateways to the Future. When you finish this section on TBI, I want you to temporarily fast forward to Chapter 14, where you can read the rest of the story on TBI. When you are done, you should be ready to demand HBOT for your family and friends with TBI.

CHAPTER 4

TRAUMATIC BRAIN INJURIES (TBI) AND OTHER MEDICAL EMERGENCIES

SINCE THE PUBLICATION OF THE FIRST EDITION OF this book, my sense of urgency over what I say in this chapter has increased exponentially. I cannot stress enough that the evidence for the effectiveness of HBOT in traumatic brain injury of *all* severities, and at *any* time after traumatic brain injury is so strong that you must seek and demand this treatment for yourself or family member. That's why I wrote: *"TBI? No Need to Die!"*

Every year in the United States, millions of individuals sustain traumatic brain injuries. The official figure is about two million, but given that over 75 percent of the injuries are concussions and the great majority of these never make it to the emergency room, where these statistics are generated, the actual number may be double. Approximately 50,000 of these patients die, but there is no need for even 30,000 of them to die.

The medical profession brags that it adheres to "evidence-based medicine." You have no doubt heard this sound-byte phrase; it's commonly used in the press, if not by your own doctor. It means that doctors use the best available science to guide their decision-making. In fact, evidence-based medicine is the use of the best scientific evidence *combined with* the doctor's clinical expertise and the patient's choice. It is not the use of scientific evidence alone.

The strongest form of scientific evidence is what doctors call the "randomized prospective controlled clinical experiment or trial." In such an experiment, the researcher gathers patients with a common diagnosis and then uses a computer to randomize them to either treatment: either HBOT (in this case), or no HBOT. Before the computer randomizes the patient, the patient has no idea which treatment he will get. The HBOT group then gets HBOT, while the other group (the control group) gets no HBOT, or else the standard of care for the diagnosis under treatment. Ideally, neither the patients nor the doctors know which treatment they are receiving (which is where the term "double blind" refers to. However, this is nearly impossible to do in the case of HBOT, since the patients must actually enter a chamber. Currently, we haven't shown that we can give the patient a fake HBOT and have them believe that they received an actual HBOT, when in fact they didn't. As a result, the acceptable "control group" in a hyperbaric study is one that receives no HBOT and continues to get the standard of care treatment for that disease.

At the end of the treatment, researchers compare the results between the two groups of tests, given before and after the treatment. If the treatment shows a significant improvement compared to the control group, doctors and insurance companies, including Medicare and Medicaid, will want to pay for it. This has become the standard of "evidenced-based" treatment in medicine. However, it's time to wave the red flag for caveats. A number of problems with these types of studies make them less than foolproof and thus, subject to criticism. In addition, sometimes studies can be done without a treatment control group and use certain types of tests that make a control group unnecessary; SPECT, discussed above, is an example of such a test. In other examples, doctors may show in a study with no treatment control group that the patients improve much more than patients with the same diagnosis in studies with the "accepted" treatments. Ultimately, doctors have to consider all of the evidence from all types of studies, combine it with their experience and knowledge of the patient's individual circumstances, and lastly, implement the treatment in light of the patient's intention.

What would you say if I told you that there are at least five randomized controlled trials of HBOT in the treatment of acute traumatic brain injury done in multiple countries over the past 45 years that have all had nearly identical results? And, I add that they were backed by metabolic studies that showed improvement in the underlying brain injuries? And what is most astounding is the fact that the data showed that we could reduce the number of deaths from acute, severe TBI by *60 percent!* Data also show that the outcomes of those who survive are better in the HBOT group than the control group.

As it turns out, a 60 percent reduction in death rate is historically nearly unprecedented for any medical therapy, for any condition. For example, the last time the medical field could say that a therapy had that degree of effect on mortality was when penicillin was developed and widely used. Then, during the Vietnam War, the use of combat helicopters was credited for the dramatic reduction in combat deaths, calculated at reducing mortality by 42 percent. Meanwhile, the American Heart Association has spent hundreds of millions of dollars on research to improve out-of-hospital cardiac arrest, but in more than 50 years they have made very little progress.

So, when we can show that HBOT can reduce TBI mortality by 60 percent, a development as groundbreaking and astounding as penicillin—should we not have seen this treatment implemented long ago? And yet, we are still fighting for it.

Knowing these facts, I ask you: Have you had a family member or friend who died of acute severe traumatic brain injury? I'll bet he or she didn't receive HBOT. Did he or she die in a hospital with hyperbaric chambers? I would be pretty upset if that was the case. Are you?

We also have two controlled trials of HBOT applied in moderate to severe TBI weeks to months after the TBI, plus multiple controlled studies in patients with residual effects of mild TBI, the post-concussion syndrome. Given these studies, why aren't we applying HBOT to these categories of brain-injured patients? The answer, discussed later, is mired in medical politics. However, the takeaway message and the only truly important point here is that *HBOT is the treatment of choice for traumatic brain injury and you must seek it and demand it for your brain-injured family members and friends.* The evidence far exceeds the standard of care and the evidence for the vast majority of typically reimbursed diagnoses (above) for HBOT. And, it meets the definition of evidence-based medicine.

Suppose, however, you are unable to get HBOT for yourself, loved one, child, or friend, which is too often the case. These survivors of TBI proceed through life with varying disabilities. This means that we add well over two million new head-injured individuals to the population every year in the United States alone. And just as tragic as the deaths, some of the brain-injured individuals end up in our prisons or homeless. Others commit suicide. This is exactly what is happening to a significant number of U.S. soldiers returning from the Iraq and Afghanistan wars.

Consider that if a head injury causes significant loss of cognition, judgment, motor, or other function, the person may not be able to return to work. Unemployment and poverty can follow, both of which are associated with crime. In many cases, substance abuse follows the injury, although the reasons for this remain unclear. Many are put on narcotic pain medications for their traumatic headaches or other traumatic injuries. Once started on narcotics, they can't stop using them. Look no further than to many of our brain-injured veterans who suffer from prescription narcotic addiction. Still others show personality changes after traumatic brain injury and end up short-tempered, some even prone to violence. For five years (ending with Hurricane Katrina), I worked at the massive Orleans Parish Prison (7,000 inmates; one of the largest in the United States) and I confirmed this finding as we documented a remarkable percentage of our inmates with previous head injuries and seizure disorders secondary to trauma.

Although brain injuries can and do occur at any age, reckless, impulsive behavior among young people is responsible for many traumatic brain injuries. Even non-reckless behavior, such as contact sports and cycling, can lead to head injuries, but protective head gear has helped reduce the incidence of these injuries and their seriousness when they do occur. Without question, seat belt and helmet laws have contributed to reducing head injuries among people of all ages.

Recently, we've seen concerns about brain-injured veterans, along with retired National Football League (NFL) players, significantly increase awareness of traumatic brain injury (TBI), specifically mild TBI. Because there is a misperception that nearly all patients with mild TBI recover in 3–6 months, we have discounted the effects of TBI for decades. Our brain-injured veterans from Iraq and Afghanistan are changing that.

It's a sad fact that that the underlying process in traumatic brain injury is loss of brain tissue. The brain attempts to accommodate that injury with a number of compensatory mechanisms, but the underlying injury remains. Time, aging, stress, or repetitive injury can bring out the traces of previous injury. This was shown elegantly by Dr. Ewing in 1980, when she took some young adults who had had a mild TBI with loss of consciousness 2–3 years before, and matched them to a group of young adults with no head injury[1]. The TBI patients had no symptoms and were functioning well in their life. She cognitively tested both groups and found them to be the same. She then exposed them to 12,530 ft. altitude (low oxygen) in a chamber used for flight simulation and repeated the cognitive tests in the chamber. The TBI group had a significant decrease in their performance. In other words, the old TBI was still there and its effects could be exposed under stress, low oxygen stress in this case.

We now appreciate that, in combination with post-traumatic stress disorder (PTSD), we have an epidemic of dysfunctional brain-injured veterans and active duty military personnel who are struggling to live normal lives. Fortunately, we have more than hope for them—we can now offer treatment. After presenting my experience with HBOT in chronic TBI at the Walter Reed Army Hospital in January 2004, and on many additional occasions to others within the military, I began to treat some Iraq and Afghanistan veterans in 2008. (See HBOT.com for information about the first of these cases, along with the powerful SPECT scans.)

I subsequently started a 30-subject pilot trial of HBOT in chronic, blast-induced TBI and PTSD through Louisiana State University (LSU). It was funded completely by donations from military support organizations, generous Americans, and my office. I presented the data at the 8th World Congress on Brain Injury of the International Brain Injury Association in Washington, D. C. in March 2010, and then published the results in 2011 in the prestigious *Journal of Neurotrauma*. In short, the results were astounding. Not only did the veterans achieve a dramatic reduction in their concussion symptoms, but they showed significant improvements in memory, thinking, anxiety, and depression. They were able to decrease or discontinue their psychoactive brain medications and eliminate suicidal intentions. In addition, their PTSD symptoms were lessened. The reduction in PTSD symptoms is the greatest reduction in PTSD symptoms in a four week period of any therapy to date. (You can find this article linked at HBOT.com.)

You also can view short videos about this pilot study, some of the veterans that were treated in the study. They are segments from television and Internet news services on veterans who volunteered their compelling stories for the benefit of others. These videos shed light on the positive effect HBOT had on their difficult and troubled lives and give a personal, very real side to what other can sound like isolated "data."

Tim Hecker, an Army Master Sergeant, is featured in the following videos (available for viewing at HBOT.com):

1. American Legion documentary: *The War Within*
2. *Brain Storm, Oxygen Under Pressure*, an international award-winning documentary, which features an interview of Tim's wife, Tina Hecker
3. NOLA Marketplace story on Tim's HBOT: Tim Hecker, NOLA Marketplace, LSU Pilot Trial

Another veteran, Margaux Vair, is featured in multiple videos (available at HBOT.com) in which she describes her injuries sustained in Iraq and her recovery with HBOT. The HBOT story of another veteran, Matt Williams, is also told in some of these videos. The story of Matt's platoon in Iraq is told in the book *Black Hearts* by Jim Frederick.

The actual footage of Margaux's injuries in Iraq has great had impact; Part II of the videos also includes comments by some Army officers on the LSU Pilot Trial.

Margaux went on to receive additional HBOT after the study, as many of my study patients have done (remember, 40 treatments is just the first phase of treatment for many patients). She and others are featured in other videos. As Margaux reports, she eventually was able to stop using the psychoactive medications she was prescribed.

In other video news/media pieces (see HBOT.com for notable examples) the preliminary results of the LSU Pilot Trial are presented and discussed along with the stories of a few more veterans:

1. Preliminary pilot trial results and SPECT brain scans (in this video, I tell patients to get HBOT as soon as you can after TBI)
2. Marine Corporal Jake Mathers
3. West Point Graduate Major Ben Richards, also the subject of a *New York Times* article
4. Marine IED hunter and canine handler Charles Rotenberry
5. CNN interview of Army veteran Chad Battles

Real Life is Not Simply an "Anecdote"

All of these videos are real-life stories of pain and suffering, reversed by HBOT. Sadly, some would disparage them as "anecdotes," a term often used in medicine to discount what a patient recounts. By definition, an anecdote is a short, interesting story, sometimes amusing, about a real incident or person.

In medicine, however, it's an account almost always regarded as unreliable or hearsay.

However, I urge you to view these videos, one after another, and draw your own conclusions. They're most certainly *not* amusing—and every one of them is reliable.

As word of the results of the pilot trial spread, I was asked by the Dean of LSU School of Medicine, Dr. Steve Nelson, to be LSU's Key Contact in the Michelle Obama/Jill Biden Joining Forces Initiative. This initiative included a program that challenged and invited medical schools to develop education and treatment programs for veterans. We were all invited to Richmond, Virginia in January, 2012 to meet with the First Lady (see HBOT.com for a news story about this event.)

I was able to give her assistant a copy of *The Oxygen Revolution* and I received a thank-you note from Mrs. Obama later, but thus far, nothing has come from her office regarding my recommendation to use HBOT for our veterans.

At the time of this writing, we are submitting the final report on all 30 veterans. Among other things, our report compares the wounded veterans' brain blood flow to normal people and found that the veterans' abnormal brain blood flow became nearly normal after the HBOT.

Subsequently, we launched a national study (see HBOT.com) based on the pilot trial for anyone with a mild-moderate brain injury. The International Hyperbaric Medical Foundation, primarily through the efforts of Bill Duncan, conducted the study, called N-BIRR, the National Brain Injury Rescue and Rehabilitation Study.

Five centers participated at their own expense and treated all of the veterans and civilians for free. Using computer cognitive testing and symptom questionnaires we were able to show the same results as the pilot trial. As a sequel to this study (also available at HBOT.com), Bill Duncan succeeded in having a law passed in Oklahoma that mandated HBOT treatment of veterans with TBI and PTSD, the Oklahoma Veteran Traumatic Brain Injury Treatment and Recovery Act. This was unprecedented legislation.

Bill went on to establish the Patriot Clinics, which, funded by donations, treats veterans until payment can be secured from the federal government. A similar effort in Texas was initiated by the grandfather (Rainey Owen) of a brain-injured veteran, Matt Smotherman. Matt was restored with HBOT, and although his grandfather's effort was initially unsuccessful, he will try again in the future to mandate that this treatment be available. (You can read about the Patriot Clinics and Matt's story at HBOT.com.)

Once again, we can see that people who have experienced the healing effects of HBOT are so moved by the impact it has had on their lives that they have opened hyperbaric facilities, gone to the press, and stood up to give testimonial of the benefit. This rarely occurs in medicine.

The news is not all rosy, however. At the start of the pilot trial I was invited to give a talk to the Navy Surgeon General Dr. Robinson and an august group of dignitaries, including the wives of a number of generals from the Joint Chiefs of Staff. Brigadier General Patt Maney was also present. Maney is both an Army general and Florida state judge, who was brain-injured by an IED in Afghanistan. He gave a video testimonial (see HBOT.com) about his inability to function and his subsequent recovery with HBOT, allowing him to return to his judgeship in Florida. Maney received my protocol of HBOT in Washington, D.C. Others attending included three of the five veterans I had treated to date, the former Secretary of the Army, the Honorable Martin Hoffmann, representatives from three congressional offices, the top Navy hyperbaric physicians, and other military physicians.

The purpose of my presentation to was to obtain funding to do the LSU Pilot Trial. I was assured that money was the least of my worries. Admiral Robinson said "they" had $900 million to spend on TBI research. Unfortunately, that money never materialized for the LSU Pilot Trial, but he asked me to be part of a working group of his medical experts to find "the best way forward."

As a result, in December 2008, a conference was held in Arlington, Virginia, called, "The Defense Centers of Excellence for Psychological Health and Traumatic Brain Injury Consensus Conference on Hyperbaric Oxygen Therapy for Traumatic Brain Injury." Sixty experts on HBOT, TBI, and PTSD were assembled. At the end of the conference, a group of doctors who had little to no experience treating chronic traumatic brain injury with HBOT were put in charge of a series of studies on HBOT for our veterans. They put together a group of mal-designed studies, which ended with conflicting results that have confused the lay public and medical community. The erroneous conclusions in these studies have all but precluded any brain injured veteran from receiving HBOT as part of standard treatment. You can read about the controversies in multiple articles on the Internet, including one I published in 2012 (see HBOT. com). The authors have never defended themselves against these criticisms.

Despite the flaws in their studies, the important bright spot is that in the study in which they used my protocol they obtained the same positive result we had achieved in previous research. They also were able to show effectiveness of another dose of hyperbaric therapy, while they showed multiple higher doses of hyperbaric therapy that didn't work. One of these was actually harmful. These Department of Defense studies, as poorly designed and erroneously interpreted as they were, nevertheless reinforced the principles I spoke about in earlier chapters: *the dose of hyperbaric oxygen therapy matters.* It must be the right dose for that person and the individual brain injury at the right time in the injury process. In addition, more is not better; the highest dose that they used indicated harm to the veterans. *replicated*

But, there is even more good news—the news that has made my statements at the outset of this chapter so forceful. In November 2013, Israeli researchers, Dr. Efrati and his colleagues, published a randomized controlled study (this type of study discussed above) of HBOT in chronic concussion. They used the same protocol of HBOT Doctors Neubauer, Gottlieb, Van Meter, and I had developed along with the SPECT brain imaging. Their results were nearly identical to what we had found and what I had published with the veterans. Symptoms, cognition, and brain blood flow all showed significant improvements after 40 HBOTs.

The importance of this cannot be overstated. Here were doctors, outside the United States, unconnected to me and my colleagues, who duplicated our results and the results of the animal study we published in 2007, using the same dose of HBOT. Essentially, studies performed by us, the U.S. military, and independent doctors in Israel all obtained the same results with the same dose of HBOT.

The other beauty of the Israeli study is that it was done on civilians. So, while we were showing the effectiveness of HBOT for concussion caused by explosions in members if the military, the Israeli study was treating civilians with common causes of TBI. The huge statistics on TBI that I quoted earlier are comprised of civilians who have sustained TBIs. These patients spanned all ages and had varying causes: slips and falls, car and motorcycle accidents, fights, and of course, sports. We are now aware of sports concussion because of the dementia and suicides occurring among professional football players. However, these individuals are manifesting the late cumulative effects of many TBIs. While they are important (and I do talk about them in a later chapter), here, the focus is on the single mild TBI/concussion that every person could experience, including during participation in sports.

Mild TBI differs from severe TBI, mostly in the amount of tissue damage that occurs. As mentioned above, we have a plethora of studies on the effectiveness of HBOT in acute severe TBI. If the pathology is the same, except for amount of damage, why wouldn't HBOT work in acute or subacute concussion? Well, it does: I have now treated 10 or so patients, including two of my sons, my nephew, an award-winning college football player, a pediatric ICU nurse, a delivery truck driver, and a variety of others. I have also communicated with an HBOT facility that has treated a few dozen skiers with acute concussions. Almost none of these patients were treated within hours of the event, but almost all were treated at least 1 day to weeks afterward, and the result was the same. With just a few HBOTs, these patients experienced a marked reduction in their symptoms and were able to return to work or school and resume their lives. They also never became chronic post-concussion syndrome patients. The principle, once again, is that the earlier we treat, the less treatment it takes to heal.

A few case examples of young people treated with HBOT for sports concussion are provided by patients I've treated, who later went public with their stories. Both were well into the chronic persistent post-concussion phase. The first is little Nate Geller, a 12-year-old boy who was whacked in the back of his head by the full swing of a defense player twice his size. Nate went from being the star of his middle school class to a child who was unable to leave home except for doctor's appointments (see HBOT.com for his impressive story).

Just recently, the mother of another TBI patient of mine popped into my clinic to let me know how well her son was doing. He is now 20, and is attending college and achieving good grades. He recently ran into Nate, who is back on top of the world, doing well in high school and sports. It's not uncommon for those who have been through these injuries to find common ground with each other.

Tyler Hane struggled with the residual effects of multiple rugby concussions, eventually having problems in college. I was asked to treat him by Dr. Jim Wright, a retired hyperbaric physician and Air Force colonel, who reported two cases of HBOT in veterans with post-concussion syndrome in 2009. Tyler's story is equally impressive, as he experienced a significant improvement that has helped launch him on his career path. (You can find more information on Tyler and his incredible story at HBOT.com.)

For those with the later life, cumulative manifestations of multiple concussions (what is now recognized as chronic traumatic encephalopathy on autopsy of the brain), we can offer some hope. As I mentioned, this entire history of HBOT for neurological injury in my clinic began with treatment demented divers, and boxers with *dementia pugilistica*, the "punch drunk syndrome."

The "punch drunk syndrome" is no different from the dementia we see in professional football players. I have now treated a few retired professional athletes who have dementia or significant cognitive problems; one of them is under treatment right now and showing improvement.

In 2011, Dr. Ken Stoller reported the results of HBOT treatment of a retired football player with presumptive CTE. The results were the same as all of the results I've described so far in this chapter. That football player, George Visger, went on to receive additional HBOT. (Read about him, his advocacy for HBOT, as well as exposure of the TBI problem in the NFL and Dr. Stoller's report, at HBOT.com.)

Since then, Joe Namath has added his name to the list of retired NFL players with cognitive problems who have experienced the benefits of HBOT long after their injuries. Joe Namath's, George Visger's, and other players' positive experience with HBOT, coupled with my results and the accumulating experience of HBOT treatment of dementia, suggests that we may be able to treat the end-stage of repetitive TBI just like the acute and subacute stages, and the chronic stage of mild TBI. (For more on Joe Namath, see HBOT.com.)

At this point, there should be no argument that HBOT works for traumatic brain injury of all severities at any time in the injury process. If you have lingering doubts, other case reports and videos are included here (and at HBOT.com). Later, you'll read about Chad Rovira and Curt Allen. Both stories are compelling; the Curt Allen video has now been viewed by over 185,000 people on YouTube. That video along has driven home the point I have made on TBI to countless patients and it bears repeating: *If you, your family members, friends, or relatives receive a traumatic brain injury do everything within your power to obtain HBOT for them. Do not take no for an answer.* Science and clinical experience supports you. TBI? No Need to Die!

For a summary of this history of HBOT for TBI and the application to our veterans, I filmed a four-part video narrative and chronology, which you can view at HBOT.com. The narrative of these videos and chronology takes you from the boxers and divers through other case experiences to the veterans and results of the LSU Pilot Trial. I have deliberately provided the SPECT imaging, the SPECT/dive/SPECTsequence and description of the changes in brain blood flow, the texture analysis of the scans, the IQ change in the veterans, the effects on PTSD and depression, and our attempt to get the congressional TBI Treatment Act passed.

To add to this history, I will refer you to an article that appeared in the July 5, 2015 edition of *New York Times* on HBOT for veterans (see HBOT.com). (Of the hundreds of pictures the photographer took at my clinic, the banner picture chosen for the article is a rather dour-appearing me, which is not consistent with the passion I have for what this therapy can do for our brain-injured veterans!) During the course of their investigation, I all but buried the authors in the scientific articles on HBOT and TBI, mine, my colleagues, and the errant ones by the Department of Defense.

In the process of producing the article, I believe the negative information the reporters were given was questioned after one of the journalists visited the clinic and spoke with every TBI patient I was treating, including some who were in my current TBI study. The end result is fairly balanced, but it doesn't touch on the science behind HBOT. It is somewhat like a Rorschach image. You can see what you want to see in the article, based on your bias. I suppose the absence of a discussion of the science is understandable: to both master the science and defend it would be to take on the entire Department of Defense, which for non-physicians and researchers is a daunting task. Overall, I was happy, because the *New York Times* offered exposure that HBOT rarely enjoys on such a large scale.

A Phenomenal Case

While the use of HBOT for traumatic brain injuries continues to evolve, we can show many examples in which great improvement has taken place when HBOT is added to neurorehabilitation protocols. For example, in the early 1990s, I had the opportunity to treat an amazing young man. At that time, I was co-director of hyperbaric medicine in the emergency department at a small community hospital in Slidell, Louisiana. One Saturday morning, I arrived for my 12-hour emergency department shift and found that our only patient was a 19-year-old comatose male on a ventilator. The nurse on duty said that he'd sustained a severe traumatic brain injury, having fallen out of a car traveling at high speed on the interstate.

Since our small hospital was situated at the confluence of three interstate highways, we saw many patients with fairly severe injuries resulting from car accidents. I felt sad when I realized there was little I could do for this young man because, much to my regret, medical politics prevented me from treating him with HBOT. I was familiar with some of the literature on hyperbaric oxygen therapy in acute severe traumatic brain injury, and I believed that enough evidence had accumulated to justify using HBOT with severely brain-injured individuals. However, since the treatment was not approved for that use, I was not free to use it in these situations.

As it turned out, this young man, Chad Rovira, was Marlon and Charlene Rovira's son. Marlon was a local veterinarian who had many friends among our staff physicians. He consulted with many of these doctors looking for the best possible treatments for Chad.

Chad's accident resulted from what we all know as "youthful imprudence." He and some friends were high on an inhalant known locally as "Blast," and the accident resulted from Chad's attempt to climb out one window and across the top of the moving car while in this chemically induced euphoric state. The incident ended up in tragedy, with Chad unconscious on the highway after landing directly on the right side of his forehead. His friends loaded him into the car and raced seven miles up the interstate to our hospital. The physician on duty had significant experience treating severe trauma and was able to intubate Chad very quickly (inserting a tube in the trachea to keep the airway open) before beginning tests, including a CT scan performed while Chad remained in a deep coma, unable to respond to any external stimuli. The scan of the brain showed bleeding between the skull and the covering of the brain and also between that covering and the brain itself. He also had small hemorrhages throughout the brain, which already showed signs of swelling. In addition, the scan revealed a fracture at the base of his skull.

Despite his lack of judgment on that particular night, Chad was a bright college freshman with aspirations of becoming an orthopedic surgeon. But the brain damage sustained in the accident severely limited his chances of living any semblance of a normal life, let alone becoming an orthopedic surgeon. In truth, his chance of dying was significant. In this state, Chad might also have lingered in a coma for months or years, and had he regained consciousness, it's entirely possible that he would have been unable to talk or even think.

I wasn't aware of it, but one of the doctors Marlon consulted mentioned that he had heard me give a talk on hyperbaric oxygen therapy the previous week. That year's talk had been particularly noteworthy because I had started successfully treating divers for brain decompression illness, but in delayed fashion, meaning weeks to months after their diving incidents.

Recalling my presentation, one of the doctors consulting on Chad's case suggested that I might be willing to consider treating him with HBOT. That same day, Marlon and a number of the consulting doctors asked for all the information I had on HBOT and traumatic brain injury. I quickly assembled it and passed it on to them, and by the end of my shift, Chad's parents and a few of the doctors came back to see me. Even after I told them I couldn't offer any guarantees, the parents asked me to treat their son.

Within three hours, my chief technician and I had Chad in the hyperbaric chamber on a ventilator, approximately 22 hours after his accident. We used a lower pressure than that typically used for decompression sickness or for chronic wounds. Once we reached the depth of pressurization intended, Chad began to vigorously over-breathe with the ventilator, and what we call "bucking" occurred. When he was placed in the chamber, he hadn't been breathing on his own and was totally dependent on the ventilator. But at depth on oxygen his brain began to function and he started to come out of his coma by breathing on his own. Unlike sophisticated ventilators used in other emergency situations and intensive care, the hyperbaric ventilator is a crude device that doesn't respond to a patient's attempt to breathe. When Chad started breathing on his own, he and the ventilator were, in simple terms, out of synch. He was fighting the ventilator and to the untrained eye, it can look like a seizure to non-medical people, but this "bucking" is actually more like coughing (a video of this reaction is available on HBOT.com.)

His response meant that neurological activity developed while in the chamber at depth, which indicated improved neurological function. We brought the bucking under control by heavily sedating Chad through an IV. Moving forward, Chad had two HBOT treatments a day, which brought about rapid improvement and eventually enabled us to remove his breathing tube. Within a week, while Chad was still comatose, we did a brain blood flow scan using the hospital's low-resolution machine. The radiologist read it as normal, but this made no sense. How could comatose Chad with acute severe traumatic brain injury have normal brain blood flow? He couldn't; it was impossible. The problem was that the scanner didn't have the ability to show the injury. Although this caused consternation amongst the doctors in Chad's case, it had no impact on his HBOT, since the decision to use HBOT was not dependent on the SPECT scan. In chronic brain injury, however, where the residual effects of injury are often disputed, a falsely "normal" SPECT brain blood flow scan can be devastating to a patient's credibility. It is equally damaging if the radiologist has very little experience reading SPECT brain imaging and reads an abnormal scan as "normal." I mention these problems with SPECT brain imaging because they're not unusual. Should you ever find yourself in a situation in which you need accurate answers about a loved one's condition, I want you to be familiar with the nuances of SPECT scanning. (See Chapter 3 and Appendix B for information about SPECT.)

In Chad's case, we transported him to a different hospital that had a high resolution scanner, which I had used to evaluate the successful treatment of two divers the previous year. Those cases had formed the basis of the lecture I presented at our hospital and which had convinced Chad's parents to try HBOT in the first place. Chad's second brain scan revealed a profoundly abnormal brain, which made sense to me, given the nature of the trauma. This meant that we had objective laboratory testing that was congruent with Chad's clinical condition.[2] (Chad's brain scans appear on page 2 of the photo insert.)

We continued HBOT and Chad made substantial gains, including emerging from the coma. We eventually transferred him to a local rehabilitation facility. Chad's neurosurgeon, Dr. Lou Provenza, remarked that he had never seen a patient with this degree of brain trauma recover so rapidly. Chad also received weeks of additional treatment at my hospital's hyperbaric facility, and during these weeks he began to walk and talk.

I nicknamed him "Lazarus" because his rapid recovery was nothing short of amazing. In four to six weeks, he'd gone from comatose and unresponsive, to a walking, talking individual. Eleven weeks after starting his therapy, Marlon decided to transfer him to the most highly respected head injury program in the New Orleans area. But before resuming HBOT at my clinic, Marlon wanted Chad to settle into this new rehab hospital.

A month went by and I heard nothing more. I wondered what had happened, but I also knew that it was highly likely the physicians in charge of Chad's case had filled his parents' heads with all sorts of inaccuracies about HBOT. Eventually I called Chad's father and he said they'd decided not to do anymore HBOT. When I asked what had brought him to that decision, he admitted that the physicians at the new facility had disparaged the treatment to the extent that he believed he couldn't override their objections. Reluctantly, I said that I understood, but I asked Marlon to periodically let me know how Chad was doing.

A couple of months went by before I heard from Marlon, and when he called, he admitted that he was disappointed in the neurorehabilitation program. Except for a slight improvement in neurological abilities, which occurred during the first week or two of treatment, the subsequent 11 weeks had brought no further gains. By this time, Marlon was fed up with the other doctors' objections to HBOT and wanted to start treatment again. However, about 15 percent of patients with the same type of injury as Chad's (sub-arachnoid hemorrhage) develop a condition in which the fluid circulation system in the brain is blocked by blood that has plugged the pores that resorb the fluid in the covering of the brain (obstructive hydrocephalus). When this happens, the neurological improvement stops and the patient's condition eventually worsens. I assumed that if Chad had made almost no improvement in three months at the best brain injury rehabilitation center in the city then obstructive hydrocephalus was likely the cause. So, before resuming HBOT, we needed a neurosurgeon to evaluate him for hydrocephalus.

I wanted to ensure that by the end of Chad's treatment, we would have indisputable proof, with no questions remaining, that hyperbaric oxygen had led to his neurological and cognitive improvements. I explained that Chad's treatment results needed to be documented with SPECT brain scans. Chad's father agreed to all my requests and notified the staff.

After the neurosurgeon cleared him of any possibility of hydrocephalus, we proceeded with a set of functional brain-imaging scans of the type that had previously tracked Chad's rather amazing improvement. I repeated his brain blood flow scan under near-identical conditions as those of his previous scans. This scan now showed some deterioration in the right frontal and right back sides of the brain. This was not surprising; one of Chad's biggest problems was his lack of insight or understanding of his condition. For example, Chad didn't believe he had a brain injury, so despite a spastic right hand, he still firmly thought he was going to be an orthopedic surgeon. This lack of understanding was a major impediment to his further rehabilitation. In the human brain, the frontal lobe areas are involved with our ability to plan ahead and evaluate facts and impressions. This area also controls social interactions and socialization in general.

After doing a brain blood flow scan, Chad had one HBOT treatment, and I repeated the scan. We saw improvement in many areas, including the right frontal area. Because of that improvement, I told the care team that this was the evidence I wanted—it demonstrated that I could still help him and that we would be able to document the improvements with a picture.

About five weeks into the HBOT therapy, I received a phone call from one of the staff at the rehab institute. According to this staff member, Chad showed negative side effects. Specifically, profuse sweating, elevated blood pressure, and depression. I hadn't noticed any of these negative signs during Chad's daily trips to our clinic, but I immediately stopped the HBOT and called for an emergency conference with his care team at the hospital.

During that conference I learned that Chad had begun playing tennis, a sport in which he'd excelled before his accident. I was amazed he was able to play tennis at all and asked if he'd been playing tennis before we started this round of hyperbaric oxygen.

As it turned out, his balance had been so poor he couldn't play any sport, so I pointed out that this recent development showed an important neurological gain. (I learned 16 years later that, unfortunately, this improvement was not permanent). I kept asking questions and learned that Chad's balance had improved to the point that he could ride a two-wheel bicycle. Only a short time before, he'd struggled with a three-wheel bike. Clearly, Chad's balance had improved overall.

When I asked about Chad's sweating, it turned out that this occurred during his tennis matches. Since it was late May in New Orleans, where temperatures were approaching 90 degrees and the humidity was 90–95 percent, anyone would sweat a great deal while playing tennis. Besides, as Marlon pointed out, Chad had sweated profusely during all his life in New Orleans.

The elevated blood pressure puzzled me, but after asking a few questions, I learned that they measured his blood pressure at the same time he was sweating, which was while he played tennis. Since everyone's blood pressure rises during exertion and sporting events, taking a blood pressure reading at that time didn't make much sense. In fact, no one took his blood pressure in the morning or at the same time of day on a repetitive basis. (As humor columnist, Dave Barry, often says, "I am not making this up." You can't write fiction better than this!)

Finally, we addressed the depression issue. Chad had apparently started talking about his brain injury—he finally realized what had happened and he also spoke about the problems with his right hand. He was in the process of fully grasping that his handicaps resulting from the accident would likely prevent him from becoming an orthopedic surgeon, his life-long dream. As you are no doubt thinking, Chad's response and his grieving was actually a sign of progress. "Wasn't his lack of insight hindering his neurorehabilitation?" I asked. It was normal that Chad grieve a loss that he had been unable to perceive during the previous seven months. Finally, the care team acknowledged that this was the gain they had been waiting for.

Over the previous few years, I had devised treatment protocols, and Chad received blocks of 40 treatments. We were getting close to 80 treatments when Chad said he wanted to stop HBOT because it was interfering with his plans to go back to college. I was dumbstruck. Returning to college had not been part of my original expectations for Chad. I had hoped he'd gain insight, physical balance, and some intellectual improvements, but I hadn't envisioned college. When I asked if he felt intellectually capable of college work, he answered with clear irritation in his voice. "Dr. Harch, I have been trying to tell you now for weeks and weeks that my math ability has improved so much that I know I'm able to handle math classes again."

At that point, he stopped treatment, and I told him that with all the testing we were doing, we could demonstrate his recovered abilities. Chad enrolled at the local junior college, and the neuropsychologist on the care team administered repeated psychometric testing that showed a number of cognitive improvements, the greatest of which was a 40 percentile improvement in written computational math. This was a huge change, highly statistically significant, and unquestionably not a chance event. Only three months earlier, Chad had been "locked" in a five-month clinical plateau. Before we reinstituted HBOT, he showed no neurocognitive improvement. Overall, we had clinical and testing improvements that seemed to match. The SPECT brain scan repeated at the conclusion of HBOT showed an improvement in brain blood flow throughout the brain, but especially in Chad's right frontal lobe.

At Chad's final visit to my clinic, we videotaped an exit exam and interview. I repeated the sequence of exam items and questions that I'd done three months before (and many months before at the time of his transfer to the rehab institute), the point at which we'd started this final round of HBOT. At one point I asked Chad if he still believed he had not sustained any brain damage.

Chad's response was quite unexpected. He began to squirm and look almost angry at the impropriety of my question. But it was the same question I had posed to him many times, three, six, and nine to ten months before.

"I need to correct you," he said. "I am not brain-damaged, I have a brain injury, and I think you need to use the proper terminology."

So, not only did he have insight, he was intellectually capable of interacting with me about my pejorative term for his condition. Well, I stood corrected and immediately apologized.

To me, this exchange was the proverbial icing on the cake. His simple statement provided proof of his remarkable cognitive improvement, brought about with a few months of hyperbaric oxygen therapy delivered nine months after the initial injury and five and a half months after the cognitive therapy and other rehabilitation strategies had failed.

Chad went on to complete some college courses and he found a job at a New Orleans area bank. Although initially hired under a special program, he's received multiple promotions. A few years ago he happened to see me on a television segment about other patients treated with HBOT. Chad recognized me and his father called and invited me to visit. Although Chad is not completely normal, he functions at levels beyond what anyone ever expected.

Furthermore, HBOT had a quite unexpected result that his father reminds me about every time I speak with him. Since Chad's injury and subsequent HBOT, he has not had a single day of illness—in 16 years, not one cold, intestinal infection, cough, episode of flu, or any other illness. This is quite remarkable. Interestingly, this phenomenon has also been reported by the mothers of some of the brain-injured children I have treated. Many of these children are very sickly in addition to their brain injury, but after HBOT their immune system begins to work more normally.

We know that the immune system and brain are very closely connected and we know that HBOT has profound effects on the acute inflammatory reaction and additional effects in chronic immune problems. It is not so farfetched to assume that HBOT is having beneficial effects on a deranged immune system in these children, as well as in Chad.

What Chad's story—his case history—tells us is that hyperbaric oxygen has enormous potential in treating acute, severe traumatic brain injury, even in delayed fashion. In Chad's case, we were able to immediately intervene. And in a very real sense, the course of his 10-month treatment provides important information and data. It is like a study in itself, in which:

- We introduced a therapy from which the patient, Chad, benefited.
- Then, when the therapy was stopped Chad made no further improvement.
- When we reintroduced the therapy, Chad made noticeable gains we could show from various types of testing.

Chad's case is now 24 years old. About 10 years ago, I reconnected with Chad at a brain injury fundraiser in New Orleans when we happened to end up in the same booth. Chad attended to support a brain injury survivors' group, and we had a gratifying reunion. It was great to see him doing so well after all of these years. Years passed, and we connected again in another state during the summer of 2014. It was wonderful to see him and observe that his quality of life remains good.

Multiple studies have shown that we can reduce the death rate if we treat this type of injury with HBOT within the first few days after the injury. Cases like Chad's illuminate the potential of HBOT to transform the entire field of emergency medicine. For the most part, brain-injured individuals are emergency department patients first, as are roughly 500,000 annual survivors of stroke. In many cases, those with chemical poisonings (discussed below) were also first treated in emergency departments, although many were not. By placing hyperbaric chambers in emergency departments, doctors who are most knowledgeable about treating medical emergencies will be able to "marry" standard therapy with HBOT, thereby improving the outcome for countless patients.

We can only begin to speculate about the outcome for well over two million individuals of all ages who sustain traumatic brain injuries. Emergency specialists treat numerous life-threatening injuries, but for many patients, lingering damage may leave them with varying degrees of disability. The body's inflammatory reaction, described in Chapter 2, is responsible for this damage, which is the same regardless of the injury; this is where HBOT can play its beneficial role in emergency medicine. Emergencies for which HBOT may be useful include: heart attack, stroke, near drowning, near hanging, acute severe hemorrhage, severe bodily trauma, shock, sepsis, overdoses, birth injury, lightning injury, and so forth. (Because stroke and birth injury are so common, I have devoted a chapter to each.)

Consider: You've just had a hefty dose of HBOT for TBI. Now, take it and run with it. Advocate for the use of HBOT in TBI. Don't hesitate to strongly recommend HBOT for every person you contact who has a TBI and is acutely in need of treatment, or living with the consequences. HBOT can literally change the trajectory of their life.

The Unseen Threats

Emergency situations also include exposure to neurotoxins, which are potentially damaging agents or substances. These toxins are specifically toxic to the nervous system, particularly neurons: the thinking, motor, and sensory cells of the nervous system.

We're surrounded by neurotoxins in our environment, and we aren't generally aware of our exposure to them. We usually think of chemical poisoning in terms of massive environmental releases, like a train-transported tank car carrying chemicals that derails, spilling open and releasing a toxic chemical into an area, perhaps even into a residential neighborhood, in which case, an emergency evacuation follows. Large fires and explosions are dramatic examples of toxin exposures—we can actually see the source of toxic fumes when these happen. Depending on the substance involved, the exposure poses varying degrees of threat to nearby populations.

In reality, however, neurotoxins are often much more subtle. For example, perhaps you develop a headache after shopping in the pesticide department of a garden shop or home improvement center. Most of the time, you wouldn't even link your headache with the shopping environment, but in fact the headache is a manifestation of the pesticides' toxic effect on the brain.

The Special Case of Carbon Monoxide

As mentioned earlier, I followed West Virginia's Sago Mine accident in late 2005, during which millions of viewers watched cable networks and waited for news about thirteen coal miners, twelve of whom died of carbon monoxide poisoning and injuries from an explosion. The sole survivor had hyperbaric oxygen delivered some days after the poisoning. As I read the early accounts, I was perplexed by the reporters' statements that the young patient was in a coma but that the doctors didn't think there was neurological damage. He had been in a coma due to carbon monoxide poisoning and low oxygen levels for a prolonged period of time and we know that carbon monoxide causes death of brain cells, so there had to be damage.

It was unfortunate that the miner received hyperbaric oxygen in markedly delayed fashion. And, he had to be transported to another state for treatment, rather than receiving immediate treatment at the scene. Had he been given HBOT immediately, I suspect his recovery would have been speedier. Apparently, he is continuing to recover and do well and a letter he wrote to the families of the non-surviving miners supports the fact that he is functioning cognitively. Likely this is partly a "reserve capacity" issue (described in Chapter 12). Randal McCloy Jr. was the youngest of the miners in the accident, and apparently a fitness buff. His age and excellent health gave him the reserve capacity to withstand such a devastating accident, one that killed all of his fellow workers.

But an additional problem emerged in this case. By the time this young miner was treated, the one, two, or three-treatment protocol for acute carbon monoxide poisoning no longer applied. At that point, they were treating a denser, chronic form of brain injury, so this young man required additional hyperbaric oxygen treatment. At our facility, we have treated a similar case (to the extent that I can determine similarity) in which we were able to treat the patient continuously from coma to clinical plateau. We administered dozens and dozens of treatments, eventually over 100 treatments. The Japanese and Chinese have also found neurological improvement with prolonged repetitive treatment.

Carbon monoxide (CO) is one of the most insidious of neurotoxins, specifically because we often have no idea that we've been poisoned. It's been estimated that during the winter months, a significant percentage of patients who go to emergency departments with a chief complaint of headache are in fact poisoned by carbon monoxide[3]. Doctors who draw carbon monoxide blood levels on patients complaining of headaches documented this phenomenon.

Fossil fuel-burning appliances generate carbon monoxide in exhaust. This includes cars, furnaces, heaters, generators, diesel engines, propane-powered appliances, and so forth. We can have significant carbon monoxide exposures but never realize it while it is occurring, in part because carbon monoxide impairs judgment. So, in other words, while the chemical poisons your brain it also impairs the process by which you would be able to determine that you've been poisoned.

So many seemingly innocuous activities can bring about this impaired state. Grandpa might take his grandchildren out on his fishing boat and sit for a long period of time while the motor idles. Perhaps he and the kids stop in a place with low air circulation, such as under a canopy of trees at the water's edge. In this type of circumstance, carbon monoxide emissions from the engine can accumulate and cause significant injury.

For example, in the last few years, we've reached greater understanding that multiple deaths on Lake Powell in Arizona have been caused by carbon monoxide exposures. At Lake Powell, children and adults dove from pontoon houseboats and then swam underneath them. These houseboats contain motors, generators, and other gas-burning appliances that discharge their exhaust and carbon monoxide under the boats between the pontoons. Kids, and adults, too, typically swim under the boats and come up in the airspace between the pontoons where the carbon monoxide has accumulated. Once they took a breath or two of this highly toxic air they lost consciousness and drowned.

During Hurricane Katrina in 2005, many millions of people living on the Gulf Coast lost electrical power. Some operated gasoline-powered generators to run household appliances and then, as the power outages lasted for weeks into months they used them for heat, cooking, and so forth. Immediately after the storm, we saw a number of carbon monoxide-poisoned patients, some severely exposed and, unfortunately, some who had died.

I treated one of the survivors with HBOT immediately after the storm had passed. His case was unusual in that he tested our resources in a time of disaster. Due to extenuating circumstances we had to stop his treatment, during which time he languished. A number of days later we restarted treatment, and he responded dramatically with return of speech, motor, and cognitive function. Many individuals suffered mild headaches, and reported that they felt like they had the flu. As it turns out, this is the most common diagnosis in missed cases of carbon monoxide poisoning. A 1987 study looked at carbon monoxide poisoning in patients who came to emergency departments with "flu-like" symptoms and found that a small but important percentage of these patients had carbon monoxide levels above 10 percent, whereas normal is about 1 percent[4].

As happens in most situations, especially in the upheaval that occurred in the aftermath of Katrina, stressed individuals don't have time to worry about a bothersome flu, so they shrug off what they consider nuisance symptoms. As a result, Katrina survivors muddled through the days and weeks, believing that they had for the most part recovered from this episode of "flu," although they still didn't feel very well. In many of these situations, carbon monoxide poisoning from the outset of a significant exposure, or after repeated low, persistent exposures, actually caused the symptoms.

Research has shown that HBOT delivered even in cases of these seemingly minor episodes of carbon monoxide poisoning can prevent or minimize the impact of "downstream damage" seen in patients who don't receive this treatment. By downstream damage, I mean a lack of well-being that lingers on, or a secondary deterioration in patients that occurs starting days, and up to six weeks or so, after the initial carbon monoxide poisoning. The damage may show up as problems functioning at work, deteriorating family and marital relationships, including notable decrease in libido, irritability, and emotional-psychological symptoms (depression, anxiety, and an overall sense of unhappiness). Although the carbon monoxide exposure may be "silent" and even considered minor, it can permanently dull the brain.

HBOT to Minimize Damage in Acute Situations

Increasing evidence accumulated from animal and human studies has shown that HBOT delivered at the time of acute toxic overdose or poisoning can have dramatic effects. This is true for carbon monoxide poisoning, hydrogen sulfide, and cyanide. We aren't completely sure how hyperbaric oxygen mitigates the effects in all these poisonings, but we can see the improved cellular function and know that the injury is thereby minimized.

Again, the inflammatory reaction or reperfusion injury is involved in these poisonings, and HBOT significantly inhibits this secondary injury. Logically, if the majority of toxins cause a secondary reperfusion injury, then it makes sense to deliver HBOT during the acute stage of a toxic syndrome. But, most of the time, we can't deliver HBOT at this optimal time because of current hospital policies and other factors, including the lack of widespread knowledge of its value in acute situations.

We often see these injuries months to years later. I have treated series of patients, especially those with carbon monoxide poisoning, and even in a post-acute situation HBOT has shown important and reproducible improvements. These patients have responded in ways similar to those I've treated with chronic stroke, chronic traumatic brain injury, and other neurological diseases. In many of these patients, HBOT was the only therapy that worked months to years after everything else had been tried and failed. This again tells us that injuries from a variety of causes apparently show the same type of damage to the brain.

An HBOT Case in Point

In 1995, a very large release of an extreme oxidizing agent, nitrogen tetroxide, occurred in a location approximately 100 miles north of New Orleans. This chemical, whose hazards are well known, rapidly releases oxygen, so it accelerates fuel burning, which is why it is the "liquid" fuel used to burn the "solid" fuel on many of our rockets and nuclear missiles. The chemical was released because water was added to a rail car that still had nitrogen tetroxide in it. The heat that was generated in the mixture of nitric acid and other oxides of nitrogen caused an explosion of the rail car and a massive release of chemicals.

Tragically, most of the first responders who rushed in to help those nearby were severely poisoned with lung and brain injuries. Months to years later, I treated a number of these severely poisoned individuals. Over the years following this catastrophic event, HBOT was the only therapy tried that significantly relieved their symptoms. Those who had been poisoned showed a variety of symptoms, including headaches, dizziness, trouble thinking, problems with memory and new learning, difficulties with concentration and paying attention, extreme fatigue, sleep disturbances, and so forth.

We were able to see the evidence of the poisoning on patients' brain blood flow, but then also saw improvement on the scans as the patients' outward symptoms improved. (A sample of the SPECT scans of one of these patients appears on page 2 of the photo insert.) In other words, they felt better, and the scans showed that the negative effects of the chemical exposure improved. The effects of HBOT on these individuals were identical to the divers and others whom I had treated in the same way.

As an aside, a group of these patients treated by one of my colleagues appeared on the Maury Povich television show in a segment entitled: "The Most Unusual Place You've Watched the Maury Povich Show." These individuals had called in to say that they routinely watched his show while they were in the hyperbaric chamber receiving treatment for their brain injuries.

We have an opportunity to learn an important lesson in this mass poisoning because the entire nation's first responders—paramedics, fireman, policeman, and on-the-scene volunteers—so often rush to the aid of others while, often unknowingly, they put their own health at risk. This was the case in the Bogalusa chemical spill described above and, notably, in the September 11, 2001, disaster in New York.

Aside from the many deaths among firefighters that occurred inside the World Trade Center towers, numerous first responders and volunteers developed acute respiratory illnesses, and many have experienced persistent breathing problems, including asthma. The Red Cross, the Centers for Disease Control and Prevention (CDC), the World Trade Center Medical Monitoring Program, and other private and public organizations, continue to accumulate data about the long-term physical and mental health ailments that have left so many partially or severely disabled. In fact, there are 16,000 of these patients registered at one New York hospital alone.

The message for our first responders is never to dismiss symptoms that appear at the scene of a chemical release or fire. These brave men and women should be promptly evaluated in the emergency department, the same as the patients they transport. Some reports approach these problems from a financial/political viewpoint, because the healthcare (and disability) costs among the thousands of first responders and others are dramatic. But, as a physician, I see the day-to-day costs in human suffering and overall ill health—such profound loss of quality of life.

HBOT and Other Toxins

We have seen that it's possible to treat patients with carbon monoxide poisoning months to years after the event. I have done this with a substantial number of patients in the past 19 years and have also treated patients exposed to other toxins, including nitrogen tetroxide, mentioned above. Other hyperbaric physicians are also treating the effects of toxic exposure some time after the event. For example, Dr. Ken Stoller, a pediatrician and hyperbaric physician who used to practice in Santa Fe, New Mexico, published a case study of a 15-year-old child with fetal alcohol syndrome (FAS) for whom HBOT was able to significantly improve cognitive function years after the alcohol poisoning that occurred during pregnancy[5].

Dr. Stoller's work has profound implications for the future treatment of this tragic syndrome, which affects so many children in our society. When we add the multitude of cases of exposure to neurotoxins, we are looking at enormous numbers of people with these types of injuries. I believe that if we routinely included HBOT in the treatment plan, the results could be staggering, beyond what we can imagine today.

The Effects are Cumulative

Unfortunately, subtle, nearly undetectable exposures, as well as the larger ones, have a cumulative effect on brain function. Each has its own impact, but each also starts the inflammatory reaction, which damages brain cells and results in the formation of scar tissue, a characteristic of which is reduced blood supply to the damaged area.

At the time of exposure, especially in the case of toxins such as carbon monoxide, the machinery of the cell itself can be damaged. Carbon monoxide in particular, as well as cyanide and other toxins, bind to the energy-making components of the cell, which cripples the cells ability to do its work. However, as previously mentioned, these damaged cells may not be so severely damaged that they are destroyed, or die. Rather, these cells may live for long periods of time in a dormant state.

In many situations, we have injured cells coupled with damage to the blood supply. Information that has accumulated over the years shows that these wounded areas can exist for years and years. HBOT has the potential to target these wounds occurring in the brain and other areas in the body, even when HBOT is delivered years after the chemical exposure.

It May Never be Too Late to Treat

It's important that you understand the potential value of delayed treatment. Treating an injury with HBOT at the time it occurs may be only the first step. In the best of all possible worlds, emergency department specialists and personnel would explain the importance of follow-up evaluation and care. However, even if you or a loved one has experienced an injury in the past, and it is no longer an emergency, HBOT may still be of great help to you.

This point is underscored by my friend and colleague, Dr. William Duncan. Dr. Duncan contributed the introduction to this book because of the profound effect HBOT has had on multiple members of his family. Some of these cases are presented on the IHMA website under the Government Testimonies section (you can also find links to many of these stories under the "Oxygen Revolution" tab on HBOT.com). One of these family members is Dr. Duncan's younger brother, Michael Duncan Page, who suffered a brain injury when his brain-injured abusive father threw him against a wall during a fit of crying two weeks after he was born. (Dr. Duncan's father had had rheumatic fever as an eight-year-old and experienced extremely high fevers. The prolonged fevers caused brain damage to Dr. Duncan's father that caused a change in personality from "the kindest, sweetest boy any father could ask for" to a highly aggressive individual who was prone to violent rages as an adult.)

Dr. Duncan brought his brother to me a few years ago, 44 years after his brother's head injury, and after only a month of HBOT he began bathing daily. We saw that his insight and speech improved significantly. In addition, the frequency of his seizures decreased. (His brain scans are included on page 3 of the photo insert). When he went back home to California, he showed up for work every day, which resulted in a promotion. Because his conversation skills had improved, he interacted in ways that were appropriate to each situation and he was able to remember what was said minutes before. Arguably the greatest improvement was the end to the repetitive, unchanging conversational loops that would continue hour after hour, adding up to days, months, and years, which drove family members crazy. The end of these loops alone made him much easier to live with and be around—only the love of a mother could endure that type of interaction.

The improvement we saw in Dr. Duncan's brother affected everyone involved in his care and raised his quality of life. To the family, the change in their loved one was nothing short of a miracle. But, medically, miracle or not, it shows the importance of considering delayed treatment.

Acute vs. Delayed HBOT

In 2005, I treated a girl who had sustained a lightning injury that had rendered her unconscious, but she eventually revived. Her head was the entry site for the lightning bolt, and it caused a significant injury that was visible on CT scan and later brain blood flow imaging. Had HBOT been available at the time of the acute injury, it is likely that much of the damage would have been averted. However, months later, her parents sought treatment for her abnormal gait, weakness, and mild cognitive problems.

After one month of HBOT, her gait had noticeably improved and we began to see an improvement in her speech and mental quickness as well. After she returned to her hometown, she continued HBOT and experienced further gains. When I last spoke to her mother, this young girl's gait was nearly normal and her strength had improved, and I was happy to learn that she was doing well in school. I mention this case to illustrate again that while administering HBOT at the acute stage of the injury is optimal, I often see cases that prove it's never too late to treat. In this case, the injury had reached the chronic stage, but the patient achieved good results with hyperbaric oxygen.

Curt, Our "Phenomenal" Teen

I'll finish this brief survey of cases by describing one of the most gratifying patients I have ever treated. Curt Allen, Jr. was a typical teenager, with his share of the usual recklessness we see in many young people. Unfortunately, he was injured one night in a car accident while intoxicated. His brain injury was equivalent to Chad's (described earlier in this chapter), but Curt's family didn't know a bunch of doctors, nor were they aware of HBOT. Even if they had known, they had no access to a chamber. Because of those circumstances, I didn't see Curt until he was nearly four months into his "non-recovery."

Three weeks after his injury, Curt had been transferred from north Louisiana to the same neurorehabilitation facility in New Orleans at which Chad and a number of my other patients had been treated. However, he'd made essentially no progress—zero—after three full months of intense therapies. He was on the brink of being sent home in a severely impaired state.

Through a series of events, Curt's mother ran into a former patient and physician colleague of mine. I'd treated this doctor following his stroke and traumatic brain injury, and I'd treated other members of his family as well. This doctor advised Curt's mother not to go back home before talking with me, which is how I happened to begin treating Curt.

Unable to get SPECT imaging, I videotaped Curt, and the comparison between the videos is simply startling. At our first encounter he was extremely slow and responded to none of my commands or attempts to stimulate him, and he was mute. By the time we reached 20 treatments his mother was discouraged because she hadn't seen any noticeable change in Curt. I told her that this was the toughest time, but she needed to hold on a little longer. A good number of patients don't see improvement until they are past 25 treatments in a block of 40.

By 25–26 HBOTs Curt began to respond to the technician's banter, and appeared animated and laughing. He continued to become more bright and alert through 40 treatments, after which I scheduled my perfunctory re-evaluation and re-video. What happened was remarkable: through the entire exam, he feigned injury, duplicating the condition he was in before we started HBOT. As I finished the video I exclaimed that he was just being an obstinate teenager, refusing to show the improvements that he had made. Then I bent down to look at his face, which was angled downward. He was smiling, almost laughing. I told my tech, Sean Bal, to turn off the video, and once that happened, Curt popped up like a jack-in-the-box, guffawing and relishing the fact that he had pulled a fast one on me. Sean quickly flicked on the camera and we caught his delight.

We then took a one month break, and during that time, Curt began to speak at the neurorehab facility where he was still going for outpatient therapy. The entire staff thought his progress was amazing and they called in staff from other floors to come in and observe him. Then, shortly after starting the next round of HBOT, he began to stand, and eventually walk with assistance. Again, the staff at the facility marveled. At my final exit video, after 80 HBOTs, Curt was conversant, in great spirits, and showed his old personality. While he wasn't what we'd call "normal," and was even a little inappropriate at times, he was a far cry from his pre-HBOT state. The change in this young man in a matter of a few short months was astounding.

The final chapters of this young life have yet to be written, but the last time I checked, Curt had a job at Wal-Mart as the front door greeter. He drives and lives in his own home. Of course, government officials will be happy to know that he is a taxpayer now, instead of a tax recipient.

Sometimes I feel almost compelled to apologize for using words like dramatic, amazing, profound, incredible, and so forth, but I don't know any other words to convey what happened. I'll let you decide for yourself after you have viewed Curt's video (available on my website, HBOT.com). As of October 2015, over 186,000 people have viewed Curt's video on YouTube.

Drawing Your Own Conclusions

The cases I've presented in this chapter represent only a sample of the hundreds of patients I've treated over the last 26 years. What began with almost serendipitously treating divers has evolved to include reproducible results in over 90 different neurological diagnoses. A few of my patients have left treatment essentially healed, in the most complete sense of that word. A few patients improved minimally, or not at all (5–10 percent). But in most patients, HBOT had a positive impact on their quality of life, and the imaging of these almost always documents these improvements. In the majority, HBOT made a change in their life for the better, and in many it led to the return of personality, individual uniqueness, and the sense of self, and along with these, dignity. I so often hear patients say, "Thank you for giving me my life back." This so aptly describes what happens when patients with neurological injuries receive HBOT. What I have seen happen to these patients reminds me of the motto at West Jefferson Medical Center: To Cure Sometimes, To Relieve Often, To Comfort Always.

With such impressive cases as Chad, Curt, and a multitude of others inside and outside of my practice, you're probably wondering why you haven't heard more about HBOT. I can only say that we are approaching the tipping point. A profound transformation is taking place in hyperbaric medicine. Research is burgeoning and we see doctors who have spent their careers in denial or negativity about HBOT changing their opinions. More importantly, widespread awareness of HBOT is increasing.

In large part, we can credit the growing awareness to the advocacy of patients and their families. Patients and their families are no longer willing to sit passively and allow the medical profession to deal them their cards. They're demanding a reshuffling of the deck; they want to see the other cards in the deck, and they insist on learning what cards are concealed under the table.

Some of the change occurs at fairly unlikely hospitals. For example, a family secured HBOT for their son, severely brain injured after a drug overdose. Ironically, the hospital that agreed to the treatment is both one of the birthplaces of modern hyperbaric medicine, and also the home institution of one of the most outspoken critics of HBOT for brain injury.

More and more patients and families are fighting Medicaid and insurance companies to obtain reimbursement for HBOT—and they are prevailing. The tools provided by the Internet—forums, YouTube, and chat groups, along with the traditional medical journal—provide sources for increasing accumulation of information on the beneficial effects of HBOT. As Winston Churchill said, "Never, never, never, never give up."

CHAPTER 5

BIRTH INJURIES AND CEREBRAL PALSY

THROUGHOUT HISTORY, HUMAN BEINGS HAVE HAD to accept the reality that both giving birth and being born are high-risk, capricious events. In fact, the trip down the birth canal is probably the most high-risk journey any of us will ever take, and it is risky for the mother as well. And while we can define and delineate the stages of labor and the course of delivery, that does not mean we can predict with certainty what will happen moment by moment.

Ironically, the advances of modern medicine have led to a peculiar arrogance about birth. What I mean is that we have come to expect "foolproof" childbirth. Between well-trained obstetricians and up-to-date hospitals, with their ultrasounds and fetal monitors, it would seem that coming into this world should be stupidly simple. However, I have joined those who call our modern expectation the "myth of the perfect birth." As this myth goes, mothers are "well trained" for childbirth and the children come out pink and active. I'm not entirely sure how this myth developed, but too many of us believe that modern medicine guarantees a good outcome.

This myth is far from the reality of birth, and our failure to understand this actually complicates the situation. If we look back only a few years or consider the impoverished countries of the so-called "Third World," sobering statistics on maternal and neonatal mortality tell us that we still have a long way to go to provide the most basic care for mothers and infants. But, so as not to overstate this, it's true that in the mid-nineteenth century, Ignaz Semmelweis, an Hungarian obstetrician, discovered the cause of what was called childbed fever (puerperal), a leading cause of maternal death. He discovered that this infection could be prevented if doctors and midwives involved with women at the time of delivery would wash their hands. In fact, one of the biggest leaps in medical progress came through our understanding of the relationship between infections and bacteria, which led to improved hygiene in all medical settings. Dr. Semmelweis remains one of the most important medical pioneers, because his discovery began the drastic declines in infant and maternal mortality that continues to this day, currently due primarily to improvements in prenatal and postnatal care.

However, even with expanded knowledge, and even with our considerable safeguards in place, the birth process adversely affects a significant number of children. Once labor begins and a woman proceeds to the final stages where the child enters the birth canal, it remains a roll of the dice whether or not that child will be injured in the process.

As a doctor, I've studied pediatric and adult brain injury in depth for over 26 years, and I've treated hundreds of brain-injured children. I'm also the father of six children, and by the time my last child was born I don't mind admitting that I was a nervous wreck.

Our First Journey

It's important to understand what happens during birth. As you know, a baby's head is the largest part of the infant to proceed through the birth canal. Obviously, in evolutionary terms, women's bodies have adapted to accommodate this, but we still find a wide range of birth canal dimensions, based on broad genetic variation among all populations.

In addition, the same woman can have babies with different size heads. Logically, a baby with a smaller head proceeds through the birth canal more easily than one with a larger head. An infant with a larger head may be subject to a greater degree of compression in the birth canal. In addition, if labor is induced, the woman's body may not be ready to accommodate the baby's head. For example, even if the birth canal has not yet dilated, the induction agent (oxytocin) causes strong uterine contractions, which means that the baby's head pushes through anyway. This was likely the cause of injury in a patient of mine in 1992, a boy we'll call Tim (not his real name), the first child with cerebral palsy (CP) treated with HBOT in North America. Cerebral palsy refers to a number of chronic neurological disorders that affect body movement and muscle coordination, and is usually the result of brain damage that occurs at any time from fetal development through infancy. In this case, labor was induced with Pitocin (oxytocin), the female hormone that causes uterine contractions. When the first dose failed, Tim's mother was given a "double dose." She then proceeded from no labor to complete delivery in 45 minutes. So, after what she described as "violent" contractions, she delivered a jittery little boy with low body temperature and low blood sugar. Tim also had a bleed between the coverings of the brain, likely resulting from being forced through a birth canal that had not properly dilated. Tim's mother noted that he seemed floppy and had trouble sucking.

Early on, Tim began to show developmental delays. After an extensive workup at age two, he was finally diagnosed with hypotonic (meaning that he had low muscle tone) cerebral palsy. This child had enormous difficulties, including constant drooling, inability to speak, very poor coordination, and such low muscle tone that he could not stand or walk. In order to keep him in an upright position, adult arms had to brace his abdomen and chest. If the adult let go of him, he would flop to the ground.

In 1992, Dr. Sheldon Gottlieb, then–Professor of Biology at the University of South Alabama in Mobile, Alabama, and director of research for Dr. Van Meter's not-for-profit Baromedical Research Institute of New Orleans, attended a cerebral palsy support group meeting in Mobile. Dr. Gottlieb told these parents that he had a treatment suggestion for children diagnosed with CP. Then he called me and said I'd soon hear from a mother who wanted me to treat her CP child with HBOT.

Frankly, this call upset me greatly—you could say I almost blew a fuse. I had just discovered that I could treat divers, those with chronic traumatic brain injuries, and stroke patients with HBOT. I also had begun treating a child after a near-drowning incident, and I'd treated a few patients with spinal cord injury. I had put my focus on divers and trauma patients. I couldn't figure out why Dr. Gottlieb would tell a group of parents that I could treat their cerebral palsy–afflicted children.

When I asked Dr. Gottlieb what he knew about CP he said he essentially knew nothing, and I told him I knew "next to nothing." But after I got over being upset, I realized that the only way I'd made advances with the divers and others was by keeping an open mind. Going back to what I've been saying in this book all along, children with CP sustained brain injuries not too different from the trauma and stroke patients I treated. My concern was that parents might see the willingness to treat their children as a promise of some kind, and I certainly couldn't offer assurances about the outcome of treatment. We then discussed how we could evaluate Tim with brain blood flow imaging.

To make a long and exciting story a little shorter, I ended up seeing Tim in late 1992 and did the sequence of SPECT scan, single HBOT, and repeat SPECT. What I noticed on SPECT was damage to a key part of the brain that serves motor function. This area seemed to show a little improvement in blood flow after the first HBOT, so I told Tim's mother that I would treat her son (Tim's case was reported in 1994).

This case launched the movement for using HBOT in pediatric brain injury. As Tim received HBOT we noticed less drooling, he seemed more alert, and he gained strength. After 40 treatments his improvements were noticeable, including increased muscle tone. After a short break, we brought him back for another 40 treatments. By the time we hit 60 or so HBOTs, Tim was walking with fingertip support for balance. Everyone involved was astounded! While he didn't acquire speech, the progression in his muscle tone that allowed him to walk was nothing short of phenomenal. My immediate response was to shout this as loud as I could. And over the next couple of years I accumulated videos of the children I subsequently treated; meanwhile, cases of CP children treated with HBOT emerged elsewhere, too.

In this case, Tim was injured because the mother's body was unable to make the accommodation for a normal birth. These injuries are often prevented, because the baby can make accommodations, too. In other words, just as women's bodies have adaptive mechanisms to accommodate an infant's trip down the birth canal, infants have mechanisms to adapt to the many possibilities and vagaries of the birth process, including the confining conditions of the birth canal. In particular, the baby's hemoglobin (the protein in red blood cells that carries oxygen to the tissues of the body) is adapted to latch onto and carry oxygen in low oxygen conditions much better than adult hemoglobin.

In an infant, the skull bones are not fused, which is why they can be compressed, moved, and overlapped without causing much damage to the baby. You may have seen for yourself that some newborns have grossly misshapen heads because of prolonged compressions in the birth canal. Within hours to days, however, the head readjusts and things seem normal. The overall medical assumption is that compression and reshaping of the head alone don't cause injuries. However, we really don't know if some babies are more susceptible to compression-related injury than others.

The issue of compression is one of the areas of the birth process about which we've tended to be cavalier. When the skull bones are compressed on the brain, brain blood flow drops. In addition, the brain becomes temporarily deformed and misshapen—while shear forces are exerted upon it. Shear forces result from two surfaces sliding against one another; in this context, the outer surface of the brain and the white and gray matter of the brain, without any other tissue between to act as cushioning. It is possible that what happens to the infant brain during compression can cause some lasting injury. Another common example of a potentially dangerous situation at birth is umbilical cord wrapping around the infant's neck (nuchal cord). This deprives the infant of needed blood flow and oxygen to the brain. However, unless the infant is profoundly and persistently affected with poor breathing, movement, color, and so forth, a nuchal cord, like head compression, is believed to impart no permanent injury.

One tenet that has remained throughout the history of Western medicine is that a baby can withstand almost any insult at birth. But in 2001, the British medical journal *The Lancet* published an important article[1] showing that events around the time of birthing figure much more prominently in causing neonatal brain injury than events occurring during the nine months of gestation. More importantly, the data suggested that there may be a greater degree of hidden or subtle brain injury in neonates than previously thought.

The researchers came to this conclusion by comparing two groups of babies. One group included infants born in severe distress, with an obvious decrease in blood supply and oxygen. These babies were born barely alive or had to be resuscitated. Researchers compared them to another group of babies ostensibly born totally normal and with high APGAR scores, but who had their first seizure within the first three days of life. (The APGAR is a quick test of a baby's vitality immediately following birth. It applies a numbered score for skin color, i.e., pink or bluish, respiration, movement, and so forth, and is meant to alert medical staff to any immediate problems with the baby.) Prior to the seizures, no evidence of any abnormality appeared in this second group of babies.

Both groups of babies were given MRIs of the brain during their first two weeks of life. In both groups, minimal evidence existed of brain damage that occurred prior to the birth. In the babies born in conditions with low blood flow and oxygen, approximately 80 percent had signs of acute brain injury. Similarly, in the second group of babies, very little evidence of injury during gestation was found, but the MRIs showed acute brain injury in 70 percent.

We can't ignore the importance of this study and its suggestion that the birth process is not as innocuous as we've always thought. This data may also offer a glimpse into the wide diversity we see in children. For example, some do not speak until well beyond two years, others develop motor skills later than considered normal. Variations in vision, including crossed eyes, for example, may in fact be due to subtle birth injuries. The same may be true for things such as speech abnormalities or aberrations for which we have no explanation.

In the past, we have assumed that these individual developmental differences are based on genetic variation or occur during development in the womb. I submit that given what we know about hyperbaric oxygen therapy's effects on acute brain injury, the potential for ameliorating damage at birth is vast, greater than we have ever imagined.

In the most extreme cases (these are often the families I see) parents suffer great emotional and financial distress, not to mention the enormous cost to society. So many birth-injured children are dependent on medical care paid for at least partially by taxpayers, but beyond the financial concerns, when these injuries are severe, society loses a potential productive and participating member—and we are all the poorer for that. In addition, the stress on the family is another undertold story, and sadly, the divorce rate among the parents of severely birth-injured children is extremely high.

Sometimes It Comes Down to Luck

I said earlier that we like to think of the birth of a child as a joyous—if arduous—event. But for me, it eventually took on a nightmarish quality. Because I knew what was at stake and how quickly a normal birth could take a dangerous turn, at the time my last child was born, all I could think of were the many dozens of children I had treated for whom birth had resulted in neurological injuries. As a father, I wanted my child out of the birth canal immediately. I know my anxiety was not unusual, and is probably shared by most labor and delivery nurses and obstetricians when they either give birth or are the partner-fathers.

Just at the point when my baby was about to emerge, the nurse instructed my then-wife to stop pushing because the doctor was not present. I was horrified. My son was stuck in the birth canal, ready to be born, with his head compressed and brain blood flow at a minimum. And his mother was told to "do her part" to delay expelling him until the doctor could get there! Luckily, the obstetrician showed up rather quickly and my son was born intact.

One reason I was so nervous was that one of my older children's births had not gone very well. To be brief, a "cavalierly administered" increased epidural dose of anesthetic resulted in what is known as ascending paralysis, meaning that the effects extended beyond the lower area of the body, so my wife was unable to breathe properly as she pushed to give birth to our daughter. Unfortunately, the obstetrician wasn't paying attention. Normally, the uterine contractions coincide with the mother's pushing action. But, because the doctor wasn't fully alert to the paralysis, this threw off the normal coordination, and as a result, my daughter was stuck in the birth canal. We waited many minutes, and when she was finally born she was purple and did not respond to stimulation. She moved very, very slowly and would not breathe. Needless to say, her APGARs were very poor.

I mention this situation because, as a doctor who was very, very familiar with this situation, and a physician who practices emergency medicine, I knew what was needed. But I was a father in that room, not a doctor, and unfortunately, I stood frozen with horror as I looked at my barely alive daughter.

Finally the obstetrician said, "Let's get some oxygen."

I screamed out loud, "Yes, oxygen! Please, anybody, get my daughter some oxygen!" Here was the obvious solution. My life is dominated by the use of oxygen, but I couldn't think to get my daughter additional oxygen. Eventually my infant daughter was revived, but she required care in the neonatal intensive care unit (ICU). I'll never forget her blank stare as I looked at her, and agonized about pulling her out of that hospital and putting her in a hyperbaric chamber. At that time I was not as knowledgeable about hyperbaric oxygen therapy and its profound effects in such a situation, so I didn't remove her. Had I known then what I know now, I might have made a different decision.

Eventually she recovered and is a normal child today. However, I can't help but think that a single hyperbaric oxygen treatment would have revived her much more quickly.

Even with truly good doctors and hospitals, the journey a baby takes into our world can be very frightening for new parents. My own experiences have sensitized me to parents who struggle to understand the birth process, but find it frightening, too.

When HBOT May Be Useful

The type of problem my daughter experienced during birth is complicated by the secondary inflammatory reaction we previously discussed, called reperfusion injury. If you recall from Chapter 2, reperfusion injury is the secondary injury that results with the resumption of blood flow following a temporary interruption. We define it as a "paradoxically harmful" aspect of blood flow return that further injures the tissue.

The "paradox" arises from the concept that you would normally expect the return of blood flow after a temporary interruption to *salvage* the tissue and the patient. For example, the return of blood flow to a person after cardiac arrest should be all roses. But it isn't. A secondary injury to tissues occurs, one that is greater than the initial absence of blood flow and oxygen. This reperfusion injury is essentially the inflammatory reaction discussed earlier, plus some other nuances that involve additional mechanisms of injury.

What we know today is that HBOT at high pressures significantly inhibits reperfusion injury. This is why, looking back, I know that a single hyperbaric treatment could have made a dramatic improvement in my daughter's condition at birth. However, at the time, we didn't have the ability to efficiently and easily provide that treatment.

Three years after my daughter's birth, I had occasion to do an extensive search in the medical literature on HBOT in birth injury. I was then asked to summarize this in a textbook chapter for the *Textbook of Hyperbaric Medicine* by Dr. K. K. Jain. During my search, I came across an amazing article from 1963, this one also published in the British medical journal, *The Lancet*[2].

This article reported a study involving 65 babies who were born not breathing. When these babies failed standard resuscitation, they were placed in an incubator-sized hyperbaric chamber. Understand that these babies were nearly dead; they would have been officially dead, had the doctors stopped all resuscitation efforts. In a dozen of these babies, doctors had inserted a breathing tube, but they had stopped the mechanical ventilation, because the tiny chamber didn't have a ventilator.

What the researchers described was absolutely remarkable. Within minutes of placing these children in the chamber and taking them to two atmospheres of pressure, many "pinked up" and started breathing. Vital signs began to improve. The babies who did not revive were then taken to four atmospheres. In all, 75 percent of the babies who had failed standard resuscitation began to breathe and were taken from the chamber in a revived state. This in itself didn't ensure survival, however. One-third of the babies regressed, underwent an additional treatment, but in the end didn't make it.

Remarkably, however, 54 percent of these infants were discharged from the hospital "apparently well." Those who did not survive died of major malformations, were stillborn (born dead), or had other conditions that precluded sustained life. The revived babies were those who likely had a birth-related insult of low oxygen/blood and who just needed the "jump-start of HBOT" and the inhibition of reperfusion injury provided by HBOT.

This *Lancet* article caused a firestorm of controversy. The authors of the study were accused of experimenting on the children, not having done enough animal research, not intubating (inserting a tube to keep the trachea open) enough of the children, and so forth. The doctors responded by doing a randomized controlled study comparing the hyperbaric chamber resuscitation with intubation and mechanical ventilation. When the results of this study were published, they showed no difference between the two methods of resuscitation[3]. What was remarkable was that without anyone touching the babies who were placed in the chamber, the simple physics of HBOT was able to save these children in equivalent numbers to the children who received maximal human intervention.

I need to make two important points about this second study, however. First, the authors did not compare HBOT plus intubation to intubation alone. With the results of the first study and what we now know about HBOT effects on the inflammatory reaction, the combination of HBOT and intubation likely would have added effects. Second, intubation of a newborn baby takes great skill. The babies are tiny, the airways are tiny, the instruments and tubes are tiny, and the baby's tissues and airway are easily injured. Last, but most important, is the stark human factor. If you have ever been in an emergency room or delivery suite when medical staff must resuscitate a newborn, you would have seen the panic in the room. Unlike adult cardiac resuscitation, where you are dealing with patients who may have lived a full life, a baby is a brand new life: so perfect, so innocent, so full of potential, and dying in your hands. It is a horrible experience. Trying to intubate in such a panic situation is extremely difficult. The author of the second *Lancet* article, Dr. J. H. Hutchison, argued that, in contrast to this intubation procedure, it is easy to just compress a baby on oxygen and let the benefits of HBOT take place.

Dr. Hutchison also pointed out that the only reason they were able to carry out this study was that the doctors highly skilled in intubation volunteered their time to be immediately available to intubate these babies 24 hours a day, seven days a week. To this day, this service is available in a miniscule number of hospitals in the United States. The most skilled in this procedure, neonatologists and neonatal intensivists, are only available at some hospitals and usually do not remain in the hospital 24 hours a day.

As a result, the doctors compared a procedure that is *not* readily available to neonates in distress with one that is fairly simple to deliver and immediately available at all hours of the day or night. The authors, writing back in the 1960s, pointed this out in the article, but it fell on deaf ears and HBOT was not adopted as standard for delivery rooms.

Another reason that the results of these studies were not applied was that in subsequent years a scare about using supplemental oxygen in newborns made the issue moot. At that time, it was believed that supplemental oxygen could cause an eye disease in infants, resulting in blindness. However, this was not the case, but rather could be attributed to the way in which the oxygen was used and then rapidly withdrawn, not the oxygen itself. A recent study confirmed this, but an incorrect assumption meant that for the next 40 years the medical community ignored HBOT use in this particular acute setting.

Finally, in the late 1990s, a doctor in Mexico, Dr. Cuau Sanchez, began to treat a few infants in an effort to duplicate what had been done in England in 1963. While he treated just seven newborns, and only two or three had brain injury, his results were the same: an immediate improvement in neurological status.

To be clear, using HBOT in the delivery room setting today is not simple. The standard of care today is to intubate any baby that needs resuscitation. Such a baby subsequently placed in a hyperbaric chamber must be ventilated through that tube. Since there is no hyperbaric chamber ventilator that can give the 60 breaths per minute these babies need, the baby must go in the chamber with a highly skilled inside attendant—an attendant who must be available 24 hours day.

Within the delivery room setting, the only way to meet all these requirements is by having hyperbaric chambers available in the emergency room. The combination of labor and delivery staff, plus the emergency physicians and nurses would make it possible to offer hyperbaric resuscitation to neonates. Based on current trends, which will make HBOT available in emergency departments, it will soon be possible to meet these requirements.

Surprisingly, in the past 10 years this "advanced" use of HBOT for birth injury has been used in what is historically one of the most underdeveloped countries: China. In 2006, Dr. Liu published a modern review of 20 clinical studies with control groups on HBOT treatment of low oxygen/low blood flow birth injury[4].

While the studies were not of the highest rigor (according to standards in Western medicine), the results were nearly uniform. They showed a reduction in death rate and improvement in neurological outcome. That probably comes as no surprise to you, since that outcome is completely consistent with the science described in this book. However, the authors of the review didn't address this point; they merely recommended that doctors perform more studies. Unfortunately, brain injured children cannot afford to wait for more studies.

The "Miracle" Child

At the end of Chapter 1, I mentioned the importance of families defining their own miracles. I also mentioned a woman who brought her severely brain-injured child, who had sustained his injuries during birth, to my facility for treatment. I could offer this mother little in the way of reassurance or hope, but having experience with the realities of brain injury, this mother arrived without raised expectations.

After treating this child, I gained greater perspective about the kind of expectations and hopes parents, particularly mothers, have for their brain injured children. Through HBOT, this boy achieved major improvements that had a profound effect on his life and the life of his family. (See the SPECT scans taken before and after the first HBOT on page 3 of the photo insert.)

First, the HBOT had a tremendous calming effect on him. Prior to his hyperbaric oxygen therapy, trips out of the house were limited to 15–30 minutes or so since he was so uncomfortable in a stroller or car seat. The only thing that comforted him seemed to be his father's jostling and playing with him vigorously. After HBOT he was much more relaxed, was able to tolerate sitting, and could go out with his mother to the store and other locations for hours at a time.

HBOT also gave him vision. His mother had been told countless times that the child was blind, but she thought he might have minimal vision. After about 15 treatments I noticed that when he was in the chamber he would quickly orient to me as I approached the chamber from the head end. I realized that he was acquiring peripheral vision. After more HBOT, he went on to develop better vision, and his personality emerged because he was better able to interact socially. The last time I spoke with his mother just prior to the publication of the release of this book; I caught her in the midst of his birthday party. (His picture at that party is on my website, HBOT.com.) In this case, the miracle came in the form of much improved quality of life. His mother called me in the summer of 2009 to tell me that he was riding a Waverunner (jet-ski), horseback riding, and speaking. I was dumbfounded to hear that Tim was now functioning at that level. It was almost unbelievable. Not only did he exceed his mother's expectations about the Happy Meal, but he surpassed all expectations of medical professionals in charge of his care.

The Impact of HBOT on Birth Injury

As we noted earlier, the term "cerebral palsy" is used by some as a general term that includes the effects of brain injury at birth. Sometimes birth injuries are obvious, but often they are not, and a diagnosis of CP is typically made by about two years of age. CP generally refers to children whose predominant problems are related to motor skills. However, in terms of birth injury, we see a variety of problems, from developmental delays to learning disability/cognitive problems, decreased vision and hearing, failure to gain weight, oral motor problems with drooling, chewing, swallowing, irritability, inability to sleep, muscle spasms, seizures, mental retardation, speech delays, and so forth. Virtually any and all disabilities are related to the particular damaged areas of the brain.

These brain injuries have a tremendous impact on the child's life, of course, and they nearly overwhelm many parents, especially when the family has other children. I have met some women with multiple special-needs children. They lead difficult lives, sometimes enduring what is beyond imagination, yet they trudge forward with a sense of duty, driven by their love for their children.

I've seen children afflicted by constant, painful muscle spasms that caused severe back arching, which made it impossible to sit for more than 15 minutes in a stroller. In these situations, family outings are limited because the child is in pain and so irritable that it's nearly impossible to live normally—almost by any standard. These children often have severe oral motor problems, and they may choke and sputter with each small mouthful of pureed food or liquid. This situation means that it may take as long as 6–8 hours a day just to feed children with these difficulties.

So, when HBOT leads to improvements, even those that might seem small to others who haven't experienced these problems, it's easy to see why it seems like a miracle. When a child can chew and swallow or the painful muscle spasms improve, along with improvement of dozens of other symptoms, these changes greatly enhance quality of life for the whole family.

HBOT also has an effect far beyond the immediate treatment of the child's obvious deficits. Once injured brain tissue has been "re-energized" by HBOT and restored to more normal function, the injured area now can begin to develop. The injured area, which has been accommodated by development in other uninjured areas, is now free to begin the developmental process. The injured area is then allowed to evolve and mature over many subsequent years. I have seen this many times with children who go on to develop far beyond the limits of what was expected at their current stage of arrested development. (You can see a few of the cases in their associated news clips at HBOT.com.)

Augmenting Standard Care

In the Resources section in this book, you will see the MUMS Network (Mothers United for Moral Support), a support and advocacy group for families with brain-injured children that is now functioning as a resource site. The group's founder, Julie Gordon, sent four women to New Orleans to check me out. (For obvious reasons, they didn't want to put their faith in a treatment that claimed to miraculously "cure" their children.) The four mothers decided to give HBOT and SPECT brain imaging a try, and their children responded very well to the treatment. At that point, the MUMS Network began to vigorously support and advocate for HBOT as an additional treatment for pediatric brain injury.

Standard therapies for brain-injured children include physical therapy and in some cases, speech therapy. In addition, children also receive treatment for medical conditions, such as seizure disorders. Other professionals may help parents cope with their children's injuries, which are on a continuum of severity. Almost all the parents I've seen have been "lectured" about the dangers of false hope, and detractors have cautioned against HBOT. While this advice may be well meaning, it often ignores the areas where hope is indeed alive.

As a specialty, pediatric neurology has not shown great interest in HBOT; thus, many parents become aware of the therapy through other channels, particularly parent support groups. It's important to note, however, that HBOT does not replace any of the therapies children would normally receive, such as physical therapy or certain medications if needed. HBOT is an additional therapy.

MUMS has had great value as an important advocacy organization that has worked for many years to educate parents of brain injured children. They have disseminated information about HBOT and have helped parents obtain treatment, with or without the recommendation or even grudging approval of their children's team of doctors.

I recommend that you see for yourself the scope of what they used to do and the information they have compiled. (See HBOT.com for a collection of links to their more pertinent research and findings.) I was on their Medical Advisory Board when the organization was active, and had a long association with the group. Some of my youngest patients came to my facility because of their network. As I've said before, medical breakthroughs require doctors to step out of the paradigm that guided their education. But if we don't have patient-pioneers—men, women, and, yes, their children—also willing to break new ground, sometimes at great cost, then we would never have significant medical breakthroughs.

Documenting Results Through Our Research Project

Because I'd treated a group of patients with chronic brain injury, which is by definition "delayed treatment," I began to see that many patients responded positively to HBOT. This led to setting up an experimental program through our hospital institutional review board that oversees human experiments. (This was

Since that review, other studies have been published on HBOT in CP. The results have been mixed, positive, and neutral—but none were negative. One of the neutral studies may be explained by other factors not relevant here, but the important point is that no therapy and no placebo experiment has ever produced the positive findings achieved in the HBOT CP studies.

When the Injury Occurs Before Birth

HBOT may be useful when treating injuries and complications that occur during pregnancy. For many years now, Russian doctors have treated intrauterine growth retardation and other problems related to pregnancy and fetal development, especially those occurring in the last three months of pregnancy. In general, we usually do not know what causes these problems to develop during gestation, though drug and alcohol intake on the part of the mother is one cause we can identify. The Russian doctors have reported that many of these abnormalities can be reversed and the outcomes of certain pregnancies improved.

Expanding on this, let's consider that throughout the world, babies are exposed in utero to alcohol, cocaine, and other substances. Russian doctors have used HBOT in adults to treat overdose/poisoning and help ameliorate drug toxicity withdrawal symptoms. Putting this together, it makes sense to speculate that hyperbaric oxygen therapy delivered early for fetal alcohol syndrome and drug exposure could profoundly affect neurological outcome. While a single HBOT could not be expected to reverse nine months of damage, multiple treatments would likely impact the long-range disability of these syndromes, much as it has in a fetal alcohol patient treated by one of my colleagues. The single treatment protocol doesn't apply here due to the lack of reperfusion or birth injury related to interruption of blood supply or brain trauma. Of course, the personal and financial cost of treating, rearing, and educating children damaged in utero by drugs and alcohol is staggering.

Unfortunately, we don't yet have the ability in the United States to treat many of these injured children at the time of their birth. At best, we can treat them in delayed fashion at a freestanding hyperbaric facility, and that's dependent on awareness of the treatment among the appropriate health care providers. This is another reason why we—all of us—must get the word out about HBOT.

The Global View

Other countries are not as restrictive as we are in the U.S., and their medical societies function differently, too. For example, in Russia, China, Japan and other countries, HBOT has been increasingly used for a variety of neurological disorders with continued success as described above. Progress is slow in the U.S., but the momentum is shifting in favor of this treatment. It is my hope that in the near future every obstetrical department, or at least the emergency department, in every hospital will be equipped with a hyperbaric chamber. That way, we can place babies in extreme distress in a hyperbaric chamber, possibly for only one treatment. This single treatment may help treat the inflammatory reaction, oxygenate a brain starved for oxygen, and prevent the devastating brain swelling from developing.

Before we get to this point, we might need additional studies with evidence that finally convinces decision-makers in hospitals and doctors that the treatment is appropriate. At this point, a growing number of facilities are documenting treatment of younger and younger children and are showing good results. However, this hasn't translated to treatment of the injury in the hospital at the time of the birth. It is likely going to take another 5–10 years to make an impact, and even then the evidence alone may not be enough to turn the tide. This means the lay public may have to get involved (as the members of MUMS did). But, until that time, parents will have to seek treatment as soon as their children are released from an acute care hospital. This is happening increasingly in my practice.

CHAPTER 6

STROKES

SIMPLY PUT, A STROKE IS A NEUROLOGICAL SYNDROME characterized by interruption of blood supply to the brain. A number of different types of strokes exist. Some strokes are caused by a blood clot that forms in a blood vessel in the brain at the site of hardening of the arteries. This type of stroke is a thrombotic, or blood clot, stroke. Other strokes are caused by a blood clot traveling from the heart, or air that gets in an artery, and goes to the brain and plugs a brain blood vessel. These are called embolic strokes. Still other strokes result from rupture of a blood vessel and bleeding in the brain. Called a hemorrhagic or bleeding stroke, this can occur within the brain substance itself. If a blood vessel ruptures on the outside of the brain (as with a ruptured aneurysm), then it is called a subarachnoid bleed.

Regardless of type, all strokes deprive an area of the brain of blood flow and oxygen. Within the brain, collateral blood supply is limited (by that, I mean blood supply from surrounding blood vessels that can supply blood to an area when there's a temporary blockage of blood flow in a particular artery). So in a stroke, as a blood clot forms or travels to an artery and blocks it, the downstream area of the brain supplied by that artery becomes deprived of oxygen and nutrients.

To illustrate, picture the area deprived of oxygen and blood as a balloon on the end of a string, with the string as the artery supplying this imaginary balloon. At the center of the balloon is the area where the absence of blood flow is the greatest, and it dies. If we extend progressively out from that center dead area, we see increasing amounts of oxygen and blood flow that have trickled in from surrounding arteries. That outwardly expanding area has a gradient of oxygen and blood flow; along that gradient, the cells can live but not function as normal brain cells sending out electrical messages. As you keep traveling farther out away from the center, you reach areas where circulation is normal and the brain cells work adequately.

The region of brain where the brain cells are alive but not functioning normally is called the ischemic penumbra. HBOT probably has its greatest effect on this ischemic penumbral area. This is also the case with all other treatments for stroke. If any intervention can occur quickly enough at the time of acute stroke, even the dying or central area may be salvageable. Since strokes are in large part caused by blood vessel problems, as we age and develop vascular disease the incidence of stroke increases. With the Baby Boomers approaching retirement age and our population living longer, we are going to see steadily increasing numbers of stroke patients in the coming decades.

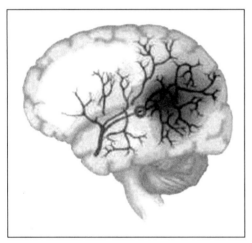

FIGURE 4. The figure depicts the blockage of an artery during a stroke. Each side of the brain is supplied by three major arteries, whose distribution of blood supply does not overlap. When a blockage occurs in a major artery the area of brain tissue to which the artery supplies blood is deprived of blood flow. The reduction in blood flow is at its maximum at the center (the darker shaded area) of the larger shaded area and this is the tissue that dies unless something is done within a few hours. The surrounding larger circle is the area of low blood flow and partial damage that can exist for years and that is potentially responsive to delayed application of HBOT.

The Risk Factors

Besides aging, risk factors for stroke include anything that accelerates vascular disease, most notably smoking, high cholesterol, hypertension (high blood pressure), and diabetes. We can't forget that we inherit our genes, and we may be predisposed to developing hypertension, diabetes, or elevated cholesterol. On the other hand, a genetic tendency does not mean we are doomed to suffer a stroke. Other factors, such as our diet and the chemical exposures we experience, contribute to our risk level as well.

Overall, about 800,000 strokes occur every year in the United States[1]. About one-third of those patients die as a result, while the remaining two-thirds live for years after, but often experience additional strokes. A previous stroke becomes a risk factor in and of itself. To be sure, stroke is one of the most financially costly of all diseases because most patients live with their disease, but suffer varying degrees of disability, even after a large investment in initial care and later rehabilitation. That said, the human costs are even greater; you may know this first hand, either because you have suffered a stroke or you have cared for a loved one following a stroke.

While most of us have seen or heard about remarkable recoveries from stroke, the rehabilitation process may take many months or years. And while the range of damage a stroke inflicts is wide, with the more fortunate experiencing relatively minor disabilities, many patients are permanently robbed of their previous productivity and activity, thus dramatically decreasing their quality of life.

First Signs and Early Treatment

Every adult should be aware of early signs of stroke, and although they are found in many books, they bear repeating. Early signs include sudden:

- Weakness in an arm or leg or both on the same side of the body
- Dizziness or confusion
- Headache
- Disturbances in the visual field, such as blurry vision
- Difficulty swallowing
- Slurred or distorted speech, or the loss of the ability to speak, or inability to understand another person's speech
- Other sensory difficulties, including altered ability to feel or touch, manifest as numbness or tingling

These symptoms occur because, depending on what area of the brain is involved, we see an acute loss of the neurological activity provided by that area. Although these symptoms may appear with other illnesses, if you or someone you're with shows any of them you need to get to a hospital immediately, either by calling an ambulance or, if it is your companion and the person is mobile and conscious, by immediately driving to the nearest emergency room.

When you arrive, the first question you will be asked is: When did these symptoms begin or first appear? This is a critical question; a three-hour window exists in which the worst damage in the largest thrombotic strokes can be reversed. If the symptoms have occurred over more than three hours—and sometimes symptoms are mild and occur over a period of days—then the treating doctors will slow the pace of their initial diagnostic evaluation. However, if the symptoms began less than three hours before arriving at the emergency room, then we make a frantic effort to diagnose the type of stroke that is in progress, and we make sure the patient does not have a bleeding stroke. If the case of a bleeding stroke, we cannot administer clot-dissolving drugs, as it will cause the bleed will enlarge.

However, if the patient does *not* have a bleeding stroke and we are still within the three-hour deadline, we speed up our evaluation. We quickly draw the patient's blood, take a chest x-ray, and rush the patient for a CT scan of the brain. Today, most emergency physicians are adept at reading the CT scans, but most hospitals have started a practice of sending the image to a special unit at the radiologist's home, which can be accomplished in a matter of minutes and immediately provide an expert reading.

Since many strokes are caused by blood clots, the clot dissolving drug TPA (tissue plasminogen activator) has been approved for use within the first 4.5 hours of the stroke. This drug is the first stroke treatment that improves function in the stroke patient. After the first 4.5 hours, extensive damage has occurred to the blood vessels and to the protective blood-brain barrier that exists between the blood vessel walls and the brain tissue itself. That means that dissolving a blood clot and reestablishing blood flow is associated with an increasingly high rate of bleeding into the brain tissue through the damaged blood vessels and blood brain-barrier. This is why the 4.5 hour window has become so critical today, even to the extent that public service information about stroke emphasizes this timeframe.

Unfortunately, our effective use of TPA is limited because the great majority of stroke patients do not reach the emergency room within that narrow time frame. For example, it is not uncommon for a person to wake up with a stroke in the morning, thus making it impossible to tell the exact time of onset. Most other patients just don't realize they're having a stroke until it's been present for quite a number of hours.

If you are beyond the 4.5 hour window or your blood pressure is extremely high (in which case you can't receive TPA), you will soon learn that there is no definitive treatment for the stroke. While studies show that acute care stroke units have better outcomes in their patients than hospitals that do not have such units, specific interventions designed to preserve brain tissue have not been identified.

Ten percent of surviving stroke patients require long-term care in nursing centers. The remaining survivors begin rehabilitation targeted to the area in which they suffered the damage. If the stroke affected motor skills, then physical therapy is undertaken. Some patients must learn to walk or write all over again. Other patients undergo speech therapy and others receive occupational therapy that integrates motor and cognitive skills. As you may well know if you or someone in your family has suffered a stroke, recovery may be slow and incomplete. In fact, the degree to which a person recovers is quite variable and not easily predicted.

HBOT and Acute Stroke

How can hyperbaric oxygen help in acute stroke? Since the primary reason a stroke causes injury is oxygen deprivation to the area, then it only makes sense that increased amounts of oxygen can prevent further brain damage. It may be that increased oxygen can also reverse some of the non-lethal brain damage. This is the thinking behind acute administration of hyperbaric oxygen.

Over the past several years, about 30 animal studies have shown a nearly universal benefit of HBOT in this situation. Another 30 studies in humans have mostly been positive. In medical research terms, the animal studies are convincing, but the human studies have not been of the highest rigor. So, coupled with the controversy over hyperbaric medicine that influences so many medical decisions, we're prevented from routinely administering HBOT to patients with acute stroke.

In recent years, it's become clearer that in acute stroke situations, at least in those for which we don't use the clot dissolving drug, the stroke may respond to much lower pressures of hyperbaric oxygen than previously believed. Unfortunately, we've been repeatedly stymied in our efforts to obtain funding for evaluation of acute stroke. However, Dr. Dietmar Schneider and his group in Leipzig, Germany, whom I recruited to join our stroke project in 1998, have gone on to achieve positive results with acute stroke, HBOT, and TPA. I expect them to continue leading the way in this area, as we in the U.S. have not seen major progress. Fortunately, patients don't have to wait for more clinical studies.

Seeking Treatment

I advise stroke patients to seek HBOT at freestanding facilities as soon as the acute evaluation in the emergency room is completed. Benefits for countless stroke cases have been documented and it's simple enough to evaluate. If the patient is placed in a hyperbaric chamber and there is seemingly no benefit, you can either adjust the dose of HBOT or discontinue the therapy. What frequently occurs is that patients respond very quickly and it's obvious that the treatment is beneficial. Treatments done on a daily basis for 10, 15, 30, or more treatments can show impressive results.

You may have heard of the late Edward Teller, the scientist known as "the father of the hydrogen bomb." He happens to be a notable example of the benefit of HBOT for sub-acute or post-acute stroke. In a 1994 conversation, Dr. Teller told me he had been undergoing hyperbaric oxygen therapy for a number of years at Dr. Richard Neubauer's HBOT clinic in southern Florida. He chose the treatment in an attempt to improve a hip condition he'd developed after an injury. When he found that the hyperbaric oxygen markedly sped up the healing process and ameliorated the pain in his hip, he began to investigate a little further. Based on what he learned about HBOT, he began going to Dr. Neubauer for periodic treatment. Dr. Teller then gave an evening address at the 1994 meeting of the American College of Hyperbaric Medicine. At the time, he was 85 years old and still had a brilliant and sharp mind.

His mental acuity was evident during the question and answer session after his talk. Just to give one example, a man in the audience asked a complex three-part question. Dr. Teller not only answered the question without notes, he moved seamlessly from each section without skipping a beat. Now, I've been asked three-part questions, and maybe you have, too, and I often have needed to ask the person to repeat one part or another—and I may take notes, too! Frankly, his ability to speak so clearly, without the backtracking and repetition so common in extemporaneous speech, dumbfounded us all.

The next day, I spoke with Dr. Teller about his experiences with hyperbaric oxygen therapy. I had an idea why he had continued HBOT for a number of years after his hip had healed, and when I asked him, his answer confirmed it.

"We have every reason to believe that HBOT benefits the brain," he said. "And we have little or no evidence that it harms the brain." Then he concluded with, "So, what do I have to lose?" In three succinct sentences, Dr. Teller summed up all the reasoning to use HBOT for the brain—and he provided his rationale to use HBOT to maintain his incredible intellect.

In 1995, Dr. Teller had a stroke, which primarily affected his short-term memory. Unable to obtain hyperbaric oxygen immediately, he had to wait until Dr. Neubauer sent a chamber to his home. He began treatment as soon as the chamber arrived, about six weeks after his stroke, and went on to say that he had a complete and total recovery from this stroke. The benefit of HBOT in yet another illness, this acute stroke, led Dr. Teller to treat himself daily for the rest of his life, another eight years. He continued to work at the Lawrence Livermore laboratories until his death in the fall of 2003. Dr. Teller died of a massive stroke from which hyperbaric oxygen could not revive him, but daily exposure to hyperbaric oxygen for the previous stroke kept him functioning at his high level, thus allowing him to remain productive through his 95th year.

Dr. Teller's case is important for a variety of reasons. First, he found that HBOT helped his hip. It is likely, but not certain, that in the process of treating his hip he experienced simultaneous improvement of his mental abilities, which provided the impetus to continue to use HBOT on an intermittent basis. Of course, he may have decided to continue using HBOT purely on the basis of his own argument that it had all the upside and very little downside. Second, starting HBOT within weeks of his stroke was still effective. This supports what I said earlier about the general adage in medicine and my belief about hyperbaric medicine that the sooner we can treat the better the results. Third, the results of treating his stroke with HBOT were so dramatic and profound that he continued HBOT for the rest of his life, maintaining his productivity and quality of life.

Fourth, Dr. Teller was not some crackpot, half-wit, demented, or quirky old man who was deluded into thinking that HBOT was a magic elixir. This was one of the brightest men in recent history, with an intact intellect with which he studied the physics of oxygen delivery, assessed available information, and came to a rational conclusion—that this therapy made sense. Moreover, he believed that it offered the best possibility of helping him. He then subsequently proved this on himself until a massive stroke caused his death.

The other important, yet unfortunate, point is that in order for Dr. Teller to obtain this treatment he had to have his own private chamber and attendant who delivered the treatment. Very few people have this luxury and I don't recommend it at the moment because of the possibility of complications and side effects. After all, HBOT is a medical treatment, regardless of whether it is delivered in a hospital, a doctor's office, or in private home.

To summarize Dr. Teller's contribution to hyperbaric medicine, I want to leave you with this quote, the last sentence from his Foreword to the third edition of the *Textbook of Hyperbaric Medicine*: "It is not entirely impossible that, perhaps sometimes in the next decade, professors of medicine will have difficulty in explaining why the treatment with oxygen was not widely adopted much earlier."

What Exactly Are We Treating?

We haven't yet identified all of the targets of hyperbaric oxygen therapy in stroke. However, the cells occurring on the marginal areas, those outside the center (as described in our balloon example above) are damaged, but do not die. Dr. K. A. Hossman has referred to this state as the ischemic freeze[2]. This ischemic freeze temporarily shuts down part of the new protein-making capability of the cells, such that the cell cannot perform its specialized functions. Where this block on new protein synthesis is located is unclear, but it appears that it is at the level of the DNA.

Neurology, the field of medicine that has investigated stroke, has held the opinion that this ischemic freeze only lasts for a few hours. However, over the last 20 years, it's become increasingly apparent from Dr. Neubauer's and my work, and now the experience of countless other physicians, too, that the ischemic freeze can last for years.

In other chapters I've used the term "idling neuron," and this is essentially what we are talking about when we discuss ischemic freeze. Low or absent blood flow causes a "freeze" on some of the metabolic functions of the neuron, likely at the DNA level, which results in an "idling neuron."

In the 1960s, some of the early HBOT researchers acknowledged this "idling" state. For example, Dr. Neubauer shattered the concept that these idling neurons could exist for a limit of six hours. In 1990, he sent a letter to The Lancet showing SPECT brain blood flow images of a woman severely neurologically disabled by a stroke 14 years earlier.[3] After a single hyperbaric oxygen treatment, she showed improved blood flow in an area of the brain thought to have been dead. He continued treating her with both hyperbaric oxygen and oxygen by facemask in her nursing home bed over the next 16 months, during which she showed progressive neurological improvement. While she was still severely handicapped, her overall level of care and quality of life had improved noticeably.

As so often happens in medicine, the coincidence of Dr. Neubauer's case with one in my practice was uncanny. I'll call our patient Mr. H. He'd been referred to our hyperbaric unit by a plastic surgeon to help aid surgery that was going to be performed on both of his heels for ulcers. The ulcers had occurred secondary to a serious stroke 12 years before that left him mute, unmotivated, and sedentary. Essentially, he had no RPMs left. (See Chapter 12 for a discussion of what I call "RPMs and the brain.") As we entered the second week of his treatment we noticed he cried as he arrived at the hyperbaric unit each day. I began a physical exam and laboratory evaluation to find a source of pain or the cause of his emotional distress, but I found nothing that explained his reaction.

The following week, he arrived at the unit and waved hello to our staff and had a noticeably improved mood. It dawned on me that Mr. H. was experiencing a gratuitous benefit of HBOT on his stroke. By the fourth week he was not only waving to the staff, he spoke his greetings—a remarkable change.

By the fifth and sixth weeks, however, the impact of this case hit home. Mr. H. began speaking in sentences and expressing himself. One morning, as he arrived in the unit from the nursing home, his wife burst through the doors and demanded to know what I done to her husband! Mr. H. had shocked her by initiating a conversation for the first time in 12 years. Naturally, Mrs. H. wanted to know what we had done to bring this about. I told her that the oxygen we were giving his feet also was working on the wound in his brain inflicted by the stroke.

So, what Dr. Neubauer's patient and Mr. H's case showed was that these damaged cells—idling neurons—could exist for at least 14 years. Other patients mentioned in this book also attest to the fact that idling neurons can exist for years. This evidence is important because it overturns a long-standing assumption in medicine, an assumption that has held back advancement in neurorehabilitation. It certainly held back research into new treatments for stroke.

Exactly how HBOT may be overriding this ischemic freeze is unknown, but we now know that the main target of activity of hyperbaric oxygen is the DNA of the cells. It's likely that the first HBOT treatment, or at least the first few exposures to HBOT, act to override this ischemic freeze on the DNA or protein synthesis areas in the cell. Once these cells begin to function, they demand greater blood supply and begin to sprout and touch other cells. Simultaneously, the repetitive exposure to hyperbaric oxygen can grow new blood supply into the damaged areas. This is what we saw in my animal research using laboratory rats, and it is what we see in wound healing using hyperbaric oxygen. Again, healing a wound in the brain is not so different from healing a diabetic foot wound.

The important point here is that HBOT effects on brain injury now begin to make sense. Low blood flow causes an ischemic freeze on the protein synthesis areas of the cell—part of which may be the DNA—that prevents the cell from performing its specialized function. HBOT acts on both the DNA and the cell's ability to make new protein in unknown ways. The new proteins include growth-type hormones and the receptors on the cells that respond to the hormones. The final result is new blood vessel and tissue growth and an improvement in the cell's ability to perform its special function. Essentially, this translates to an improvement or return of neurological function.

Current Thinking and Critical Points

Unfortunately, the medical community remains divided on the subject of hyperbaric oxygen and stroke. If you raise the subject with some, they will be quick to exclaim that there is no evidence supporting HBOT in acute or chronic stroke. If you find yourself asking the question, you may get a negative answer, even from a doctor who has not looked into the issue. You may be far more curious and have read more evidence about HBOT than the doctor you're consulting.

As a patient or a patient advocate—which is what you become when a loved one suffers a stroke—it's important to remember that you should not seek HBOT in order to replace another already established, proven treatment. This isn't an either-or situation. It's better expressed as "both-and," meaning that you would be adding HBOT to currently existing rehabilitation therapies. Again and again, whether it was young Chad, discussed in Chapter 4, or the joint replacement surgeries discussed in Chapter 10, we have seen HBOT enhance other therapies and speed healing.

The same is true for chronic stroke, where the person has been declared as rehabilitated as he or she is likely to be. Ideally, HBOT is best delivered while the patients are still receiving occupational, speech, and physical therapy. However, these therapies are often discontinued by the time I see these patients. In most cases, HBOT is delivered as the only therapy. Their doctors often tell these patients that HBOT is useless, but my response is always the same: how will you know if you don't try? What if your loved one regained some thought processes or motor skills, or his or her mood improved? Frankly, advances in medicine often are made because patients are willing to try new things. At this point, until HBOT is part of acute and chronic stroke treatment protocols, which may take decades or generations, the choice really is up to you.

A notable example of successful HBOT in chronic stroke is the story of a man I treated in 1992, and whose case I presented at a 1994 hyperbaric meeting. He was referred to me because of intractable dizziness, imbalance, and impaired use of his left leg years after multiple small strokes. He confided that if not for his grandchildren, he would like to die. He was now housebound, too proud to be seen with a cane or risk falling in public and needing help to get back up. However, over the course of three months he made a substantial improvement in his gait, strength, and reduction of dizziness to the point where he could walk without his brace or cane in public. These improvements began during his HBOT, and changed him into a new and happy man. (His brain scans are on page 3 of the photo insert.)

Fortunately, as I mentioned before, the international community is often far more open-minded about medical treatment than we are in the U.S., especially when it comes to using more inexpensive therapies. The U.S. healthcare industry is dominated by patent-protected drugs and devices that generate high incomes for doctors and the medical industry. In many less wealthy countries, healthcare dollars must be used more judiciously. As a result, relatively inexpensive therapies like HBOT are used more frequently.

For example, in January of 2013 Israeli doctors published a controlled study which also treated the control group with HBOT after their control wait period. They treated 74 patients 6–36 months after a stroke using 40 HBOTs. They were able to show neurological, cognitive, quality-of-life, and brain blood flow improvements in nearly all of the patients, while no improvement occurred in the control group[4]. This study duplicated the results that I, Dr. Neubauer, and countless other doctors found when applying HBOT to chronic stroke—and it did so with a rigorous study design that is hard to criticize. If you ever seek HBOT for chronic stroke (for yourself or a loved one), take a copy of this study to your doctor and hyperbaric physician.

What I've found over the years is that the larger the stroke and the later we intervene, the less function we are able to recover. But, we can still recover a degree of function in nearly every patient. The individuals who have done the best over the years and the ones that I strongly encourage to obtain HBOT are the patients with chronic small vessel strokes, which affect the white matter of the brain. Interestingly, this is the brain tissue that is most injured in brain decompression sickness, traumatic brain injury, and carbon monoxide poisoning, all diagnoses that respond to delayed HBOT with substantial success.

Dr. Neubauer has also documented HBOT's responsiveness to small vessel stroke, and in 2006, the same finding was shown in an additional small study. So, what I have seen among my patients is being duplicated by other physicians.

More recently, I have had confirmation of small vessel stroke responsiveness to HBOT in the treatment of CADASIL Syndrome. CADASIL, or Cerebral Autosomal Dominant Arteriopathy with Subcortical Infarcts and Leukoencephalopathy, is an inherited stroke disorder that affects the small blood vessels in the white matter of the brain—the connecting tracts. Remember, it is disease and injury to the connecting tracts of the brain that are amongst the medical conditions most responsive to HBOT: brain decompression illness, traumatic brain injury, carbon monoxide poisoning, CP, multiple sclerosis, and so forth.

The patient referred to me, Charmaine Neville, was a singer and member of the famous Neville family of musicians in New Orleans. She was known for doing high-kick stunts as part of her act. One of her good friends, Meg Farris of WWL-TV (CBS) New Orleans, a reporter who has covered HBOT in innumerable newscasts, was a friend of Charmaine's and asked me if I would treat Charmaine pro bono. This was in the fall of 2011, a few months before the 2012 New Orleans Jazz Fest, in which Charmaine would no longer be able to perform.

I agreed to treat Charmaine, but insisted that she stop smoking first. She gave up that lifelong habit, and a few months later I SPECT scanned her and began her treatment. With the blessing of CBS, Meg produced a documentary of the treatment which appeared on television (available on HBOT.com). The video shows the improvement in Charmaine's gait and balance, as well as great improvements in her cognitive function. Not only was she able to perform at Jazz Fest 2012, she went on to continue her singing career, and is still performing to this day.

Since that time, I have treated two additional CADASIL patients. The first patient was wheelchair bound, but began to show the same type of improvements as Charmaine. Unfortunately, her treatment was cut short by intervening medical problems that meant she had to return to her primary care doctors, located in another state. The second is currently under treatment and also showing improvement. What these cases have done is reinforce for me the effectiveness of HBOT in small vessel stroke, primarily in the white matter of the brain.

The Goal of Neurorehabilitation

In neurorehabilitation, the approach to treatment reflects the biology of repair. So, if many brain injuries result from low blood flow, swelling, low oxygen, inflammation, and the related factors that cause the ischemic freeze, then it is critically important to reverse the ischemic freeze. And, once the freeze has been reversed, the damaged neurons that have drawn back or lost many of their connections to other neurons must be stimulated to grow new connections and reestablish the diversity and richness of the brain that make us complex beings who can think and express our individual personalities.

In order to stimulate new connections, we expose stroke patients to a variety of stimulative therapies, including physical therapy, aquatherapy, and acupuncture. But stroke patients also undergo therapies designed to stimulate other areas of the brain, such as creative centers, through music and art therapy; speech and language therapies also stimulate memory and the ability to learn new material. Aromatherapy may trigger memories, but in addition, many odors have the ability to stimulate or relax us. So, we use these complementary therapies to achieve our mosaic of treatment. That image of the mosaic shows us what integrated care "looks like." And, in many cases, HBOT should be part of the total care plan. I believe this is particularly true for stroke patients.

In the last couple of years, we have made some progress with stroke and HBOT. In 2009, the HBOT Committee of the Undersea and Hyperbaric Medical Society put central retinal artery occlusion, a "stroke of the eye," on the "approved indications" list. While this is a rare condition that affects a small number of people in the population, it *is* a positive step in the right direction. The Israeli study mentioned above should provide further impetus to use HBOT more widely for stroke treatment in the U.S.

CHAPTER 7

AUTISM

YOU ARE NO DOUBT AWARE THAT WE'RE IN THE midst of what many call an "autism epidemic," although the exact cause of the rise in autism diagnoses in children has yet to be determined.

It also surprises many people that the condition itself, with its many forms and severities, was described only about 60 years ago. Many doctors, including chemists, academic obstetricians/geneticists, pediatricians, and others firmly believe the epidemic is primarily due to the heavy dose of vaccines delivered to very young infants. Specifically, those who link autism with vaccines believe the preservative thimerosol in the vaccines is the cause because of its high concentration of mercury.

In the early 1990s our neonatal vaccine schedule changed so that we now begin with a hepatitis vaccine given in the nursery. When my last son was born, I happened to be in the nursery when a nurse came in with a syringe. I asked what it was for and when I learned that my newborn son would be receiving a hepatitis vaccine I reacted immediately and stopped her from giving it. But, after a long discussion with the pediatrician, I reluctantly gave in and allowed the hospital to administer the vaccine. I was assured that it was safe and had no side effects—and all the professional pediatric associations approved it.

Looking back, I realize that I was grossly ignorant. To begin with, what was the rationale for this vaccine series in the first place? I've practiced emergency medicine for over 20 years, and in that time I've seen thousands of children, but I don't believe I have ever seen a child with hepatitis. So, what is the need for a hepatitis vaccine in a newborn whose chances of contracting hepatitis are about zero? His mother and I were not IV drug users, nor did we engage in unprotected high-risk sex. Yet, millions of infants whose parents also don't engage in high-risk behaviors are given a vaccine for a disease they, too, have almost no chance of contracting.

I now deeply regret that I allowed the hospital to give my son this vaccine; furthermore, I've begun to seriously question our intense vaccine schedule, which, as I understand it, starts vaccinations considerably earlier than current European practice. Despite multiple studies now claiming that vaccines have no involvement with autism, I am not convinced.

I have listened to too many mothers vividly describe dramatic changes in their children that began within hours to a few days of vaccine administration. Some began with high fevers, followed by loss of speech and other neurological functions, resulting in a later diagnosis of autism. The temporal relationship is undeniable. In any other situation in medicine in which clinical deterioration immediately followed some kind of medical intervention or other event, a cause and effect explanation would not be denied. That being said, the situation with autism is much more complex. Epidemics are usually caused by infectious outbreaks or environmental agents. And given the abundance of potential environmental factors that are present in modern life, it is likely that there are many causes for autism.

While my son is normal, I am painfully aware that many children are not. The autism experts claim that baby boys have a genetic predisposition to preferentially take up and retain the mercury in the vaccines, but I am not an expert on the causes and so have not formed a strong opinion. Epidemics, however, do not have genetic causes. I do have my doubts about the argument for mercury as the sole cause of the autism epidemic because I have seen a number of cases that seem to contradict this idea, especially the number of cases due to birth injuries.

While the controversy continues over the causes of the autism epidemic, one thing is unequivocally true: autism is a biological disease. Ample evidence from multiple scientific papers shows brain abnormalities (seen on MRI), genetic predispositions, a variety of biological risk factors, hormonal abnormalities, and other organic or biological components to, or associations with, this disease. It is clearly not a psychiatric disease, as many insurance companies classify it, thus limiting the payout for treatment.

My reason for introducing a discussion of autism in this way rests in the fact that I have treated more than 40 autistic children with HBOT. I treated my first case in 1996, and later learned that a physician in Florida had earlier treated his son with HBOT and reported success. The vast majority of these children have shown improvement in their autistic behaviors, and since 1996, others have now duplicated my experience and the initial experience of the doctor in Florida. At the AutismOne conference, held in Chicago in 2004, Dr. John Cassidy, a former cardiologist and colleague of mine who used to practice hyperbaric medicine in Los Angeles, and I presented 14 cases, many with SPECT brain imaging to provide illustration[1]. A number of these cases are presented on the IHMA website at www.hyperbaricmedicalassociation.org, under the Government Testimonies section.

Very recently, a number of physicians prominent in the treatment of autistic children and at one time critical of using HBOT for the disease have begun using hyperbaric oxygen with their patients. These physicians have now become ardent advocates of HBOT for autism, because they found that HBOT was one of the only biomedical treatments for autism. Their support for HBOT was largely driven by the experience of a family practitioner and his wife, herself a nurse practitioner, who conducted HBOT research based on their experiences with their autistic sons. This is a familiar theme in hyperbaric medicine: a doctor or family member tries HBOT for a loved one and the personal experience is so powerful it leads the person to open an HBOT center or to a change in career focus.

Such was the case for Dr. Dan Rossignol and his wife Lanier. After their sons showed encouraging improvement with HBOT they published a series of articles and studies on HBOT in autism. (You can find their material in the journals, *Medical Hypothesis* and *BioMed Central Pediatrics*). They reaffirmed my experience and other widespread reports. Unfortunately, conflicting reports have recently been published that have further increased the controversy of HBOT in autism.

My experience with HBOT in autism is important because a good number of my autistic patients had sustained obvious insults during birth. Coupled with the *Lancet* article about birth injury referred to in Chapter 5, this strongly argues that birth injury caused the autism in some of my patients. The SPECT imaging of these children showed that they seemed to have common injured areas of the brain, especially the temporal lobes, also supporting the idea that their autism was a neurological condition resulting from what happened to them during birth. Moreover, the SPECT imaging underscores that the actual pediatric neurological condition that results from some type of injury at birth is a function of the pattern or combination of regions of the brain that are injured.

These children responded to HBOT just like adults, kids with CP, trauma patients, and the patients with dozens of other neurological conditions that I investigated during the 1990s. So, at least in part, we were dealing with "generic" secondary brain damage, likely the result of the inflammatory reaction.

Successfully using HBOT for autism then leads to the question of effectively using HBOT for other types of developmental problems, including learning disorders. In so many children with these common learning disabilities, those testing the children cannot find a direct cause of the disorder. However, in my experience, when we take detailed histories from the mothers, we see problems at birth. (More alarming are the too frequent situations in which the actual birth records with the fetal monitor recordings and other critical information have been "lost" from the medical records and the parents assured that everything was "just fine.") This leads to further questions: Could there have been a low blood flow insult to the child's brain responsible for the subsequent learning disorder? Could early vaccine administration have complicated this? Was there surreptitious cocaine, methamphetamine, alcohol, or other substance abuse on the mother's part during pregnancy?

A poignant example of this occurred a few years ago. A mother brought her three-year-old daughter to me for treatment of a neurological condition of unknown cause, but it was obvious that the child had profound developmental delays. The day of her child's first visit, the mother decided to stop by the hospital to pick up a copy of her own medical records for a later appointment with a doctor. Once she received her file, she happened to ask if there were any other records related to her three-year-old. The records attendant returned with a very thin file that had newly appeared in the child's records.

The mother gave me this file to review, along with her other records. The new file contained records reporting that the child was born with a very low blood sugar level, which wasn't treated until 16 hours later. This could explain part of what was wrong with the child, but the injury was now three years old, and the HBOT would be treating the residual wounding to the brain regardless of cause. The mother asked me for direction: what should she do next? I recommended she take the records to the previous neurologists who were stumped by the baby's neurological condition and see if prolonged low blood sugar in a newborn baby changed their diagnosis.

In many cases of pediatric brain injury, it is very difficult to say what is behind the child's problems, but where these types of insults are involved it is not a stretch to assume that they could have caused organic damage to the brain. Given what we know about HBOT's effects on common secondary pathology, my experience with over 300 children, and the experience of other doctors, HBOT may prove to be effective for learning disorders and some of these other nebulous conditions of childhood. In very young children with brain injuries, it is a matter of jump-starting development at the initiation of HBOT. From the first treatment forward, the stunted and injured brain is now capable of beginning the developmental process at the injury site in the brain.

One of the First Cases of Autism and HBOT

An early patient I treated provides an example of the kind of improvements we can make with HBOT. I first saw Brian (not his real name) in 1996 when he was four years old. He showed spasticity (high muscle tone) on the right side of his body and also had repetitive autistic behaviors, including emotional detachment from his mother and siblings, a learning disability, speech problems, frequent staring spells with abnormal EEG's, and cognitive problems. He showed no socialization, meaning that he didn't relate to those around him. Brian's problems were likely permanent.

At birth, Brian weighed 12 pounds, 10 ounces, largely because his mother developed diabetes during her pregnancy. However, the diabetes wasn't treated, and she was two weeks past her due date before labor was induced. Her labor was 30 hours long and arduous, and Brian was born with a grossly misshapen head and had to be resuscitated. He had other signs of distress, as well, and was intubated in the nursery.

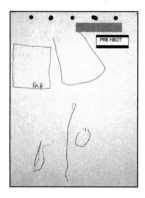

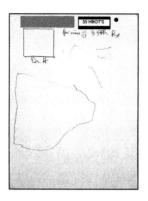

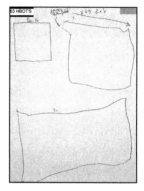

FIGURE 5A. Drawing of "square" by autistic boy before HBOT. Dr. Harch's example is labeled "Dr. H." First attempt by child is to the right of "Dr. H." Second, third, and fourth attempts are below from left to right.

FIGURE 5B. Drawing of "square" after 35 HBOTs. Child's first attempt is below "Dr. H" and second attempt are the lines to the right of "Dr. H."

FIGURE 5C. Drawing of "square" after 63 HBOTs. Child's first attempt is to the right and second below "Dr. H." The crinkled areas of the first attempt are where the paper moved as the child was copying the square.

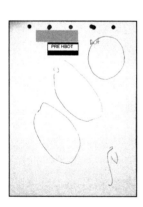

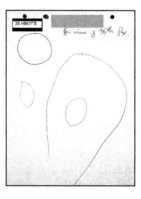

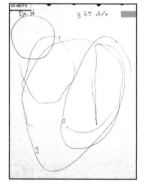

FIGURE 5D. Drawing of "circle" by autistic boy before HBOT. First, second, and third attempts by the child are in the middle, left lower, and right lower areas of the page, respectively.

FIGURE 5E. Drawing of "circle" after 35 HBOTs. Child's first and second attempts are the small circles below and to the right, respectively, of "Dr. H." Third attempt is the large circle.

FIGURE 5F. Drawing of "circle" after 63 HBOTs. First, second, and third attempts are marked. The second attempt was prematurely stopped by Dr. H to start a third attempt. The child wanted to keep drawing circles.

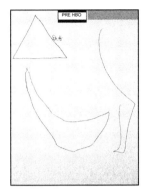

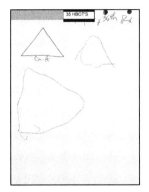

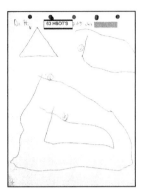

FIGURE 5G. Drawing of "triangle" by autistic boy before HBOT. First attempt by the child is below "Dr. H" and second is to the right: "Salvador Dali figure."

FIGURE 5H. Drawing of "triangle" after 35 HBOTs. Child's first attempt is below and second is to the right of "Dr. H."

FIGURE 5I. Drawing of "triangle" after 63 HBOs. First, second, and third attempts are marked. Note the third attempt placed proportionately within the first attempt.

Surprisingly, Brian went home with his mother, but his developmental problems were soon noted. He didn't crawl or grasp objects, he had tight muscles on one side of his body, he didn't make his motor milestones, and eventually had difficulty walking. Eventually, an MRI revealed a 1-cm (less than ½-inch) hemangioma, which is a small glob of blood vessels in the hemisphere of the brain. Brian's mother was told that the hemangioma explained all of his problems.

Brian's mother wasn't convinced by this explanation, and when I consulted with her, it didn't sit well with me either. I recommended that she get a second opinion from a neurologist at the nearby university medical center. There, Brian was diagnosed with a rare bone disorder called syndesmotic osteocranioencephalopathy, found in children with large hands, large feet, and a large head, all from rapid bone growth and maturation. I had to scratch my head again. All of the above abnormalities from rapid bone growth? It didn't make sense.

Eventually, Brian was examined at another university medical center. Based on their exam and physical examination, the doctor said that Brian's condition stemmed from problems occurring during labor and delivery and that the hemangioma was a red herring. This doctor diagnosed Brian with cerebral palsy and, later, autism spectrum disorder with a CARS (Childhood Autism Rating Scale) score of 29 (30 is the threshold for overt autism).

I believed I could help Brian, so he and his mother came to New Orleans for HBOT. As we treated Brian he progressively became more social, had a decrease in his spasticity, showed improvement in right body motor function, and his speech advanced. We saw decreases in his autistic behaviors, and his cognitive functions improved. Most of all, he developed and began to display emotion and attachment to his mother and siblings. The diagrams he created show—in crude terms—his progression from "Salvador Dali-esque" drawings to real triangles and squares. I've included pictures of diagrams that Brian drew before, during, and after his course of HBOT. (His brain scans appear on page 4 of the photo insert.)

When Brian went back to school, his teachers noted significant improvements in performance, and his mother was relieved to report that for the first time in his life, Brian actually played with his siblings. Of course, this added a positive element to the family dynamic. Some weeks later, Brian's mother called to tell me something he had said during a quiet moment: "Mom, it's so nice not living in the dark anymore."

This dumbfounded me, but based on his brain scans, his drawings, and his multitude of problems, Brian truly had lived in the dark—and HBOT turned on the light, permanently, within him.

The Children Tell Their Stories

Other autistic and brain-injured children have made comments similar to Brian's. One boy told me that his head was full of "alligators and chainsaws." Looking at his brain scan, his description made sense. Another four-year-old told me that when she was inside the chamber, she felt so much better inside her head. Again, when I looked at her brain scan after HBOT I could understand her statement.

In all of these instances, HBOT put their brains back in balance and these children could feel it—experience it—in the way they felt internally. And the pictures, of course, are worth a thousand words. These children aren't just cases, they are living human beings whose lives were severely compromised, and a relatively simple treatment made a difference that they could articulate.

Another poignant example of the benefit of HBOT in one of the autistic children I treated was captured in a short news piece, after the mother called into ABC television to report her daughter's improvement with HBOT. I hope viewers take note of the profound change in this little girl after just a few months of HBOT. The story of Chad Rovira, whom you read about in the TBI chapter, also appears in the video (available for viewing at HBOT.com).

The importance of my success in using HBOT for these autistic children is that it underscores that HBOT can be used as a "generic" drug for a wide range of neurological disorders. In reviewing the first 22 autistic children I have treated, I documented many different risk factors that could account for their autism. For some it was an in utero event occurring at some point during pregnancy, for others it was an insult at birth or during the neonatal or early development period, and in many it was a combination of insults at different times that resulted in the picture of autism.

Regardless of the cause, the great majority of the children improved after HBOT, and the differences in their SPECT brain imaging documented the changes. This reinforced my conviction that we were treating common secondary injury processes that are likely present in many types of neurological disorders. It also de-emphasized the importance of identifying causes and attributing liability, allowing the focus to remain on treatment. Simply put, regardless of the cause of the autism, the response to treatment was nearly uniform.

If we could combine HBOT with the various therapies available, it's likely the success rate would be much higher. For example, if a child has mercury poisoning that stunts neural tissue growth and even causes regression, then it makes sense that a combination or sequence of chelation therapy (a treatment designed to remove harmful substances from the body) plus HBOT would be effective. In other words, we would first remove the neurotoxin or possibly help speed its removal with chelation therapy, and then add HBOT for its effect on blood flow, metabolism, and tissue growth. Following chelation therapy and HBOT, we would use enrichment therapies, like cognitive stimulation or occupational/speech therapy, in order to stimulate new neural connections. So, once again, HBOT is not an either-or therapy. Rather, it is a foundation therapy which we combine with other enrichment therapies to recover the greatest brain function and maximize human potential.

CHAPTER 8

ALZHEIMER'S, PARKINSON'S, AND OTHER NEUROLOGICAL DISEASES

W E ARE FORTUNATE TO LIVE AT THIS PARTICULAR time, because we can avail ourselves of so many wonderful advances in modern medicine. As I recently heard an elderly woman comment, "My parents would never have imagined taking out an old, worn-out joint and putting in a new one, like replacing a worn-out roof on a house." Of course, our ability to replace joints is only one of the many benefits we have today. We also enjoy increased lifespan and advances in preventive care.

However, we must cope with the flip side of increased lifespan. In medicine, we see that as people live longer, the brain is often the limiting organ system in their overall level of function. In other words, for many people the brain seems to give out before the other organs in the body. When we consider how much "abuse" the brain is subject to throughout life, this is understandable.

To clarify, head trauma is certainly one kind of brain insult, but so are repeated exposures to cigarette smoke, various types of drugs (recreational, prescription, or non-prescription), chemicals, high fever, and carbon monoxide. Stroke is also a brain injury. Of course, we all can and do try to avoid certain traumatic injuries. That's what the campaigns to use seat belts and bike helmets are all about.

Many of us have had a bump on the head, and it is below the level that we can measure unless we have symptoms that indicate that the brain is injured, such as a loss of consciousness, dizziness, nausea, visual symptoms, memory loss, and so forth. Depending on the severity of the symptoms, we recovered in minutes to hours and probably never saw a doctor. We just went on our way once the swelling was gone. On a continuum of brain injury, we call this type of event "mild" traumatic brain injury. Similarly, many of us have experienced certain chemical exposures, including carbon monoxide or varying degrees of air pollution that occur most everywhere in the world. Few of us live for even a day without some form of chemical exposure.

The brain is considered by many doctors to be the most delicate—and complex—organ in the body. As with all complex machines, seemingly minor disturbances or disruptions can cause significant dysfunction. These insults can be put on a continuum and range from minor, almost unnoticeable, to very significant, with obvious damage. They occur over a lifetime, and they have a cumulative effect on brain function. In addition, some of the injuries may have an immediate impact, but also a delayed effect that may take years to become apparent. The net result is symptomatic neurological disease that we see manifested because so many individuals among our older population are living longer. (I discuss this in greater detail in Chapter 12.)

Reserve Capacity

Every organ system in the body has redundancy or reserve capacity. We are born with two kidneys but we can live with one. But, if you have one kidney and then sustain a significant injury that causes muscle cells to rupture and release muscle proteins into the blood stream, this could overwhelm the capacity of your kidney and cause loss of kidney function. Similarly, we are born with two lungs and can live just fine with one, but not at 11,000 feet of altitude. In fact, this is why respiratory ailments and cardiac disease are not common at high altitudes. People with respiratory and heart diseases cannot live at decreased ambient levels of oxygen and survive. However, we have redundancy in our cardiovascular system, and if you suffer a heart attack you could lose a significant amount of the heart muscle and still survive—you may even be asymptomatic and not be aware that your heart was damaged. But, like individuals with one lung, you won't be able to function well at higher altitude and it isn't likely that you could jog even a mile or two. And, of course, you certainly won't be able to run a marathon.

We could go through this exercise for every organ system in the body to understand redundancy and reserve capacity. We even have special cases, such as the liver. With that organ, we can remove a large portion of it, and it may partially regenerate.

The Brain's Reserves

The brain also has redundancy and reserve capacity, but with each insult, a certain amount of its reserve capacity is lost. This has been proven in animals where a surgically inflicted injury causes an adaptive response in the brain. The response is such that the animal's brain tries to maintain the overall surface area of every synapse.

Individual brain cells send out a single process called an axon, along which the electrical impulse travels. As babies, this axon makes contact with just a few other cells. As we develop, our brain capacity increases and is enriched, and an axon branches hundreds of times and will make contact with up to a thousand other cells. These are the connections that are lost in brain injury and that we try to re-establish with multi-modality therapies such as HBOT, physical and occupational therapies, speech therapy, biofeedback, aquatherapy, and so forth. A synapse forms on the place where an axon touches the other cells.

An electrical impulse that travels along an axon is converted by chemicals at the synapse to electrical energy that then is transmitted to the next cell. Each synapse has a certain amount of surface area. You can think of it like the pad of your finger. When an animal is injured and the axons are disrupted, the remaining axons adapt by increasing the size of that finger pad. This means that the overall surface area is now the same as before, except that there aren't as many finger pads. The other individual finger pads have enlarged to fill the space, so to speak.

The adaptation that maintains the overall surface area decreases the complexity of the brain because it has reduced the number of contacts—synapses. If the animal continues to injure the brain, then it eventually reaches a point at which the size of those finger pads or synapses has "maxed out," and the brain can no longer adapt. The animal will lose neurological function at that point.

The loss of reserve capacity is caused by many things, including stress and fatigue. Patients with any type of brain injury, whether it's stroke, trauma, or toxic exposure, are mentally and physically fatigued by the end of the day—more so than those without a brain injury. These patients also show lost capacity during situations in which sensory exposure is intense. I spoke about this in the chapter on traumatic brain injuries (see Chapter 4), in which I recounted the study done by Dr. Ewing on previous TBI patients. Remember that Dr. Ewing showed that TBI subjects had less reserve capacity than normal patients and this loss of reserve capacity (decreased cognitive function) could be measured when the TBI patients were exposed to low oxygen levels of altitude.

For example, in neurologically injured individuals, symptoms might appear if they are around small children who are active and running around in their normal frenetic state. This is why busy malls, airports, holiday crowds, and so forth may be extraordinarily stressful for brain-injured people. There just aren't enough synapses to handle all the simultaneous sights, sounds, touches, and other sensory input. The brain is overloaded. Understanding this also helps explain why your elderly parent or grandparent can't cope very well with a house filled with children and adults playing loud music and talking. When they tell you "it's all too much," they mean it!

A Lifetime of Exposure

We essentially go through life accumulating small injuries or exposures. It's easy to see how in one active lifetime we might be exposed to carbon monoxide, lose consciousness from a fall, inhale toxins while refinishing furniture and then again at the beauty shop, perhaps suffer a small stroke later in life, and so on. Some chemical exposures, such as those in oil refineries or mines, are occupational hazards. Those who work in or live around chemical factories may be constantly exposed. And with each exposure or injury, we lose a little bit of reserve capacity.

The magnitude of the insult matters, of course, so an early accumulation may mean experiencing neurological symptoms earlier in life. This is the nature of dementia.

A Very Public Example

I often think of what happened to Ronald Reagan. As you know, when elected president, he was an extremely fit man in his 70s, but he suffered a gunshot wound to the chest during an assassination attempt. He experienced low blood pressure before he was resuscitated, then low blood counts, surgery, anesthesia, and infection before he was discharged from the hospital. Once he resumed his public life, many noticed that he was not as sharp as he was before the gunshot incident. In fact, a biographer has noted this in a book written about President Reagan.

A few years later, he sustained a brain injury when he was thrown from a horse.

Six months afterward he underwent surgery to remove a blood clot between the skull and the brain. Within a few years after this surgery he was declared to have Alzheimer's disease. This will sound odd to many, and may even anger a few, but to me, that diagnosis never made any sense. Alzheimer's is pre-senile dementia, meaning that the symptoms of dementia occur before the expected time in old age. Reagan was 83 and had sustained two known brain insults. He had low blood flow, low blood counts for a while, general anesthesia (we now know from recent studies that surgery alone in elderly patients results in loss of cognitive function), low oxygen levels, infection, a diffuse traumatic brain injury, and bleeding between the skull and brain which causes dysfunction of the underlying brain. The low blood flow and low oxygen insults are important because they affect the areas of the brain where the three arteries on each side meet called the "watershed" areas. They have the lowest flow to begin with, and they are areas where Alzheimer's disease often manifests.

What appears to have happened is that through these multiple insults President Reagan lost the remaining amount of his reserve capacity. In other words, the acute injuries left his brain without "hidden reserves" and rendered him demented. In his case, his brain no longer had the vitality that the remainder of his body possessed, a fact remarked upon by everyone who witnessed his physical strength and otherwise good health.

I mean no disrespect to the family by discussing these injuries and the diagnosis of Alzheimer's disease. I simply believe we are better off looking at the underlying causes of dementia rather than applying a label because it offers what looks like an understandable explanation. If we assume this man would have lived to be 100, then he had pre-senile dementia or Alzheimer's disease. But, this tells us nothing other than that he died of an unfortunate disease for which we have no cause, that robs people of their retirement years, and for which we have no cure. I think we're served better by understanding that his dementia was the result of a global decrease in blood flow and other insults followed by traumatic injury to an elderly brain.

Other examples exist of significant brain insults that later manifest themselves as premature dementia due to loss of reserve capacity. As the World War II generation of veterans aged, physicians noted that those who suffered significant blood loss on the battlefield or had moderate to severe head injuries[1] were more at risk for Alzheimer's disease later in life. What happened? In medical terms, hemorrhagic shock from blood loss lowered the blood pressure and affected the watershed areas in the brain, which are very sensitive to systemic reduction in blood pressure. Head injury similarly compromised the reserve capacity of the brain but by a different mechanism.

Because these soldiers were fit young men, the brain injury they suffered (from blood loss) may not have been immediately apparent. However, the injury was sufficient enough to compromise their reserve capacity. In effect, it advanced their aging process 20 years or so. As a result, they developed dementia earlier in life than expected, and hence, received a diagnosis of Alzheimer's disease.

The problem with the diagnosis is that it can obscure the cause and mislead people into thinking that Alzheimer's is just something that happens to people out of the blue. This has frightening implications for family members who then worry themselves sick over the thought that one day they will slowly lapse into Alzheimer's disease.

This situation occurred with a patient I saw a few years ago, a woman in her late forties who was fully demented. I saw her through her family, because her neurologist at the medical school in their home town referred them to me. This patient intrigued me because full dementia at age 48 is exceedingly rare. What's more, her doctors had no cause for this. The family had no history of dementia. At first, she was diagnosed with Alzheimer's, and then given other types of dementia diagnoses, but none really fit. I knew, however, that there just had to be some organic insult that occurred at some point earlier in life that accounted for her dementia later on.

I spent a considerable amount of time on the phone with her daughter and kept asking when she first noticed that her mother's cognitive abilities began to slip. The daughter kept going back in time, to earlier and earlier dates in her mother's life and continued to mention all sorts of bizarre behaviors. What actually prompted me to start this line of questioning was the fact that this woman had been married nine times. This patient's daughter eventually described a plethora of behavioral difficulties first noticed by age five, the time when children begin to develop their personalities.

I then asked if anything happened in her mother's infancy and she recalled hearing about an episode that occurred when her mother was six months old. It seems that as a baby, my patient, now in her forties, was taken to a drive-in

Figure 1. Here is an example of a "normal" scan for a 26-year-old woman. On the right-hand side of the figure, you see SPECT scan slices. The slices are the "transverse" orientation where the computer slices from the top to the base of the brain, with the patient's right side on the left side of the image and the front of the face at the top of the slice. The slices proceed from the top of the brain in the top left corner of the slices to the base of the brain in the bottom right corner.

In a "normal" brain, the slices are smooth with very little alternation of colors. In other words, you see the same color (yellow-orange) for most of the scan with very little alternation to purple or blue in the outer ribbon of the brain (the cortex). The color map proceeds from highest brain blood flow to lowest in the following order: yellow, orange, purple, blue, and black.

The computer takes the outermost perimeter of each slice and reconstructs it into the three-dimensional color image you see on the left-hand side of the figure. The

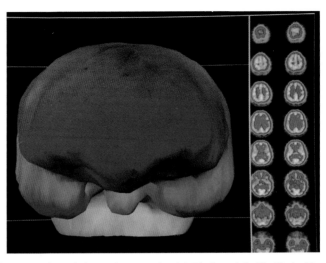

colors are purely artistic. The image is the "face" look of the patient's brain where the patient is looking directly at you. The large broad area in the front is the area of both frontal lobes and is situated directly behind the forehead. The two protuberances on the lower right and left are the temporal lobes. The surface should appear smooth and all of the lobes should be well-formed.

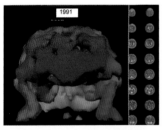

Figure 2A. Here is the 3-D SPECT scan of Dan Greathouse, the 34-year-old male diver with brain decompression illness four months after his diving accident and three months after three ineffective HBOTs (as discussed on page 49). Note the multiple holes on the 3-D and the spotty irregular color pattern on the slices. The vertical "posts" on the 3-D at the front and base of each side of the brain are artifacts due to blood flow in the great vessels of the neck and are not part of the brain.

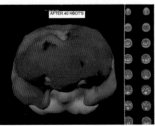

Figure 2B. 3-D SPECT scan after the 43rd HBOT (40th HBOT in the new series of delayed HBOTs). You can see that some of the holes on the 3-D scan have been filled in.

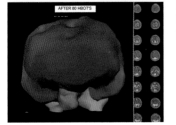

Figure 2C. 3-D SPECT scan after the 83rd HBOT (80th HBOT in the new series of delayed HBOTs). Note the smoothness of the 3-D scan, indicating improvement.

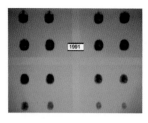

Figure 3A. Here are transverse images of Chad's first SPECT scan two days after severe traumatic brain injury (as described on page 81). The images are somewhat fuzzy due to multiple reproductions, but they were obtained on a low resolution scanner and were read as "normal" by the radiologist. Note the apparent lack of any defects despite the fact that Chad is comatose on a ventilator. The four images in the lower right hand corner have a hint that something is wrong, but they are not definitive. Compare this to the next scan, Figure 3B, which was taken one month later. The higher resolution scanner shows the significant injury to the brain, especially on the left front.

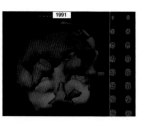

Figure 3B. 3-D surface reconstruction of Chad's SPECT scan on high resolution scanner at West Jefferson Medical Center one month after severe traumatic brain injury. At this point, Chad had had HBOT once or twice a day since the day of his injury and is off the ventilator and doing much better clinically. Despite this, note the marked reductions in flow to the entire left side of the brain (the viewer's right side). This reduction in flow is seen on each image in rows 4, 5, and 7 on the right side of each image. The scan is tipped up slightly to give a better view of the underside of the brain. This same view is present on the subsequent two scans.

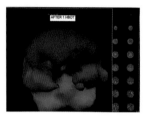

Figure 3C. 3-D surface reconstruction of Chad's SPECT scan on the same high resolution scanner 9 days and 5 HBOTs after the scan in Figure 3B. Note the improvement in blood flow to the entire left side of the brain. This was my proof that HBOT could further improve Chad and his brain injury.

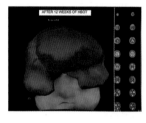

Figure 3D. 3-D surface reconstruction of Chad's SPECT scan 11 weeks and 108 HBOTs after his brain injury. He is now walking and talking. Note the further improvement in brain blood flow consistent with his improved clinical condition. However, he has now developed contre-coup defects (injury opposite the original area of impact; this is a well-known phenomenon in brain injury). These defects are apparent on the viewer's left side of each image on rows 6, 7, and 8.

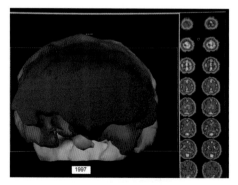

Figure 4A. Here's the 3-D SPECT scan before HBOT and 2 years after exposure to nitrogen tetroxide in the middle-aged first responder referred to on page 92. Notice the irregularity (alternating colors of the cortex) of the scan slices on the right. Similarly, the 3-D shows multiple areas of significantly decreased blood flow (holes) throughout the brain.

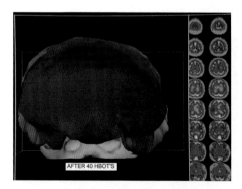

Figure 4B. 3-D SPECT scan performed after 40 HBOTs and three months after Figure 4A. Notice the smoother appearance of the slices on the right and the 3-D image.

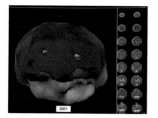 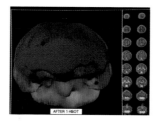 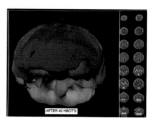

Figure 5A. Here is the 3-D SPECT scan of Dr. William Duncan's brother before HBOT and 44 years after traumatic brain injury (see page 94). Note the irregularity and presence of holes.

Figure 5B. 3-D SPECT scan after one HBOT.

Figure 5C. 3-D SPECT scan after 40 HBOTs.

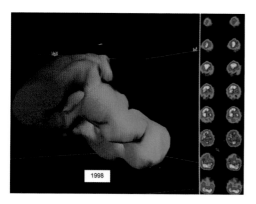 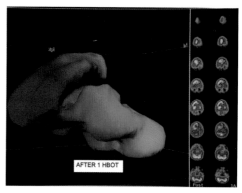

Figure 6A. 3-D left frontal view of SPECT scan before HBOT of a four-year-old boy with severe birth injury (described on page 109). Notice the irregularity of the slices to the right and the absence of blood flow to the entire back half of the brain on the 3-D.

Figure 6B. 3-D left frontal view of SPECT scan after one HBOT. Notice the smoother appearance of the slices and generally increased size of the areas of blood flow on the 3-D.

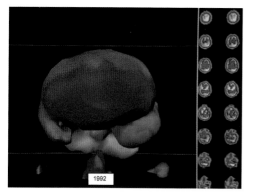 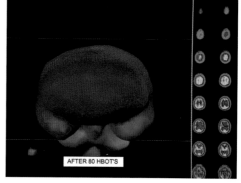

Figure 7A. 3-D of elderly man before HBOT and over two years after multiple small strokes (as described on page 127). Note the irregularity of the slices, coarseness of the 3-D, and marked decrease in the size of the right temporal lobe.

Figure 7B. 3-D after 80 HBOTs. Note the smoother appearance of the slices, surface of the 3-D, and symmetry of the temporal lobes.

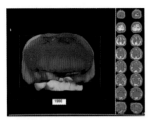

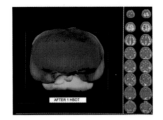

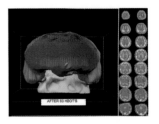

Figure 8A. 3-D of Brian, the five-year-old autistic boy (described on page 138) before HBOT. Note the irregularity of the slices as well as holes in the frontal, temporal, and cerebellar lobes. The cerebellar lobes are the blue band at the bottom of the 3-D.

Figure 8B. 3-D after one HBOT. Note the generalized improvement of the slices and 3-D.

Figure 8C. 3-D after 63 HBOTs. Note the smoother appearance of the slices and generalized improvement of the 3-D compared to Figure 8A.

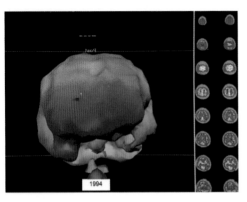

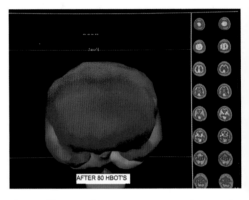

Figure 9A. 3-D of the middle-aged man with multiple sclerosis (described on page 152) before HBOT. Note the irregularity of the slices and the multiple holes on 3-D, especially on the left side of the brain and left temporal lobe.

Figure 9B. 3-D after 80 HBOTs. Note the smoother appearance of the slices and overall improvement of the 3-D.

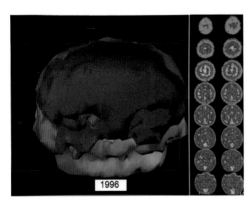

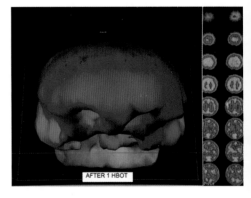

Figure 10A. 3-D SPECT scan before HBOT of Jason, the 19-year-old drug abuser (described on page 193). You can see multiple holes on the 3-D and diffuse patchy blood flow on the slices.

Figure 10B. 3-D SPECT scan after one HBOT. Note generalized improvement.

movie with her parents. Since it was cold, the family kept the engine and heater running during the movie, but at one point, my patient's mother opened the car door, which turned on the dome light, which is when she noticed that the baby was blue and barely breathing. After rushing her to the hospital, she was diagnosed with severe carbon monoxide poisoning. She was kept in an oxygen tent for a number of days before her parents took her home. A few years later they noticed some unusual behavior, which developed into a lifelong problem.

So, what is the diagnosis here? It is dementia for sure. The picture on her SPECT brain imaging, however, was not Alzheimer's, but a diffuse abnormality that the radiologist said was consistent with a "toxic exposure." So, as a child, my patient suffered a severe carbon monoxide episode at a critical time in development that erased much of her reserve capacity by killing a fair number of brain cells and white matter connecting tracts. Essentially, she aged 30 years with this poisoning, and started her life at 6 months of age with the brain of a 30 year old. Then, 45–48 years later she ran out of brain gas at the typical time in cumulative years (78) that most of us begin to lose cognitive ability.

I treated this patient with HBOT, but it didn't have a dramatic impact. The family saw initial improvement that was encouraging and her referring physician thought she was less agitated and generally clinically improved. My physical exam, testing, and SPECT brain imaging also showed improvement. I believe she needed and would have benefited from more HBOT, but for family reasons we couldn't continue. We can sum up the greatest benefit of her evaluation, however, in two words: anxiety relief. Once I could explain their mother's dementia and the importance of the carbon monoxide poisoning at that critical point in development, they literally broke down in relief. It is only natural that both these young people worried that "mom's condition" would one day strike them in their prime and reduce them to dementia. They had even started planning for their caretaking later in life.

In the nature of neurological diagnosis, we see that if enough symptoms match a given description of an illness, a patient is "branded" with a diagnosis of Alzheimer's disease. The other problem with Alzheimer's is that it has become almost a "diagnosis du jour," or a popular diagnosis of the times. More and more of our elderly population receive Alzheimer's diagnoses because they fit part of the symptom complex. However, I don't think this is accurate; in all likelihood, what we're actually seeing with our aging population is the loss of the reserve capacity in the brain, which is occurring before the loss of reserve capacity in other organs.

I tried to address this question at a "drug company dinner." These are a common and "favored" venue in medicine where, in essence, a pharmaceutical company invites doctors to come to a presentation put on by one of their paid speakers for the purposes of introducing doctors to a new drug.

This particular dinner was held in a wonderful restaurant in the historic French Quarter of New Orleans. The topic was a new Alzheimer's drug. At the start of the lecture, I asked the speaker to address the current situation in which the diagnosis of Alzheimer's had morphed/expanded to diagnose a larger segment of the elderly population than was traditionally described. I was curtly told that I was behind the times, that I was uninformed, and that the issue itself was irrelevant. The only topic of any importance being discussed that night was to be the new drug for Alzheimer's disease. I disagreed, and still disagree; no new insights or information have changed my mind. Rather than trying to broadly lump all people together under the heading of syndromes, where we try to apply a "one treatment fits all" approach, we are better served by trying to understand each individual patient's neurological condition, the areas of the brain that are injured and responsible for the condition, and then treating accordingly. In the end, one treatment may suit just a few.

Before we end this discussion on Alzheimer's and dementia, I'll say that I have successfully treated six of the eight Alzheimer's patients referred to me; in this context, success means that while none were cured, HBOT helped bring about improvements and subsequently slowed their disease progression[2]. The brain scans of the first patient were presented in one of my appearances before the U.S. Congress (available on HBOT.com).

My current Alzheimer's patient is a former college football player with innumerable concussions. I expect he is going to receive long-term treatment and I am following his results carefully in order to provide updates on the usefulness of HBOT for patients with a diagnosis of Alzheimer's disease.

Many Neurological Manifestations

Some people manifest loss of brain reserve capacity in terms of dementia, others through Parkinson's disease, while others show different neurological syndromes.

In addition, as our vascular system ages, the chance of developing clots in our arteries increases, too. These clots cause strokes.

As a quick aside, Parkinson's is puzzling in that it is more of a syndrome than a disease. It has no known cause, but many suspected causes. It is primarily the result of a loss of dopamine in the centers of the brain that control movement. There can be several possible reasons for this dopamine loss. It can be caused by loss of the cells that release the dopamine in the movement centers (these cells originate in the brainstem); by loss of cells in the areas that control movement, the deep gray matter of the brain (basal ganglia); or by loss of the white matter connective tract between these areas and other areas of the brain. The syndrome is more complex than that, however, because these areas of the brain are served by multiple other chemical systems. Injuries to different parts of this center, an area of convergence and transmission of information from higher and lower centers in the brain (think of it like the Grand Central Station of the brain), accounts for the different combinations of symptoms and signs in Parkinson's. This area is supplied by short, straight arteries that are very susceptible to drops in systemic blood pressure. The deep gray matter is also the area of the brain often injured in severe carbon monoxide poisoning. (See HBOT.com for more information on the effects of carbon monoxide poisoning on key areas of the brain.)

I mention this detail because many different of kinds of insults to the basal ganglia can cause injury and result in Parkinson's disease. It is encouraging that Italian and Russian researchers have reported some success with treating Parkinson's patients with HBOT. My results have been mixed, likely due to the heterogeneity of this syndrome. We've also seen reports of the successful use of low-dose naltrexone (LDN) in Parkinson's disease (these reports have been made available on HBOT.com). One of my patients has combined low-dose naltrexone and HBOT with very positive results, providing yet another example of the "both-and" approach to HBOT vs. the false "either-or" choice we still see in much of medicine.

The Lifespan Dilemma

An increase in lifespan simply means that we have an increased time to accumulate neurological insults. In addition, we survive certain kinds of injuries—anywhere in the body—more often than we once did. For example, our life-saving interventions, used in emergency settings and even on the battlefield today, have meant we don't lose as many people with head injuries today as in the past. We also save more people who have heart attacks and strokes than we once did. Yet, these injuries add to the cumulative effect on our reserve capacity. Those injuries insult the brain, so while we save more individuals, we compromise the brain, and thus we see the signs of aging sooner.

Statistically speaking, as we entered 2006, the first of the Baby Boomer generation turned 60, and as time marches on we will see a significant increase in the number of people with neurological problems. You may have already noticed this in your own family.

In addition, due to the vast increase in chemical exposure that took place in the industrial world since the end of World War II, the so-called "boomers" have another problem. To this we can add the dramatic explosion in recreational drug use in the Baby Boomer generation. This also has likely taken a toll on reserve capacity of the brains of many who were involved in this kind of "experimentation." Friends of mine, including a few doctors, have approached me about developing neurological symptoms. What they really want to know is if past drug use could be the cause. And while I can't provide a specific answer in their cases, it is true that rampant drug use may have caused damage that manifests later in life.

The post-war generation shows great interest in myriad alternative health therapies, and many are willing to try therapies that may restore lost brain function and protect what is left. HBOT may offer the hope they look for.

HBOT for Neurological Disease

For the most part, we treat neurological diseases with one or more of a variety of drugs developed in the last decade or so. Until these drugs arrived on the scene, we had no treatment for most neurological disorders. Unfortunately, most of these medications treat only symptoms and the patients who take them are not permanently changed. In fact, what these individuals face is at best a lifetime of partial symptom relief.

What distinguishes HBOT is that hyperbaric oxygen is the only repair drug for neurological conditions. It stimulates DNA to produce growth and repair hormones and the protein receptors on cells that respond to these hormones. As you've seen from the discussion in other chapters, repetitive exposure to hyperbaric oxygen causes new blood vessels to grow, and it can metabolically energize the cells. As a result, we get permanent changes in brain function as new blood supply grows, and the healing effects of oxygen revive the damaged cells that have been living in these areas of low blood flow (the ischemic penumbra).

In the future, I hope we will end the sole reliance on "magic bullet pills" to reverse lifelong neurological injury, or even recently acquired brain injury. When you think about it, the whole premise of a single daily pill to reverse all of the metabolic and anatomic changes caused by lifelong insults or problems is ludicrous. This is especially true when you view all of the known chemical reactions in our body. Thirty years ago, these reactions fit on a single wall poster. They now would blanket many walls. The current approach is to target a single chemical reaction with a particular drug and then expect miraculous outcomes. This is fantasy thinking; but it *is* what we have been led to believe, have become accustomed to, and now demand from the medical profession. Ideally, we need a change in mentality to change lifestyle, eliminate toxic substances, improve our diet, and combine therapies to thereby maximize our outcomes. Because of its biological properties, HBOT is perfectly suited to be synergistic with a variety of drugs and treatments both known and yet to be developed.

What about Multiple Sclerosis?

A discussion of hyperbaric oxygen therapy in chronic brain injury would not be complete without mentioning multiple sclerosis (MS). In the past, when I've been asked to analyze hyperbaric oxygen in chronic brain injury, I avoided the topic of multiple sclerosis altogether. I made that decision because the whole MS–hyperbaric phenomenon had become so incredibly politicized that it seemed impossible for clinicians and researchers to look objectively at the effects of HBOT in MS.

Many theories exist about what causes MS, but ultimately it remains a disease with an unknown cause. We know a few things about the progression of the disease, however. As it progresses, there continue to be insults to the nervous system, primarily in the white matter, which is composed of the cable-like connecting tracts in the brain. Small blood vessels supply these tracts. For reasons we don't know, the blood vessels in this white matter become leaky due to damage to the blood–brain barrier, that functional tissue barrier between blood vessels and brain tissue. The vessels leak fluid that causes small dots or points that decrease oxygen supply to the white matter. These leaks and their damage are almost like mini-strokes.

Hyperbaric oxygen therapy can have a significant effect when given at the time of these insults. In addition, the location of these lesions is very similar to brain decompression sickness. Brain decompression sickness is primarily a white matter disease in the brain. In addition, the size of the lesions in decompression sickness is similar to MS lesions. Over time, these lesions accumulate in the brains of MS patients and the subsequent scarring that takes place forms the well-known plaques in the patient's brain. We can see these plaques on MRI scans.

These plaques are areas of confluent scars that span large tracts of white matter. Essentially, they short-circuit the white matter electrical transmission, and that malfunction results in the neurological symptoms that MS patients show.

When I started the Perfusion Metabolism Encephalopathy study, one of the first patients I evaluated was an MS patient. I had wanted to avoid treating MS, but I wasn't about to deny anyone the possibility of treatment, regardless of diagnosis. I agreed to treat this patient, and you can see that his brain shows noticeable improvement in brain blood flow after one hyperbaric treatment and even more so after a series of 80. (See the scans on page 4 of the photo insert.)

This man showed improved bladder control and his mental abilities sharpened; in particular, he was able to think and process more quickly. His motor function also improved. However, this man's ultimate goal was to get back on the ski slopes, and HBOT didn't get him that far. Nevertheless, I found the improvements he did show quite remarkable, and the scans verified the changes in brain blood flow.

One of the reasons that such a firestorm erupted over HBOT for MS involves our previous inability to "capture" clinical improvements through sophisticated scanning methods. For example, MRI and CT scans had not been able to image the changes that Dr. Neubauer saw in his patients in the 1970s, and in 1978, when he reported his observations in the *Journal of the Florida Medical Association*; the low resolution SPECT scanners were inadequate as well[3, 4]. However, I saw positive results from HBOT in our first patient in 1994.

Unfortunately, treating MS with HBOT has polarized the neurological community in the United States. And beyond that, Dr. Neubauer recommended treating MS at pressures lower than had been established by the U.S. Navy for any use. He was also doing it at a fraction of the price charged in hospital-based facilities. Dr. Neubauer's approach and actions incensed a small group of physicians trained only in limited use of hyperbaric medicine for decompression sickness and wounds.

Contentious or not, Dr. Neubauer's work was the first use of HBOT in the United States, especially low pressure HBOT for chronic neurological conditions, and the controversy that followed soon spawned a grant by the Multiple Sclerosis Society. The society chose an investigator at New York University, Dr. B. H. Fischer, to conduct a hyperbaric oxygen therapy trial with multiple sclerosis patients. Dr. Fischer went on to perform one of the most rigorous trials of hyperbaric oxygen therapy in MS to date. The results published in the *New England Journal of Medicine* in 1983 showed a beneficial effect of hyperbaric oxygen in MS[5].

Unfortunately, the situation turned politically ugly. Know that infighting in the medical community rivals anything we see in the halls of Congress! Dr. Fischer's study was wrongfully disparaged, the controversy continued, and multiple studies were subsequently done. However, one of the most critical pieces of information emerged from all the brouhaha.

By 1989, Dr. Sheldon Gottlieb had written a review of all of the MS-hyperbaric literature and found that those studies that used the lower hyperbaric pressures generally had positive results, whereas those at the typical higher hyperbaric pressures were negative. This information leads us, again, to the "less is more" principle, and we have another confirmation that we can apply this therapy in more than one way!

This experience in MS led to the work of a doctor in Scotland, Dr. Philip James, who to this date has treated and followed up with the most MS-HBOT patients. Because the U. K. medical system refused to treat MS with hyperbaric oxygen, a not-for-profit trust was organized. This sounds like a true revolution to many of us—this trust established over 60 hyperbaric centers in the United Kingdom! What is truly astounding is that MS patients run the facilities for the purpose of providing treatment to themselves and others. In England at that time, only certified physicians could prescribe 100 percent oxygen, so the centers get around that by using 95 percent oxygen instead. A recent change in the law now allows the use of 100 percent oxygen without a medical license.

This network in the United Kingdom was under the guidance of Dr. Philip James in Dundee, Scotland. He is now retired and has written a book, *Oxygen and the Brain, the Journey of our Lifetime*, a fascinating and incredibly insightful book that resulted from a lifelong devotion to the therapeutic use of oxygen. It may be difficult for those of us in the United States to believe, but over the years many thousands of MS patients have received successful HBOT. They accomplish this by allowing patients to seek their own dose, and this feature makes this one of the most individualized programs existing in medicine.

A few years ago, I came across Dr. James' and Dr. D. J. Perrin's papers which they described the protocol. I was surprised to see that it was nearly identical to the protocol I had independently discovered during our Perfusion Metabolism Encephalopathy study. What the protocol consisted of was a block of baseline hyperbaric treatments and then the patients were allowed to seek their own maintenance level. When we look at this evidence, it's clear that first, we're on to something important, and second, we should never let political forces deny patients a treatment that has shown such positive results.

The problem with doing research with hyperbaric oxygen on MS patients is that the disease is highly individual, sporadic, and unpredictable in any given patient. It is also a disease that patients may live with and adjust to over decades. Of course, research aside, this is why the individualized HBOT program in the U. K. makes sense. It pairs a set of facts with a customized solution, rather than relying on a universal protocol. Unfortunately, in medicine as in clothes, "one size fits all" sometimes means "one size fits no one."

The information gathered about HBOT and MS indicates that patients need treatment over a long period of time. Short-term studies often are unable to define a difference between the populations using hyperbaric oxygen vs. standard treatment. Part of the reason for this is that we use HBOT in an attempt to grow new white matter tracts and this takes time, longer than the duration of many of the studies. In addition, the dose of hyperbaric oxygen therapy has to be correct in short-term studies.

The final research issue involves the status of patients entering a study. If patients with advanced disease enter the study, the impact of hyperbaric oxygen is small because so much tissue has been damaged, scarred, and lost. So, in order to see a statistically significant change from their baseline level of function, we need large numbers of moderately affected patients treated over long periods of time. This is incredibly expensive and time-consuming.

As mentioned above, some medical researchers believe that MS results from damage to the blood–brain barrier. The most prominent proponent of these is the previously mentioned Dr. Philip James. In acute neurological insults, we have shown that hyperbaric oxygen therapy protects and repairs the blood–brain barrier. This may be how hyperbaric oxygen restores function and/or ameliorates acute episodes of MS.

A nurse and friend of mine, who happened to have been a vice president of the regional chapter of a hyperbaric medical society, developed MS, and in her search for therapy she came across hyperbaric oxygen. Using repetitive HBOT, her symptoms completely disappeared for long periods of time. When she had recurrent episodes, she had more treatment and thus functioned at very high levels for many years. In fact, her experience led to her administrative/leadership in hyperbaric oxygen therapy.

My own personal experience over the past 26 years has been accentuated by one of our patients, who came to us with a diagnosis of chronic progressive multiple sclerosis. This diagnosis generally means a fairly rapid progression of MS, often leading to death in less than 10 years. However, this patient underwent HBOT at our center for the better part of 25 years, and over that time his neurological status has changed very little. When he was first treated, he used a walker and had a markedly impaired gait. Over the years, when he has had acute exacerbations, I increased his hyperbaric oxygen therapy from once a week to daily for a couple of weeks at a time, which moved him past his acute episodes. (You can find out more about his story at HBOT.com).

A few years ago I had the opportunity to speak to this man's university-based neurologist, who had been following him for nearly three years. I wanted to confirm this man's exact diagnosis for his testimonial, which I intended to put on my website. The neurologist confirmed that he had chronic, progressive multiple sclerosis. Then, in reviewing the prognosis and the "natural history" of the disease, it was clear that this patient "should have died" long ago. The neurologist agreed but he couldn't recall how long the patient had his disease. When I told him that we were approaching 30 years, he was flabbergasted.

During our conversation, I told him that the patient had been receiving a single hyperbaric oxygen treatment once a week for nearly 25 years. However, the patient, O'Neal Breaux, hadn't told his doctor about the HBOT. The neurologist was somewhat dumbfounded and couldn't explain the results. This patient's clinical picture was at odds with what any doctor would expect to see based on the diagnosis. However, he agreed to continue to follow the patient with me.

We're Still Waiting for Acceptance

Most recently, various members of the hyperbaric community put out an evidence-based medicine (see Glossary) paper summarizing the research on HBOT in MS. The paper acknowledged that HBOT can improve bladder function in MS patients, but discounted that very important finding in their overall conclusions, which stated that no evidence exists for a beneficial effect of hyperbaric oxygen therapy in MS. Unfortunately, this current fashion in medicine of evidence-based analyses is extremely limited and we can miss the underlying science. I think this may be what has occurred during the long history of HBOT for multiple sclerosis.

Meanwhile, though, many MS patients find their way to HBOT on their own. Over the years, patients who could afford to, and were willing to try something their doctors didn't suggest, went to England for treatment. Others, such as my patient and those of other doctors who use HBOT, have sought treatment closer to home. In addition, I would guess that many men and women with MS simply enjoy the results, tell their friends, but keep their own counsel and don't tell their doctors about it, just like my patient.

Before concluding this section on MS, I want to leave you with an indelible image of the potential for HBOT in MS treatment. It is another personal family story, and also one of those "coincidences" described in the Acknowledgements (though I do not believe in coincidences). The patient is my wife, Juliette, a career nurse who retired at 45 years of age after a very successful career. In her retirement, she took a part-time job with her sister at a hyperbaric facility in Santa Fe, New Mexico, in order to rejuvenate after a long, exhaustive nursing career. She knew that HBOT stimulates tissue growth, and she reasoned that it might have reparative and anti-aging effects from which she could benefit. Since the hyperbaric chamber was a multiple person chamber (multiplace) she would need to accompany patients inside the chamber. Juliette also reasoned that some exposure to oxygen in the chamber might help any negative effects of living at altitude (Santa Fe is over 7,000 ft. elevated above sea level). She started breathing oxygen with the patients during the last half hour of the treatments.

She experienced a feeling of well-being that was attributed to the many other lifestyle benefits from living in Santa Fe.

Just before Hurricane Katrina struck, Juliette joined me in New Orleans. No longer receiving gratuitous HBOT, she began to develop a variety of vague and strange symptoms that were attributed to the chaotic and tiring mobile life in the aftermath of the hurricane. But even three years after the storm, she remained exhausted and had a variety of symptoms. One day, she slipped and fell. Her medical evaluation included an MRI which showed white matter lesions, later proven (through a variety of testing) to be due to MS.

Well, when the going gets tough, the tough get HBOT. She started HBOT and has continued to receive it to this day. Her symptoms have improved and become manageable, and she lives a full productive busy life without limitations. In the past eight years of treatment we have seen white matter MS lesions disappear on her brain MRI, while others remain. By carefully listening to her body, we have been able to identify when she develops new MS lesions and treat her intensively with HBOT. If you were to meet her today you would have no idea that she has chronic relapsing MS.

The point of this story is that I don't hesitate to treat any of my family members, should they develop a condition that I feel may benefit from HBOT. Juliette is only one of many examples. (See for yourself at HBOT.com, where you'll find a video featuring Juliette. Could you guess that she has MS?)

ALS, the Pseudo-Companion Diagnosis to MS

For some reason, many people associate MS with ALS (amotrophic lateral sclerosis, known as Lou Gehrig's disease) or they confuse the two. Because of that I thought I should say a few words about ALS.

As you probably know, ALS is a chronic progressive degenerative motor disease that eventually results in death. It affects and destroys the motor neurons in the spinal cord that are responsible for carrying the electrical message to muscles that causes them to move. The cause of ALS remains unknown and there is no cure. Recently, a drug was approved that may help prolong life by a few months in patients who have difficulty swallowing.

In the late 1990s I became aware of scattered reports of HBOT for ALS patients. One patient's relatives told me that their loved one had such a positive initial response to HBOT that the family donated money to fund the start-up of an entire hospital-based hyperbaric department at an osteopathic hospital in Fort Worth, Texas.

At the same time, a cousin of mine was diagnosed with ALS, and I tried in vain to get HBOT for him. He died just a few years ago. As bad luck would have it he died a few years before the first official report of benefits of HBOT in ALS was released. In the early 2000s, a number of ALS patients in southern Florida obtained HBOT and reported improvement. Then the neurologist who followed them at a university hospital decided to investigate, and in 2004 he and his colleagues published a five-patient pilot trial of HBOT in ALS and noted a benefit[6].

These doctors subsequently conducted a larger study, which was negative, and at odds with a 1985 Russian study, in which the researchers noted "a minimum and short positive effect only in some patients."[7] The Russian paper sums up the result achieved by a few ALS patients of mine using a different dose than the studies done in Miami. At this point the evidence for HBOT in ALS is not encouraging. Nevertheless, "a minimum and short positive effect only in some patients" is more than the current therapy for ALS which only hopes to slow the progression of disease slightly.

It may be that multi-modality therapy, which I advocate here and in my practice, is part of the answer. For example, an ALS patient in Idaho named Kim Cherry contacted me a few years ago. He had been diagnosed with the more severe form of ALS, bulbar ALS, which is in the brainstem. Mr. Cherry was beating the historical rapid deterioration of ALS with a combination of therapies that included HBOT, ozone therapy, diet and others. Currently, he is alive and doing well—over four years after his fatal diagnosis. (You can read more about Mr. Cherry's story at HBOT.com.)

While Kim has not cured his ALS, he has done remarkably well without the use of drugs. Most importantly, he took charge of his medical care and called upon possibly the greatest healing principle—his drive to survive. Kim Cherry's sheer will to live, to not accept the self-fulfilling prophecy of modern medicine for his condition, is most likely responsible for his survival. He told me that it was rooted in his "belief and trust in divine intervention," saying, "We believe that no doctor should ever tell us when we will die. That is between each of us and our God." Likewise, in the absence of this kind of will, there is nothing that can keep us alive.

No one knows if or how HBOT might work with ALS, but as I have pointed out before, lack of knowledge of mechanisms has nothing to do with whether a treatment works or not—and, of course, whether or not a patient should try the treatment.

Treatment Guidelines for Neurological Conditions

Today, when patients evaluate hyperbaric oxygen therapy for their chronic neurological condition, I generally recommend they commit to a 40-treatment block. They should have this block of treatments in a concentrated fashion, meaning without gaps of three or more days at a time. It appears that the threshold for permanence in most patients is a little over 30 treatments. This expanded knowledge explains in part why experiments done in the 1960s with dementia patients showed that the blocks of fewer treatments led to considerable variation in the durability and permanence of the effects.

I have confirmed this through my experience in New Orleans during hurricane season. When hurricanes began to approach the Gulf Coast, my patients from out of town quickly returned to their home states. That meant interruptions in therapy at various stages. As they either called me or filtered back to New Orleans after various gaps of time, I collected information about the degree to which their improvements were permanent relative to the number of treatments they received. Those who had fewer than 30–35 treatments had a reduced retention of the effects than those who had achieved 35–40 treatments, and moreover, the difference in retention was marked.

CHAPTER 9

DIABETES AND CARDIAC DISEASE

OVER 29 MILLION PEOPLE IN THE UNITED STATES have diabetes, but according to authorities on the disease, close to one-third of these men and women are unaware that they have it.

Like consistently elevated blood pressure (hypertension), diabetes is in many cases a silent disease that often begins to inflict its considerable damage to the body before symptoms appear. Indeed, it's estimated that over 86 million adults 20 and older fall into a category known as pre-diabetes that is, their blood sugar levels are higher than normal, but not high enough to meet the diagnostic measure for Type II diabetes.

Diabetes is divided into two main types: Type I and Type II. Type I was previously known as juvenile diabetes because it generally occurs in children and young adults. It is the most severe form of the disease and is thought to be triggered by an immune system response; recent studies show that the trigger may be the body's own insulin. Its onset is rapid and it quickly destroys the cells in the pancreas that produce insulin, which is why the affected person becomes permanently dependent on an external source of insulin.

Although Type I diabetes is a very serious disease and requires a lifetime of careful management, it is Type II diabetes that currently is the cause for so much concern. Certain risk factors are outside of our control, such as aging and particular racial backgrounds, including Americans of African, Asian, and Latino ethnicity, as well as Native Americans. But our choices play a role, too, and risk factors include obesity and a sedentary lifestyle. (By extension, regular exercise and maintaining weight within a normal range can help prevent the disease.)

In Type II diabetes, the insulin-producing cells either don't produce enough insulin or the body's cells are "insulin resistant," in that they ignore it or are insensitive to it. This means that the cells are deprived of glucose, which continues to build up and circulate in the blood.

Insulin is one of the essential hormones—it makes life possible, because our bodies can't use basic fuel, glucose, without it. Glucose (a type of sugar) must be regulated and kept within a certain range. When the level is too low (hypoglycemia), the individual may feel weak or shaky and perhaps mentally foggy. When the blood consistently has elevated blood glucose levels (hyperglycemia) they may also feel weak and dizzy, but other organ systems may also be affected and eventually damaged. This is why those with either Type I or Type II diabetes require regular monitoring for complications that can affect the cardiovascular system, the kidneys, and the eyes.

As you probably know, a vast range of diseases can result from diabetes, including kidney damage. Diabetes is also a major risk factor for stroke and heart disease. In addition, these individuals are more likely to develop complications from seemingly any disease, such as gall bladder disease, flu, pneumonia, or even a simple toenail infection. The American Diabetes Association's website (www. diabetes.org) lists the enormous human and economic costs of the disease. Consider that one of every ten healthcare dollars spent in the United States alone is used to care for diabetics. It's easy to see the impact of the disease on our healthcare system.

HBOT and Diabetic Foot Wounds

Diabetics are at high risk for foot wounds, which are serious complications of the disease. Many factors combine to cause these wounds. Part of the diabetic process is damage to peripheral nerves, which include the nerves in the feet responsible for sensation. As diabetics lose sensation in their feet, they no longer respond to pressure, touch, hot, cold, and even pain. They bear weight on the soles of their feet unevenly, causing calluses to form. The calluses then move as a block of tissue, like a piece of wood, as these individuals walk, causing wounding between the callus and the underlying tissue. A break in the skin soon develops, which becomes infected.

Unless they inspect their feet regularly, diabetics may not notice that a wound has become infected until the infection has advanced into the bone or spread up the leg to cause pain elsewhere. By the time they're alerted to the injury, a significant amount of damage may have been done to the foot. Because blood and oxygen supply is limited by the damaged nerves and blood vessels, and the diabetic's immune system doesn't function properly, these infections are troublesome and often don't heal. In extreme cases, gangrene develops in the wound. (Gangrene is tissue decay that develops under conditions of low blood flow, infection, or both.) When the damage is severe, it may be necessary to amputate the foot to save the rest of the leg. Or, the lower leg may also be amputated as a life-saving measure.

These foot wound infections often are a mixture of aerobic and anaerobic bacteria (anaerobic bacteria grow without oxygen). We have seen over many years that applying hyperbaric oxygen to these diabetic foot wounds often brings dramatic results.

The Nature of These Wounds

HBOT is an effective treatment for diabetic foot wounds because it improves the ability of white blood cells to kill bacteria. In addition, it directly kills some types of bacteria that grow in low oxygen environments, inactivates toxins produced by others, and increases the effectiveness of a number of antibiotics. So, HBOT can help the body bring foot infections under control, and then HBOT stimulates healing of skin and bone tissue and encourages the growth of new blood vessels and other tissues through its action on many genes, which then promote healing of these wounds. Rather than an amputation, surgeons need to remove only a minimal amount of tissue.

Fortunately, Medicare now—at long last—approves HBOT[1] as a treatment for these diabetic foot wounds. It received this approval after a long process that started as a part of a healthcare initiative in 1990 during George H. W. Bush's administration. (See Appendix A for a discussion illustrating the way this approval came about. It sheds light on the way we set healthcare policy in the United States. Because both Bill Duncan and I had a role in this policy initiative, this advance for HBOT has been both professionally and personally gratifying.) Specifically, Medicare recognizes the benefits of HBOT for diabetic foot wounds because it can help prevent amputations, the costs of which are severe when measured in both human and economic terms. In addition, according to 2003 figures, about 70 percent of lower limb amputations result from diabetic foot wounding.

Following amputation of a lower limb, diabetics often end up wheelchair-bound, and in many cases they can no longer work. Once in a wheelchair, their lives proceed on a downhill progression. It's as if the wheelchair itself is put on a downhill slope, one that ends in disaster. In addition, major amputations often lead to significant depression, and affected individuals may become sedentary and lethargic; their lack of productivity and ability to live normally may make them less interested in life. Medically, they very often require amputation of the other leg within a few years. This combination of factors that accumulates after an amputation contributes to premature death in diabetics.

Every year, between 2–5 percent of diabetics develop a foot ulcer. Based on available figures, that means that each year 582,000 to 1,455,000 diabetics in the United States receive treatment for these foot wounds. Because the incidence of diabetes is on the rise, these numbers will likely increase, too. With Medicare approval, hyperbaric medicine departments and wound care departments in hospitals and clinics have seen a rise in the number of patients they treat. We don't have figures yet on the absolute numbers receiving HBOT for diabetic foot wounds, but this application has been partly responsible for the increase in the number of HBOT/wound centers in the U.S. since 2003.

It's true that some insurance companies approved HBOT reimbursement for diabetic foot wounds prior to the Medicare ruling. However, since many diabetics are disabled and thus have Medicare as their medical benefits provider, they were unable to get HBOT for their foot wounds until the new Medicare approval. In addition, because of Medicare approval, more insurance companies that previously didn't reimburse for diabetic foot wounds will subsequently follow suit. That means that Medicare's decision will benefit healthcare consumers affected by these foot wounds, regardless of their age or disability status.

The Pay-Off: Good for Patients, Good for the Field

With Medicare approval, informed patients will have greater influence over treatment decisions, as well as over the treatments they're offered. As you know, patients often tell their doctors what they've learned about a treatment and its acceptance, and not necessarily the other way around! This is a good thing because even the best doctors can't possibly know about every new development in medicine. This is why informed patients are ultimately such a great asset. It is likely that informed patients will drive the greater use of HBOT for diabetic foot wounds.

Right now, those who are concerned about diabetic foot wounds should go to the Medicare website (see Resources) and arm themselves with the scientific evidence I originally assembled. You can take this information to your doctors (and you can take this book, too!).

Patients benefit from HBOT for foot wounds in many ways. For example, during and after HBOT, the blood sugar levels diabetics must monitor so carefully appear to come under better control. As a result, their overall wellbeing improves. This type of quality improvement was documented in a paper presented at a scientific meeting in 2001[2]. The author, Dr. A. Abidia, used a quality of life measure (the Short Form 36) along with the usual measurements of foot wound healing. They found that the HBOT group had significant improvements in a number of measures having to do with general health, vitality, and wellbeing. Clearly, the quality of life benefits of preserving both the feet and regaining the ability to walk normally are very significant. Mobility and independence are important qualities for normal living at any age. Some of this benefit on vitality and wellbeing may have also resulted from hyperbaric oxygen effects on the brain and any vascular disease in the brain these diabetics may have had.

Certainly, diabetics may eventually adjust to an amputation—they have no choice but to try to make peace with it. However, if they can avoid an amputation, they will also be spared all the side effects, including depression and the long period of adjustment. Some patients never fully recover from the loss of a limb, and for many it begins a rapid downhill slide to death. So, putting all the monetary considerations aside, the ability to prevent these amputations has had and will have a profound effect on patients' quality of life.

Additional exciting information emerged in 2008, when researchers in Argentina harvested bone marrow stem cells from patients with Type II diabetes mellitus. They gave these individuals five HBOT treatments and then re-injected each patient's stem cells directly into the artery that supplies the pancreas. After the injection they gave the patients five more HBOTs. At the end of one year these patients' average fasting glucose dropped by 50 percent, from 205 to 105. They also had a reduction in their insulin requirements, from 35 units/day to 2.5 units/day. This is a dramatic result, and one that holds great promise for Type II diabetics in the future. It also suggests that the combination of HBOT and stem cells may be effective for other conditions.

HBOT and Cardiac Surgery

As mentioned above, diabetics are at greater risk for heart disease than the rest of the population. Many of these patients eventually require heart surgery. As it turns out, however, diabetic or not, all patients undergoing heart surgery might benefit from HBOT. We've seen reports of a pre- and post-HBOT approach used in cardiac surgery, with results showing that two HBOT treatments delivered the day before cardiac surgery reduced cognitive deficits caused by the surgery by 30 percent. In the early 1990s, I approached the cardiac surgeons at my hospital about using pre- and post- operative hyperbaric oxygen for their patients because for some time now, a few of us in the field have believed it could help prevent some post-surgical complications.

For example, some patients wake up after surgery with neurological deficits. Over the past 10 years, multiple studies have shown that 30 percent of bypass patients have persistent neurological and cognitive problems. I have always thought this was partly due to the air bubbles from the bypass machine getting into the arterial circulation. This is known to occur, and can be seen on ultrasound studies of arteries in the neck during bypass surgery. You can actually see the bubbles going to the brain. It seems clear to me that, during cardiac bypass, patients can develop brain decompression sickness much the same way that divers do. Their symptoms upon awaking are then better understood through the lens of the decompression sickness profile.

Our surgeon-colleagues approved of a study, but we were never able to find the money to proceed. However, in 2005, results of an important study in England were reported[3]. There, researchers gave bypass patients a couple of hyperbaric treatments before surgery and found a significant reduction in cognitive problems and inflammatory blood markers when compared to patients not receiving the HBOT.

The English study used fairly minimal treatment, so the results might be even more dramatic if the patients had HBOT shortly after the surgery and for a period of time during their cardiac rehab. As explained earlier, the likely mechanism of action of HBOT in this English study was HBOT's inhibitory effect on white blood cells and thus, reduction in reperfusion injury. There may also have been an effect on bubbles and any toxic effects of anesthetic gases. The mechanism of action is the same as that previously explained, namely the inhibition of the inflammatory reaction and white blood cells that occurs during anesthesia and heart bypass surgery.

As our population ages, the incidence of both diabetes and heart disease, along with subsequent bypass surgery, will likely increase. There is an enormous benefit of preventing (or successfully treating) the neurological injury that these surgeries can cause. In all likelihood HBOT would also help heal surgical scarring in the chest and leg that are a part of bypass surgery. In addition, a percentage of patients suffer from depression, which is often attributed to the emotional impact of surgery or to some unknown factor. While emotional factors can be a significant contributor to post-op depression, I believe that this depression can actually be attributed to an organic injury to the brain caused by the bubbles, particulate clots, and low blood flow to the brain that occurs during the operation. It is identical to what we see in the patients with brain decompression sickness.

Although this is seemingly unrelated to heart surgeries, in the United States some cosmetic surgeons are using hyperbaric air and oxygen in pre- and postoperative patient care. Unofficially (meaning outside a formal study design) they're reporting that the treatment minimizes swelling and hastens healing. With more and more of these reports, there is an accumulating body of cases that shows the efficacy of HBOT treatment on damaged skin tissues. Given this information, it seems clear that HBOT would likely help heal surgical scarring in the chest and leg, which are a result of bypass surgery.

All this information adds to the growing body of knowledge about the benefit of HBOT for an ever widening field of surgical procedures and reinforces our knowledge and expectation that HBOT will work in many more surgeries.

Given what we know about HBOT and its effects on the inflammatory reaction, diving medicine, and now bypass patients (from the English study), it's reasonable and justified for a patient undergoing bypass to forcefully request HBOT before their surgery. The English study may begin to turn the tide and result in a more open-minded attitude. The pre-op HBOT can be done in either a hospital or a freestanding facility.

I have now used this approach on multiple family members and patients for an assortment of surgeries, and have mentioned several in this book. The principles are the same, regardless of the surgery. HBOT, delivered within 24 hours of a surgery (preferably in less than 8 hours), and coupled with HBOT as soon after surgery as possible, prevents some, or at least a significant portion of the inflammatory reaction induced by surgical trauma; tourniqueting procedures, where the blood flow has to be stopped to an arm, leg, heart, and so forth; anesthesia injury; severe drops in blood pressure; or any other surgical/perioperative insults. HBOT after surgery then treats the swelling and surgical injury and speeds healing of tissue.

If HBOT can't be performed before surgery and the patient and family find that neurological and cognitive difficulties are present after the surgery, then delayed treatment would still be effective. I base that opinion on the many cases of delayed treatment of brain decompression illness that I have accrued in the past 26 years.

CHAPTER 10

JOINT REPLACEMENT, ARTHRITIS, AND BONE REMODELING

FOR SOME REASON MANY PEOPLE, AND DOCTORS TOO, think of our bones as very different from the rest of the body. Maybe it's because the bones are so firm, rigid, wooden, and unlike all the rest of our soft tissues and "vital" organs. In a sense, bones get no respect. However, they are just as vital as the rest of our organs. Without our bones we would be amorphous bags of soft tissues, much like Jabba the Hutt in Star Wars, and would have to be transported around in large wheelbarrows. In fact, our bones are living tissues just like all the rest of the body's tissues, and not surprisingly, HBOT acts on the bones just like it does on any other tissue in the body.

Animal studies show that in areas of trauma, HBOT stimulates the growth of new bone tissue, and we know that hyperbaric oxygen has the ability to stimulate bone remodeling (absorbing old bone and laying down new bone) and healing. In addition, the treatment has proven effective against infection, which means it may be useful for persistent bone infections resistant to other treatments. It is also useful in acute bone infections, especially when a patient's immune system is dysfunctional. This is one of the reasons why HBOT is so successful in diabetic foot wounds. Many diabetics don't discover their once-superficial wound until it has extended into the bone, and by that time it is very difficult to treat.

Other conditions may damage bone tissue. For example, radiation delivered as part of cancer treatment is known to damage the bone, but since HBOT promotes bone healing, treating radiation-damaged bone is one of the strongest indications for the treatment. In addition, trauma, infections, steroid use, and some prescription drugs may cause damage to the bone and lead to avascular necrosis, or AVN (dead or dying bone tissue caused by lack of blood supply). Current studies show that HBOT may be useful in the treatment of avascular necrosis of the hip, and Italian and Israeli researchers have reported, and others have suggested, that HBOT may repair the damage, inhibit further degeneration of the bone tissue, and ameliorate patients' symptoms.

The last study, a randomized controlled trial on AVN by Dr. Camporesi[1] showed that all patients were pain-free seven years after HBOT and none had undergone hip replacement. Normally, without HBOT the great majority of patients with AVN of the hip go onto hip replacement. If you had your choice of 90 HBOTs over a two year period or a hip replacement that had to be redone a number of times before the end of your life, subject to potential recall of defective hip joints (as recently happened with one type of artificial hip), which would you choose?

Orthopedic Surgery, Joint Replacement, and Repair

It's likely that hyperbaric oxygen therapy before and after orthopedic surgery can markedly improve healing time and get patients back on their feet sooner. I saw this firsthand when an employee's husband, "Bubba" Knight, underwent an anterior cruciate ligament (ACL) repair. The anterior cruciate ligament is the main ligament that gives the knee stability. It is one of the most frequently and severely injured ligaments in football and other contact sports. Bubba was an ex-fireman, a smoker, diabetic, overweight, out of shape, and not in particularly good health. When he told his orthopedic surgeon that he intended to have HBOT immediately following his discharge from the hospital, the surgeon appeared amused and indifferent. At the time of his discharge his knee was very swollen. In spite of his surgeon's reaction, we proceeded with our plan to treat him, and at his first postoperative visit and all subsequent visits, the orthopedic surgeon was flabbergasted at the marked reduction in the swelling of the knee. He had never seen any of his ACL patients respond so dramatically and progress through physical therapy so quickly, not even the college and pro athletes he had treated.

We had all told the surgeon that this "amazing" healing would likely take place, but the doctor paid little attention to any of us. In a sense, the effects were more dramatic because this man was not in particularly good health, and hence, considered a poor surgical risk by any standard.

Based on Bubba's experience, I decided to try HBOT after my ACL reconstruction years later. Unlike Bubba, I went in the chamber immediately before surgery and then restarted HBOT two days after. Of course, I'd told the orthopedic surgeon I intended to do this. At the same time, I'd asked him to use growth factors on the reconstructed ligament to stimulate healing. The growth factors were going to be applied by a simple technique a partner and I had developed[2], involving processing normal growth factors in the blood at the patient's bedside or in the operating room, which makes it easy for a doctor to squirt them on a wound. All told, the process takes all of 20 minutes.

My orthopedist was wary of my tinkering with growth factors and declined to use them, but he had no objections to the HBOT. Frankly, even if he had objected, I would have gone ahead and had HBOT anyway. But I wouldn't have mentioned it to him, thus joining the ranks of millions of patients who have treatments but don't tell their doctors because they don't want to deal with the disapproval!

(Of course, I don't ever recommend withholding information from any of your caregivers; to do so could have potential dire consequences. But I felt justified pursuing HBOT, even if my doctor would have objected, because I was assuming full responsibility for any bad outcome if something went wrong. In other words, I wouldn't sue him for a bad result when I applied a therapy that he objected to and didn't have the benefit of knowing about. More importantly, with my knowledge of and experience with HBOT, and his lack of the same, I was convinced of a good outcome. If you should find yourself in the same situation, however, with respect to HBOT or any other procedure, I would recommend a second opinion, and then, change doctors if necessary.)

As it turned out, when I showed up for my first postoperative visit he was astonished at the minimal swelling in my knee and very surprised by how easily I could bend it. When he asked me what had happened to promote such fast healing I reminded him that I was undergoing hyperbaric oxygen therapy.

My personal experience with HBOT and orthopedic injuries doesn't end here, however. Since my ACL reconstruction I have used HBOT to help heal some of my other family members' injuries. The most remarkable one was, once again, my wife's. The slip and fall I mentioned earlier in the book resulted in Juliette breaking her kneecap in two pieces. After an emergency room visit she saw an orthopedic surgeon. Not knowing the gravity of this type of fracture, and having danced all of her life, she asked the surgeon if she would be able wear high-heeled shoes or even dance after his surgery. In disgust he threw his clipboard across the room and asked her if she thought he was a miracle worker. He said that she would be lucky if she walked normally again and had manageable pain.

She was devastated. But, as I've mentioned before, when the going gets tough, the tough get HBOT. The night before her surgery, after she was checked into the hospital, I took her down to the HBOT Department where I worked and treated her. After her surgery the next day, and every night she was in the hospital, I took her to have a hyperbaric treatment. Since this was not one of the typically reimbursed indications, and I did not want to cause problems with the hospital administration (or with colleagues and HBOT staff, who were uncomfortable treating an "off-label" indication), I would take her down at 10 pm or later.

The result was remarkable. Although she was told by the surgeon that she would not be able to bear weight for six weeks, because of the rapid decrease in swelling and reduction in pain, she was up and out of her bed, standing, on the third day after surgery. Going to the physical therapy (PT) department every day helped her make astounding progress. Soon she was walking with assistance, while the PT department was all over the hospital bragging about their success story. Of course, we knew the other part of the story. The surgeon was astounded, too, but likewise knew for sure that Juliette's rapid progress was due to his excellent technique!

With HBOT as one of her treatments, Juliette made progress far beyond what anyone expected, especially for a 50-year-old woman. At her last visit to the orthopedist (six weeks after surgery) she happened to be standing next to a 30-year-old woman in a wheelchair as they waited in line at the billing window. They began swapping stories. The young woman complained that she, too, had fractured her kneecap six months before and she was still in a wheelchair. Treated with HBOT, Juliette went on to wear high-heels frequently, dance at will, exercise, ride a bike, and even snow ski. In late 2014, I became an injured patient myself, as a result of an improper exercise technique while speed-lifting weights with my legs. I sustained a sudden tear in my calf muscle, and within 60 seconds I could barely walk. I limped to my car and literally hopped into my house on one leg. I applied ice and rested my leg.

Less than 90 minutes later, I was in the hyperbaric chamber treating the inflammatory reaction from the injury, knowing as I did the advantage of treating the inflammatory reaction early. I had an immediate reduction in pain. I treated myself intensively at the clinic over the next two days and was able to walk with crutches. I continued my HBOT for 10 days to two weeks after that, and was able to resume my conditioning for an upcoming ski trip. Just eight weeks after this large tear in my calf muscle, I was able to ski for a week with minimal discomfort.

These personal stories are the kind of "anecdotes" routinely disparaged within medicine. But those of us who see these results ourselves, and understand HBOT or read about the treatment, would simply view them as predictable outcomes. What makes them more than "anecdotes" is that they are underpinned by all of the basic science showing that HBOT can minimize the inflammatory reaction and reduce swelling, among other things.

Sadly, very little has been done with HBOT and orthopedics since the 2007 release of this book. The only continuing use occurs among professional sports teams that have found that HBOT speeds rehabilitation of their injured players (see pages 195-196). In the spring of 2015, I had the occasion to treat an Olympic athlete who developed a muscle tear. The results were the same: a rapid return to training and competition.

Enhancing the Great Advancements in Medicine

Musculoskeletal injuries and degeneration can occur at any age. However, the risk of developing conditions which lead to joint replacement increases with age. Not so long ago, the idea of replacing hip and knee joints sounded like futuristic fantasy. Today these surgeries are routine, and they will become more common as the Baby Boomer generation ages. If we add HBOT to the protocols, we'll end up shortening recovery and rehabilitation time, and that in turn will influence the all-important "bottom line."

The potential is great for using HBOT in any orthopedic surgery, especially where a limb is deprived of oxygen. You may not be aware of it, but orthopedic surgeries are done with a tourniquet on the extremity to provide a bloodless operative field. As explained in Chapter 2, the extremity is deprived of blood flow and oxygen for the entire time the tourniquet is up. Once the tourniquet is released, the tissues are reactivated, and the inflammatory reaction begins. But we could limit the swelling by administering HBOT both before and after the surgery.

This is especially true for joint replacement procedures in general, and knee replacements in particular, since they involve both tourniqueting and extensive surgical tissue injury. During knee replacement large incisions are made, the bones in both the upper and lower leg must be sawed/shaved to accommodate the artificial knee, and a significant amount of soft tissue injury occurs, including damage to the veins and lymphatics that drain the tissues of the lower leg. HBOT before surgery could minimize the inflammatory reaction that results in so much post-surgical swelling. HBOT after surgery would further reduce swelling just as it did in "Bubba's" case and in mine.

Since many knee replacement patients are not in the best of health and have a number of medical problems, the reduction in swelling would likely translate to earlier mobility, faster recovery, and fewer complications. Large studies will have to bear this out, but all of the information and some of the experiences are in place to suggest that HBOT will have a big impact on joint replacement surgery.

An example of the potential for HBOT in an orthopedic injury, similar to a tourniquet procedure, is the partial deprivation of blood flow that can occur with constriction or compression of an extremity. A modern-day example of this was the famous case of Jessica McClure.

Jessica captured the attention of the whole country when she fell into a well in Texas in the early 1990s. The story was covered to such an extent that a TV movie was made about the little girl and the rescue efforts that saved her life. She fell into an abandoned well and became wedged in the well where her foot was twisted and compressed. The prolonged contortion of her foot and compression/confinement against the walls of the well severely damaged her foot. Hyperbaric oxygen was administered to her within hours after her rescue. Without HBOT, she'd likely have needed a major amputation. Delivered in this timely way, HBOT minimized the amount of tissue on her foot that had to be removed and saved this little girl from losing the foot altogether.

You Just "Feel it in Your Bones"

Arthritis is an affliction that sooner or later affects all of us to some degree. Simply defined, it is inflammation of joint(s) and the tissue surrounding the joints and is composed of over 100 different conditions. Osteoarthritis, the most prevalent and the common type of arthritis associated with aging, will likely continue to be a growing health issue in the coming decades. Just two years ago, two separate groups reported that arthritis patients, particularly those with osteoarthritis, have increased joint pain with changes in barometric pressure. At the 2004 meeting of the American College of Rheumatology, Dr. T. E. McAlindon[3] reported that joint pain increased with increased atmospheric pressure. Dr. J. Verges simultaneously reported in Spain that joint pain increased with decreased pressure[4]. While the two findings are contradictory, the clear conclusion is that complaints of joint pain when the weather changes are very real. Of course, those with arthritis would say, "Duh," but sometimes we really do need to document a phenomenon, even one that is probably as old as the disease itself.

As often happens in science and medicine it will take a few more studies and many more years to sort out the conflicting findings of these two studies. Nevertheless, this hasn't stopped one of my colleagues. He has found that even a slight increase in pressure can relieve the achy joints of arthritis. Treating arthritis patients with slightly increased hyperbaric pressures has become a mainstay of his practice. Interestingly, he only uses pressurized air. The basis for this decision likely rests in the extensive literature that I happened upon after meeting with the FDA in 2012. That literature suggests that all living organisms are sensitive to pressure, even very small increases in pressure.

We also know that there is an association between smoking and arthritis, which likely has something to do with the low oxygen levels caused by carbon monoxide in the inhaled smoke. Both this low oxygen and the carbon monoxide itself may affect the joints. I would venture a guess that if my colleague added a little oxygen to his pressurized air treatments he would have more impressive results.

The benefits of hyperbaric treatment of arthritis are not exclusive to osteoarthritis. The Russians have reported a number of studies on the benefits of hyperbaric oxygen therapy in rheumatoid arthritis. Rheumatoid arthritis is one of many forms of arthritis in which the immune system goes haywire and attacks our joint tissue as if it were "foreign" tissue, like a transplanted organ. In this instance, HBOT is likely inhibiting the self-destructive immune system with its immunosuppressive effects.

What About Back Surgery and Spinal Cord Injury?

Potentially, HBOT has a place both before and after any surgery because surgical trauma involves an inflammatory reaction, which HBOT can minimize. I mentioned this earlier in connection with knee reconstruction and knee replacement surgeries. So, if the knee, why not the spine? In fact, the Russians have used HBOT after spinal surgery and have reported favorable results, and the Japanese report that HBOT helps control post-surgical infections. In addition, the Japanese have used HBOT as a limited treatment prior to surgery to help predict who will have a good outcome after spinal surgery for compression of the spinal cord. By that, I mean that they use limited treatment to help identify the injured, but not yet dead, spinal tissue that can still be salvaged.

This same tissue is the target of HBOT in acute spinal cord injury, and as with the surgical patients above, the Japanese have identified potential for recovery and have predicted recovery with limited HBOT after injury. In addition, with more treatment, the Japanese, the Russians, and American physicians, too, have successfully used HBOT in the period immediately following spinal cord injuries. All report the greatest benefits in patients with partial injury to the spinal cord. This makes sense and is consistent with earlier discussions about the effects of HBOT on the inflammatory reaction, low blood flow, and marginal tissue which is injured, but not yet dead.

In complete injury to the spinal cord, where the cord is cut in two pieces (or shattered by a direct bullet injury that disrupts the cord, for example), success is much less likely. The spinal cord is composed of not only spinal neurological cells that connect the brain to the entire body, but also of long white matter connecting tracts from the brain to each level of the cord. The spinal cord is like a relay station; nerve cells in the brain send messages to the cord by way of long connecting tracts. At each level of the cord the cells contact other neurons that then carry the messages in the nerves in the arms, legs, and torso.

When the cord is cut in half or shattered in pieces, the connecting tracts are cut and die back. Growing new ones takes a very long time and may not occur at all. However, with partial injury and swelling that affects part or the rest of the cord, HBOT can have a significant effect in salvaging the injured and swollen tissue.

These principles were reinforced time and time again in the late 1980s and early 1990s at the small hospital in Slidell, Louisiana, where I first treated many of the divers and Chad Rovira (described in Chapter 4). My first acute spinal cord case was a 33-year-old man injured in an accident in which he was not wearing a seat belt (and also driving while drunk). He hit a pine tree head-on at a high speed and was immediately paralyzed.

I treated him in the emergency room, and six hours later the neurosurgeon, radiologist, and I were all staring at his imaging and tests, which were completely negative. Our patient had a stretch injury to his cord or a disruption in blood supply and there was seemingly nothing any of us could do for him. Almost simultaneously we all exclaimed that he needed oxygen, and I immediately put him in the chamber. At depth, he reported that he had some sensation in his left foot, which was confirmed when we took him out of the chamber. With each successive treatment he acquired greater sensation and eventually movement. Seventeen days later, this man walked out of the hospital without neurological deficits.

After that amazing experience, the neurosurgeons I worked with asked me to treat every acute spinal cord injury with HBOT. Over the course of the next five years, we had nearly 25 of these cases, including one of the doctors on our staff. My results were nearly identical to what we have seen in reports by the Japanese, Russians, and other American doctors. The patients with incomplete injuries and the shortest delay to treatment had the best results, and the downside was minimal.

During that time, we also saw patients with chronic injuries, some many years old. Here, too, those with partial injuries received the benefit of HBOT and they also experienced minimal side effects.

Does HBOT Have a Role in Chiropractic Care?

A possibility exists that HBOT could be coupled with chiropractic care in some situations. From my own experience, I know that after doing spinal manipulation chiropractors sometimes recommend ice and various over-the-counter anti-inflammatory medications, such as aspirin or ibuprofen. Part of their manipulation involves overcoming the rigidity at joints that are locked by a combination of inflammation and muscle spasm. Overcoming this immobility of the joints and reestablishing joint play (the popping or cracking that people hear and equate with a chiropractic manipulation) involves a minor trauma, hence the occasional recommendation to apply ice and take an anti-inflammatory. For the same reasons that chiropractors recommend these steps, HBOT performed either before or after the chiropractic treatment could be useful in minimizing the minor trauma and speeding the healing process. Because of its ability to penetrate tissues deeply it might have a greater effect than just ice and Tylenol after the chiropractic therapy.

I'm glad for the chance to say good things about chiropractic medicine. The medical profession has, at least through its major associations, disparaged and even viciously criticized chiropractors, who are, after all, another recognized (and, based on the number of patients who see them, trusted) group of healthcare professionals. Much of this criticism stems from ignorance about the philosophy of chiropractic. To me, their biomechanical approach to biomechanical problems has always made sense. I've had chiropractic care myself to correct a neck injury—and several re-injuries—that involved nerve impingement.

I have a neurosurgeon friend who regularly sharpened his knife—figuratively speaking—and repeatedly asked me if I was ready for a discectomy and fusion for my herniated disk. He wanted to perform this surgery to protect my neck from further trauma. However, I chose the chiropractic route. The practitioner I chose was also the chiropractor for the New Orleans Saints, and for some NCAA teams. Together, we looked at the disk herniation (or ruptured disk) on my MRI. He agreed to treat me, and through his manipulation he had me pain-free in a matter of weeks—and I've stayed that way.

Based on personal experience, not to mention studies in numerous countries, I think chiropractic is one of the most useful medical therapies, and it complements so many other forms of therapy. Patients have voted with their feet and their dollars, too, and chiropractic is now a reimbursed treatment with most insurance companies. I think of chiropractic as a model for the way treatment becomes accepted. It's my hope that hyperbaric oxygen therapy will proceed along these same lines while we continue to generate additional research.

Chiropractors are also known for a level of wellness care not generally found elsewhere. For example, certain occupations result in "postural" problems and certain kinds of pain. Anyone who sits at a computer all day understands this, as do hair dressers, dentists and dental hygienists, those involved in heavy lifting, and others. Chiropractors can help these problems with their manipulation therapies, but also through advice about such things as ergonomics and sleep. For example, a chiropractor will show patients how to lift heavy objects and prevent injuries. They often provide recommendations for diet and exercise programs, too.

Many chiropractors show interest in new therapies that promote overall wellness, and I believe it likely that they will contribute to the expanded uses of HBOT as the treatment makes its way to acceptance. I have sometimes believed that the fundamental factor holding back significant progress for acceptance of HBOT was limited imagination. But now it appears that these limits are falling away.

Chapter 11

AIDS, Asthma, Alcohol Abuse, and Other Uses for HBOT

A S I'VE SAID BEFORE, WE'RE ONLY BEGINNING TO discover the many diseases and conditions for which HBOT may be useful. In some cases, we discover that HBOT is useful for one condition when treating the person for another. Again, when a seemingly unrelated condition improves, this gives us further evidence of the way in which HBOT acts as a "whole person" treatment. I can't emphasize enough the possibility that hyperbaric oxygen can promote healing in a vast number of conditions that afflict humankind. The diseases discussed below represent a few of the varied diseases for which we have indications, but no substantial research (as yet), that HBOT may be useful.

Lyme Disease

HBOT has shown encouraging early results as a treatment for Lyme disease, an illness caused by a bacterium (*borrelia burgdorferi*) and transmitted by the deer tick. More recent evidence suggests it might be due to a number of different bacteria, which may explain the difficulty in treating the disease. It usually starts with a flu-like illness and a rash, and then develops into a more chronic condition, with a host of symptoms that are similar to chronic fatigue. These include malaise, decreased energy, cloudy thinking, memory problems, headaches, dizziness, and other neurological symptoms.

The first study of HBOT and Lyme disease was done in Texas a number of years ago by Bill Fife, Ph.D., and the majority of patients in the study responded to hyperbaric oxygen therapy months to years after their infection. Since that time, thousands more Lyme disease patients have been treated with HBOT, mostly in the northeast United States. It remains a difficult disease to treat, even with HBOT. My experience is very limited and I don't have solid results to report. Part of the problem with Lyme is that it is difficult to know if you are treating active infection, the neurological damage done from the infection, or both. The dose of HBOT may differ for these different targets, and so more work needs to be done with HBOT for this diagnosis.

Migraine Headaches

This is another common condition for which HBOT may have benefits. I say "may," because small studies have shown conflicting results. In a migraine headache, it's believed that brain blood vessels contract and then dilate, which produces the pounding, throbbing component of migraines. The triggers for these often debilitating headaches are many and varied, but a few chemicals are known to be among them. Heredity is also a significant component of this headache syndrome.

While many questions remain unanswered, we do know that hyperbaric oxygen therapy acts on the tone of blood vessels. Naturally, some migraine patients have reported benefits. As we learn more about the different causes, it follows that we will find more appropriate ways for HBOT to play a role in the treatment of migraine headaches.

One encouraging piece of news is related to the treatment of headaches. A significant number of patients who develop headaches after traumatic brain injury have what are known as vascular headaches. Many of these patients have already been diagnosed with migraine headaches, itself a type of vascular headache. In 2014, a published study reported that nearly 50 percent of mild TBI patients have injury to the covering of the brain, which is rich in blood vessels. This makes sense; when the head hits something and stops moving, the brain keeps moving and impacts the inside of the skull. Between the brain and the skull is the covering of the brain, which in addition to blood vessels is heavily invested with pain fibers. The headache that results from TBI likely is due to an injury to the covering of the brain. However, *nearly 90 percent of the veterans I treated in the LSU Pilot Trial who complained of headaches had a reduction or complete cessation of headaches after HBOT.* This suggests that migraine headache caused by irritated, inflamed, or injured blood vessels in the brain might be responsive to HBOT.

Chronic Fatigue Syndrome

Chronic fatigue syndrome is an environmental illness whose cause is for the most part unknown. What we do know is that it saps energy, and it makes sense that the brain is a primary site of action. (In Chapter 12, I discuss "rpm" and intrinsic operating speed; for now, just know that nearly every brain disease knocks down a patient's energy level and overall speed of operation.)

SPECT brain blood flow imaging in chronic fatigue syndrome patients has shown abnormalities consistent with the hypothesis that the brain is involved. Over the years, I've treated a number of patients with chronic fatigue. Two stand out: one was a nurse, the other an attorney, and both were totally disabled and unemployed because of their chronic fatigue. One patient may have suffered an untreated carbon monoxide poisoning years before, which might have been a link. In both patients, a series of hyperbaric oxygen treatments led to significant improvement. They are both working again. With one patient, I was able to obtain SPECT brain imaging before and after a single treatment and at the end of the series of treatments. The original brain scan was abnormal, but subsequent scans showed improvement, consistent with the clinical changes we observed. Again, without knowing the actual cause of the illness, we may simply be treating residual pathology of prior injuries, which would explain why these patients responded to hyperbaric oxygen.

AIDS (Autoimmune Deficiency Syndrome)

In a 1992 study done at the University of Maryland's Hyperbaric Department, AIDS patients experienced improved energy levels after HBOT[1]. Again, we don't know the exact mechanism of this improvement; the investigators had been chasing a variety of blood markers, hoping to see a dramatic change in a component in the blood that in turn would be responsible for some of the improvement in their patients. As a moderator on the panel in the session where the study results were presented, I suggested that it was likely that the hyperbaric oxygen effect was in the brain instead, and therefore did explain the improved energy.

This is a case in which SPECT brain imaging could prove important—this imaging is the most sensitive to the early signs of AIDS injury to the brain. The injury occurs primarily in the white matter, and it's possible that HBOT positively affected the white matter in the brains of these AIDS patients. As previously mentioned, the white matter is also one of the sites of injury in brain decompression illness and carbon monoxide poisoning, both of which respond to HBOT, even when delivered in delayed fashion. The connection seems clear, and at least worth pursuing. Unfortunately, no SPECT brain imaging was done on this group of AIDS patients and no further research was performed. However, I believe this is an area where research would prove valuable.

Hearing Problems

The Germans have treated both acute and chronic hearing loss, vertigo, and tinnitus (ringing in the ears) with HBOT and have reported good outcomes, primarily for the acute conditions, with less positive results in the chronic ones. A recent review of HBOT in these conditions noted a significant improvement for patients with acute hearing loss. This is one of the only effective therapies for acute hearing loss and it has minimal side effects. A few years ago, a young doctor I knew experienced a traumatic injury to his ear from a firecracker. I treated him for hearing loss within days of the accident, and he regained a significant amount of hearing. It prompted him to review the medical literature on HBOT. What he found astounded him, as well as everyone in hyperbaric medicine: there were *seven* randomized controlled studies on the use of HBOT is acute hearing loss.

A group of my LSU hyperbaric faculty and one of the hyperbaric fellows summarized this literature and published an article on the subject, and now it is one of the "typically reimbursed" HBOT indications listed in Chapter 3. The national medical society for Ear, Nose, and Throat surgeons recognizes HBOT as a viable option for a period up to three months after hearing loss. As always, the sooner treatment is rendered, the better the results. The only caution in treating these patients occurs in those whose hearing loss or imbalance is caused by a traumatic rupture of the cochlear (hearing organ) or semicircular canals (balance organ). Changes in pressure can cause further injury unless we compress and decompress slowly or place the tiny plastic ventilation tubes used with children before treating with HBOT.

Vision Impairment

Hyperbaric oxygen may have an important role in treating vision-related problems. An acute situation exists with central retinal artery occlusion, which is essentially a stroke of the primary blood vessel supplying the eye. No effective treatment for this condition exists and patients often end up blind in the affected eye. However, in the late 1980s, the retinal specialist at our hospital began to refer patients for HBOT evaluation. Then, in 2004, one of my colleagues, Dr. Heather Murphy-Lavoie reported on a group of 14 of our patients. She matched this group to a similar group of control patients who had not received HBOT and found that more patients in our group experienced a significantly greater degree of return of vision than patients in the control group.

In June 2006, this diagnosis was reviewed by the Undersea Hyperbaric Medical Society (UHMS) HBOT Committee for inclusion on the typically reimbursed list of indications for HBOT. Dr. Murphy-Lavoie was invited to make this presentation, which was favorably received and has now become a new "approved" use of HBOT.

In early 2006, I treated a woman, Mary Danna, who had undergone a very simple outpatient facial plastic surgery under local anesthesia. However, that night she started vomiting, and by the following morning had lost vision in one eye. She had bleeding behind the eye and then increased pressure within the bony orbit that closed off blood supply to the eye. Over the course of the next few weeks, we treated her with HBOT and she had a remarkable return of her vision. She went from an inability to see any light to the ability to make out my facial features from four feet away.

During the second week of HBOT, this woman's retinal specialist described this as a miraculous return of vision, since the natural history of this type of eye problem is for zero return of vision. By the third week of HBOT, he put her return of vision in perspective with all of the cases of central retinal artery occlusion he had referred to me before and called it another routine case treated with hyperbaric oxygen. We have seen hyperbaric oxygen therapy used in a variety of acute conditions of the eye and have seen many positive outcomes.

While we have less information and data with chronic eye conditions, what we do have suggests that HBOT may play a role in treating chronic ophthalmologic conditions. These include macular degeneration (a slow degenerative condition of the focal point on the retina that leads to slow vision loss), open angle glaucoma (a chronic obstruction of the fluid circulation system in the eye), retinitis pigmentosa (a pigmentary disorder of the eye in which vision is progressively lost), and other conditions.

Unfortunately, we haven't accumulated enough experience to make definitive statements yet. However, the first comprehensive review of HBOT in ophthalmology was published in 2009. This review is important because the article, which recommended HBOT for a wide variety of ophthalmologic conditions, was based more on sound reasoning and the physiological principles enumerated in this book than on overwhelming clinical evidence. This is an important advance, especially since the article was published in a traditionally very conservative hyperbaric medicine journal.

We may gain information about the benefits without formal studies in a couple of different ways, however. It is possible that individuals with the financial resources and a willingness to try new treatments could locate a center willing to use HBOT for macular degeneration, with the understanding that it is an off-label use of HBOT. However, it is more likely that we will discover if HBOT has a role in treating diseases of the eye if it turns out to be a secondary benefit—in other words, a patient is treated for one disease, but another condition improves, too.

In fact, this scenario is exactly how I realized that we could treat chronic brain injury. In Chapter 6, I told the story of Mr. H, the elderly man I treated for heel ulcers in preparation for plastic surgery. Twelve years earlier, this man suffered a stroke that had left him mute. During his HBOT, he began to talk again. This type of return of neurological function after years of loss had occurred in other patients we were treating for wound problems around this time. I immediately saw the great implications of these secondary improvements. (Secondary sounds less important, but they were certainly not secondary benefits to the patients who experienced them!) Frankly, at the time I had a feeling I was observing medical history in the making—and I was right.

Cancer

When I first wrote this book, I hesitated to offer much encouragement about using HBOT as part of a cancer treatment plan, despite a scientific rationale and some positive reports. However, more information continues to develop, and I've also reviewed older information about which I was unaware.

From a theoretical standpoint alone, HBOT may have a role to play in cancer therapy. As it turns out, many cancers exist and thrive in low oxygen conditions, especially rapidly growing cancers. Even cancers with high blood vessel density can have low oxygen levels. Strong evidence exists showing that when a cell becomes cancerous, it does so because it has had a change in its metabolism, bringing it to a state in which it operates primarily without oxygen. In the presence of oxygen, especially high doses of oxygen, a cancer cell's metabolism is compromised. In addition, smoking is highly associated with metastatic spread of cancers, which makes sense when you consider what smoking does. With every puff of a cigarette, the carbon monoxide in smoke displaces oxygen and binds to our hemoglobin, the protein in red blood cells that carries oxygen throughout the body. The nicotine in smoke simultaneously causes a tight constriction of blood vessels to markedly decrease blood flow.

The combination of decreased blood flow and lowered oxygen carrying capacity is a one-two punch to tissues, causing a significant reduction in oxygen levels. When a cancer that thrives in a low oxygen environment is subjected to the oxygen lowering effects of smoking, rapid local and metastatic spread of cancer often results.

Radiation therapy for cancer is based on the ability to generate highly reactive chemicals called free radicals that rapidly react with tissue, especially tissue that is dividing and multiplying like cancer. This process is dependent on oxygen levels: the lower the oxygen levels in the tumor, the lower the killing effect of radiation on the cancer. Conversely, the higher the oxygen level, the more cancer is killed. HBOT is the best way to achieve the highest levels of oxygen in cancer. In fact, in the 1970s, a radiation oncologist in New Orleans demonstrated preliminary clinical studies showing a synergistic effect of radiation and HBOT on cancer. With this kind of synergistic effect, we demonstrate that sometimes, $1 + 1 = 3$.

In the late 1990s and early 2000s, doctors in Japan picked up the torch and applied HBOT plus radiation to patients with the most deadly type of brain cancer. The average life expectancy of these patients nearly doubled, from 13 months to 22 months. Although this doesn't sound like a dramatic change and we are not necessarily talking about a cure, these results were astounding. And it *is* a start. To achieve a near doubling of lifespan in patients with one of the most aggressive of all cancers where no other treatment has even come close was startling.

At the same time, the study allayed other concerns and misconceptions. The primary misconception goes something like this: all tissues, including cancerous tissue, need oxygen to grow, and hyperbaric oxygen provides high oxygen levels; therefore, HBOT should stimulate cancer growth. This has long been a concern of patients with previous or residual cancer who have undergone radiation therapy and experienced radiation injury, and then sought HBOT to repair the injury. Radiation injury is one of the indications for HBOT. Yet despite the numerous studies that have reviewed all of the medical literature on this subject, no evidence has surfaced that HBOT stimulates cancer growth. In fact, in the brain cancer study, the opposite occurred.

More recent research has suggested that HBOT may also decrease the side effects of chemotherapy. An animal study in 2008 showed that when HBOT was administered with a chemotherapeutic agent known to permanently damage the heart, the heart damage was markedly reduced.

I saw this potential for HBOT reinforced by a similar effect in a friend and colleague of mine. Ken Locklear is an ex-Navy diver, a hyperbaric technician, publisher, and hyperbaric services business owner/provider. He's also a co-founder of the IHMA, along with Dr. Duncan and me. He was stricken with Stage IV metastatic colon cancer nearly three years ago at the age of 37. His life expectancy was about six months. Ken underwent surgery, after which he began chemotherapy. However, after he scoured the medical literature on HBOT in cancer, he discovered articles from the 1950s suggesting that HBOT may have a role in cancer treatment.

Ken began HBOT during his chemotherapy, and not only did the cancer become undetectable in four months, he experienced none of the nausea, vomiting, hair loss, peripheral neuropathy (nerve damage in the extremities), and low red and white blood cell counts or platelet counts. He was even able to maintain and even expand his businesses, and he and his wife had a child during this time.

The HBOT was so successful in reducing these typical side effects that his oncologist significantly increased the doses of his chemotherapy and gave him over one and a half times the number of treatments with the most toxic chemotherapeutic agent. Ken subsequently has been granted a patent to use HBOT to minimize side effects of chemotherapy in cancer. He is currently funding animal research in an attempt to duplicate his experience.

Unfortunately, after the cancer disappeared and Ken stopped chemotherapy and HBOT, the cancer returned. He has reinstated the HBOT and chemotherapy and he is again controlling symptoms and growth, and possibly reducing the size of the cancer. He is making cancer a chronic disease, much like AIDS has become for many people over the last two decades. Obviously, I hope to post on my website another positive addendum to Ken's story. In the meantime, Ken and I are compiling a resource containing scientific articles on HBOT in cancer treatment.

More recently, Dr. Dominic D'Agostino and his colleagues at the University of South Florida combined the high oxygen environment of HBOT with a diet that had no carbohydrates (sugar) to treat mice with widespread metastatic cancer[2]. While the HBOT had no effect on cancer progression, the combination of HBOT with this diet, the ketogenic diet, increased average survival time in the mice by nearly 80 percent. In other words, it nearly doubled the lifespan of the cancer-ridden mice.

The combination of removing the low oxygen environment that promotes growth of cancer, along with a diet that starved the cancer of its food source, had a significant effect. The diet therapy alone is similar to elemental diets recommended for humans with cancer. Imagine combining these simple non-toxic treatments to treat people with cancer—what an exciting future for cancer treatment, especially with the addition of chemo or radiation.

Asthma

Active asthma or *reactive airways disease* and emphysema represent additional diagnoses which may respond to HBOT. Part of the disease process in these conditions is inflammation. As mentioned in earlier chapters HBOT has been shown to have beneficial effects on inflammation. Doctors, however, have been extremely cautious with HBOT in these conditions and even tell patients they must not undergo HBOT. The reason is that asthma and other forms of reactive airways disease cause constriction of the small air tubes in the lungs. When this happens, you can have air trapped in small segments of the lung. If you are in a hyperbaric chamber at depth and have a segment with trapped air, as you ascend to the surface that air can expand, rupture into the pulmonary blood vessels (air embolism), and proceed to the brain or heart, causing stroke and heart attack. Fortunately, this is exceedingly rare, mostly a theoretical problem, and avoidable. If it were a considerable risk we would see air embolism extremely commonly in divers. In a large survey of asthmatic divers done in the 1990s they were found to be at no greater risk that the non-asthmatic divers.

The theoretical difficulties involved with asthma patients may be overcome with careful treatment techniques, such as very slow compression and decompression rates and using lung dilator medicines just before HBOT.

For example, earlier I mentioned the large chemical spill of nitrogen tetroxide in Bogalusa, Louisiana. As a result of the toxic exposure, these individuals developed an extreme chemical reactive airways disease that was difficult to control. When these patients underwent hyperbaric oxygen therapy, we were very careful when compressing and decompressing them. A physician-colleague in Bogalusa, Dr. LeRoy Joiner, also saw improvement in the patients' pulmonary symptoms. They had fewer episodes of shortness of breath and required less medication. Around that time, Dr. William Maxfield mentioned to me that he'd had success treating asthmatic patients with HBOT. I subsequently saw reports from an international symposium in Russia about the use of hyperbaric oxygen therapy in chronic asthma.

Shortly thereafter, Dr. Maxfield told me about Mici Teller, the wife of Dr. Edward Teller. (I discussed Dr. Teller in Chapter 6: he had used HBOT, first for a hip injury and then for a stroke.) In 1995, Mici Teller was deteriorating from emphysema and was bedridden. She had lost a significant amount of weight (she was down to 76 pounds) and was on supplemental oxygen. She suffered from anoxic dementia (caused by lack of oxygen) and her doctors had given her two to three months to live. At that point, Drs. Maxfield and Neubauer directed Mici's HBOT in the chamber that Teller had recently installed for the treatment of his stroke.

The two doctors recommended a very low pressure hyperbaric protocol, and within weeks she began to respond. Soon she was no longer using supplemental oxygen, her appetite improved, and she gained 36 pounds. She regained her bright, active, energetic state, and was no longer bedridden. Mici Teller lived another five years, and had almost daily hyperbaric oxygen therapy during that time. This case is consistent with the reports from the Russians and now others on the use of hyperbaric oxygen for chronic pulmonary problems.

HBOT and the Effects of Alcohol and Other Drug Abuse

Between 1986 and 1987 I completed a year of radiology training at Charity Hospital and Louisiana State University School of Medicine, New Orleans. The VA hospital in New Orleans was one of our training sites, and while rotating there I met a Japanese doctor who had for many years practiced hyperbaric medicine at a large facility in Osaka, Japan. She once said that the most effective treatment for hangovers resulting from their sake parties was a single hyperbaric oxygen treatment the following morning.

Reports like this always sound mildly amusing, but I find them intriguing, too. After all, it isn't difficult to project the potential of HBOT for detoxification of alcoholics and others in drug-induced states. Russian doctors have actually investigated these uses. When I thought about this potential application in greater depth, it made sense. Hangovers are thought to be caused by a combination of dehydration and the effects of various contents of the particular alcoholic beverage, plus the incomplete combustion of alcohol in the brain.

According to this theory, some of the incomplete combustion products of excess alcohol consumption are responsible for hangovers. By supplying additional oxygen, it is reasonable to assume that we would hasten the combustion of these intermediary compounds; namely, the aldehydes and acids that accumulate in the brain. By lessening their time in the brain, we would lessen the toxicity effect and resolve the hangover.

This is just a conjecture at this point, but it makes some sense. It also makes sense based on our knowledge of HBOT's beneficial effects for other forms of toxic brain injury such as carbon monoxide, cyanide, or hydrogen sulfide poisoning, where the targets may be toxin-damaged tissue or impending cell death. For example, we know that alcohol kills brain cells and HBOT has been shown to prevent cell death that occurs after low blood flow/low oxygen or carbon monoxide and low blood flow/low oxygen insults. It's very possible that these same targets are present in the hangover brain. In support of this idea, the Russians have used HBOT in acute overdose, acute toxic ingestions, and acute drug withdrawal. A hangover is not so different, just a different drug/toxin.

In 2009 and 2010, I reviewed the world's medical literature on HBOT in the treatment of drug and chemical intoxication and detoxification for a scientific meeting of the International College of Integrative Medicine. I was surprised to find the amount of information I uncovered. It's astonishing that HBOT has been used for a variety of acute drug and chemical poisonings/ detoxifications. In many cases, it appeared that HBOT was treating the inflammatory reaction after the poisoning, and other times it treated the actual poison itself.

Looking to the future, I believe HBOT could play an important role in our treatment of alcoholism, drug addiction and drug/chemical intoxication/ detoxification, both during and beyond the acute withdrawal and recovery period. HBOT could be a beneficial step for recovering alcoholics/addicts to take as part of their long-term rejuvenation and repair of brain tissue. We've all known people who have recovered from long-standing addictions and have gone on to live great lives. However, some are frustrated with their progress, as if they aren't able to live up to their full potential. This is likely the result of brain damage from the years of alcohol, tobacco, and drug abuse. These patients have essentially a "tired brain," or prematurely aged brain. HBOT may have a serious role in rejuvenating and rebuilding these patients brains, and hence, their lives.

Two examples of this are presented in my congressional testimonies and another case is described in the chapter on dementia (Chapter 12). One case included in the congressional testimony is particularly poignant and relevant to this discussion on drug damaged brains.

Jason (not his real name) was a 19-year-old disaffected and deeply troubled adolescent. At the time of his referral by a colleague of mine he had global life dysfunction, and his parents were long past the ability to help him. He had been in trouble with the law, school authorities, had problems with his relationships, and was generally out of control. He was heading for certain incarceration, but at that point his doctor asked me about the possibility of HBOT, because he had seen positive effects of HBOT in a number of his patients treated for toxic brain injury.

Jason admitted that he'd ingested well over 1,000 doses of Rohypnol (the date rape drug), possibly as many as 2,000 doses, and admitted using it to bring about loss of consciousness. He had also taken myriad other drugs in the span of the previous five years, including marijuana, LSD, hallucinogenic mushrooms, cocaine, crack, alcohol, glue, Valium, and even typewriter correction solvent.

However, even in the absence of drug use over the previous seven months, he still had cognitive, behavioral, and emotional problems, and chronic severe headaches.

I performed a history and physical exam and then the sequence of a SPECT brain scan, a single HBOT, and repeat SPECT scan. His remarkable brain images are included on page 4 of the photo insert. For a 19-year-old young man his brain looks nearly as bad as the 48-year-old woman suffering dementia following carbon monoxide poisoning, mentioned in Chapter 8, and the 74-year old demented man, Earl, described in Chapter 12. Such damage so early in life is astounding—and all from drugs.

The image after a single HBOT is even more profound, showing a marked improvement in blood flow. We commenced a course of HBOT and Jason experienced improvement in his symptoms as the second SPECT scan predicted. Unfortunately, I can't report a happy ending. Due to the distance he had to travel for treatment and other personal problems I was not able to treat him as much as possible and coordinate this with intensive substance abuse rehabilitation. The last time I spoke with his doctor he was in trouble with the law over a number of charges. In all likelihood he had returned to his drug abuse and criminal behavior. I strongly feel that, had he been able to obtain additional HBOT with substance abuse treatment, it might have made a difference in his life.

If this case and the others I have treated with brain injury secondary to chronic drug abuse are any indication, the potential for HBOT in substance abuse is huge. I believe further studies and cases will bear this out.

Chronic Pain Syndrome and Complex Regional Pain Syndrome

Chronic pain syndrome is comprised of a wide range of disorders, in many of which inflammation plays a key role[3]. As you have seen, HBOT has profound effects on the immune system and inflammation, so it's not surprising that HBOT can be effective in chronic pain syndromes.

The anti-inflammatory and pro-inflammatory genes are among the largest clusters of genes respectively expressed and suppressed by HBOT. A few years ago, a group of Turkish hyperbaric physicians published an article summarizing the positive effects of HBOT in some chronic pain syndromes: fibromyalgia syndrome, complex regional pain syndrome, myofascial pain syndrome, migraine, and cluster headaches[4]. (A similarly favorable review of the literature followed from other doctors[5].) I have treated patients with chronic pain from a variety of different causes, often in the treatment of other conditions, and have had positive results. Generally, patients experience decreased pain, especially when the inflammation was likely the cause.

One chronic pain syndrome deserves special mention: *complex regional pain syndrome*. Most people are familiar with the syndrome, even if they haven't heard its label. It is the condition that results from a type of trauma to an arm or leg, and is believed to be caused by a nervous system injury or malfunction. The nerves, blood vessels, and immune system are primarily involved, but as the acute injury heals, the pain does not recede. Instead, it stays, even increasing over time, to the point that the person can't tolerate touch, the weight of clothing, or even wind blowing on the skin of the affected area. Persistent swelling, temperature changes, circulatory changes, and incredible sensitivity characterize the injured area. The longer it is present, the more difficult it is to treat. It can even spread to other areas. While a variety of treatments and drugs have been used, we are seeing increasing evidence that HBOT may be effective.

I have treated a number of patients with this syndrome. The most recent case was particularly gratifying—and impressive—most likely because I was able to treat the woman before the condition became chronic. This patient was helping her husband remodel their house, when a 90-pound scaffolding metal rod was dropped onto her foot, causing a crush injury with fracture. Once in the emergency room, she was misdiagnosed, and multiple healthcare practitioners vigorously and repetitively pulled on her injured toes attempting to treat a suspected dislocation. The pain was excruciating. Needless to say, with this additional trauma the acute pain did not subside. Eight weeks after the fracture she was unable to put a shoe on her foot or put her foot on the ground, leaving her dependent on crutches to get around. Her ability to care for her children and function on a daily basis was significantly affected.

During the very first HBOT I could see the color improve in her foot, along a noticeable reduction in her symptoms. Over the next four weeks she had a remarkable reversal of her condition. (You can watch the amazing video documentary of her treatment at HBOT.com.)

HBOT for Athletes?

Hyperbaric oxygen has entered the public consciousness in a few "non-tabloid" ways. For example, the Vancouver Canucks (a Canadian hockey team) became one of the first professional sports teams to use HBOT for their players' injuries. In the June 13, 1994 issue of *Sports Illustrated*[6], writer Richard O'Brien reported that in the 1993–1994 hockey season, when the team began using HBOT, Canucks' players had the least amount of lost ice time due to injuries of all of the National Hockey League teams.

To be clear, I don't recommend using HBOT as a performance-enhancing drug. Too much oxygen in normal people can speed metabolism and have effects that I describe to patients as "oxygen fatigue." This oxygen fatigue could have been an issue at the home games, but not the away games, where the Canucks didn't have access to HBOT.

Since the mid-1990s, other sports teams and individual athletes have used hyperbaric oxygen therapy. I became involved with the All-Pro linebacker for the Denver Broncos, Bill Romanowski. Bill's primary physician referred him to me during the later years of his career. Bill was far ahead of his peers in the investigation and application of performance enhancement techniques such as diet/nutrition, vitamin supplements, and exercise techniques. To these, he added HBOT.

Bill had incorporated HBOT into his training regimen, but wasn't having the success he'd hoped for. After pointing out some principles of HBOT, I also suggested a change in the timing and application of HBOT in his regimen. Bill soon experienced improved results and firmly believes it is one of the primary reasons he was able to successfully extend his career in Denver. After his trade to the Oakland Raiders, Bill had a highly publicized precipitous retirement, which attributes to his inability to obtain HBOT in the Bay Area to treat his weekly head injuries.

Since retirement, Bill has become actively involved in developing nutritional therapies for concussion while also advocating for the use of HBOT for acute and chronic sports concussion.

Another football player, linebacker Zack Thomas of the Miami Dolphins, routinely has used a portable chamber as part of his training and recovery program.

The most dramatic recent case involved Terrell Owens, who suffered a fracture in his lower leg when he played for the Philadelphia Eagles. He combined HBOT with other treatments to accelerate healing. He specifically used the treatment as part of his preparation for the 2005 Super Bowl, and he was able to play in that game seven weeks after his sprain and fracture. At the time of the injury, it was projected that it would take 8–12 weeks for him to heal, and it was a certainty that he would not play in the Super Bowl. The fact that he was able to perform at all in such a short period of time was testament to the effect of HBOT, and was consistent with what we know about the reparative effects of HBOT in injury.

A Trip to the Oxygen Bar

In terms of popular awareness, oxygen bars have brought the issue of oxygen into the public consciousness—you may even see such a "bar" in a mall, where you can pull up a chair and order some oxygen. In the New Orleans area we have one in a real bar so that patrons can enjoy a number of alcoholic drinks before retiring to the oxygen bar. Do they provide any benefit to users? Who knows for sure? We do know, however, that even small amounts of increased oxygen, such as what occurs in the portable air compressed chambers, are beneficial. It follows that adding surface oxygen makes sense. The key to its benefit may well be intermittent administration.

As previously mentioned, one of the reasons we don't see the drug-like effects of oxygen in the hospital is that we routinely apply oxygen in a tonic state, meaning for a prolonged period of time. Patients are placed on supplemental oxygen for many hours, and sometimes days. In this use, we don't increase and decrease oxygen pressure, which constitutes oxygen signaling to the DNA and other tissues. In hospital settings and in the home, where supplemental oxygen is used (often on a continuous basis) by those with emphysema or congestive heart failure, we are trying to bring oxygen levels back up to a level that maintains normal metabolic functions.

At an oxygen bar, however, a person inhales oxygen for a short period of time, sometimes for as little as 30 minutes or an hour or two, sometimes for longer. So, this might have some signaling effect, especially if done to "repair" prior brain damage. If it's done in an actual bar while drinking alcohol it may act as a tool for delivering greater amounts of oxygen to the brain, since alcohol dilates blood vessels. In the process the oxygen intake may counteract the negative effects of alcohol and even help combust the alcohol to prevent hangover, as discussed above. Given my Japanese colleague's story about HBOT and sake hangovers in Japan, using oxygen while ingesting alcohol doesn't seem so ridiculous. At the same time, it could also prevent delayed cell death due to alcohol.

Athletes, particularly football players, routinely use oxygen on the sidelines in order to rejuvenate during a game. This makes sense when you consider that football is a non-aerobic sport. In other words, it's characterized by high energy and rapid bursts of exertion, followed by rest periods between each plays. This type of intense activity relies on a combination of aerobic and anaerobic metabolism. Anaerobic metabolism results in combustion products that we believe are responsible for the muscle pain and achiness, as well as muscle fatigue. Supplemental oxygen to counteract the oxygen debt built up by anaerobic metabolism makes sense. When muscle activity demands more oxygen than is available the muscle burns fuel without oxygen. This is very inefficient and results in the production of large amounts of acid.

This is talked about in terms of oxygen debt, or the amount of oxygen you have to pay back to burn the byproducts of incomplete combustion, similar to a hangover.

Athletes also use supplemental oxygen at altitude when they aren't acclimated. If you're an NBA player who lives at sea level, but must fly into Denver to play a basketball game, for example, then you're likely to be tired earlier in each quarter than usual. Just ask any visiting NBA coach or player about how long their game feels while playing in Denver.

One of my patients was a perfect example of someone whose residual injury could benefit from just supplemental oxygen. This patient was treated acutely for a stroke of the eye and experienced substantial improvement in her vision. Her vision did not return to normal, however, and she was left with vision impairment. Ten months later, when we pressurized her during a television videotaping for a promotion of an experimental stroke trial with HBOT that I was commencing at the university, she experienced further improvement in her impaired vision within a matter of minutes. At the time, the gas in the chamber was air, and while we began to infuse 100 percent oxygen it takes time for the oxygen concentration to reach 100 percent. In essence, I was giving her supplemental, non-pressurized air and oxygen and that was responsible for her improvement in vision on the eye chart 10 months after her stroke of the eye. This experience was captured on videotape.

The Possibilities Expand

As we accumulate research in the United States and abroad, I have no doubt that even more conditions will benefit from HBOT. Some of these diseases may be revealed as HBOT is used with other unrelated conditions. In the coming decades, we will have further confirmation about the enormous range of both acute injuries and long-standing conditions that may benefit from hyperbaric oxygen.

CHAPTER 12

HBOT: AN ANTI-AGING TOOL

T HROUGHOUT THIS BOOK, I'VE MENTIONED THE ISSUE of our aging population, which is rapidly becoming a big issue in healthcare as the tens of millions of Baby Boomers head into their older years. The increase in the numbers of men and women over 60 will continue to grow because the parents of Baby Boomers are living longer as well. It's not unusual for those in their 50s and 60s to be caregivers for elderly parents.

Of course, we need to qualify the concept of longevity, because being alive more years than previous generations is not the same thing as living well while growing old.

In 2004, I was invited to give a talk on hyperbaric oxygen therapy in anti-aging at the American Academy of Anti-Aging Medicine Conference, held in Las Vegas. I was happy to present at that conference, because it has been my "secret conviction" that HBOT delivered on a long-term basis could either slow the aging process or else reverse some of the changes involved in aging. I've been somewhat reluctant to speak out about this application, because it would draw still more controversy to HBOT. However, the evidence points to the validity of my contention.

HBOT and Its Effects on DNA

Based on the hundreds of brain-injured individuals I've treated, especially those with the cognitive deterioration we see in dementia, it's become clear that we can often improve or even reverse damage that's occurred in old insults to the brain. In addition, my research has led to the discovery that the aging phenomenon is primarily based in the DNA. To clarify, we know that hyperbaric oxygen acts on and affects the DNA. It does so by causing the genes to be "read," or copied into messenger molecules that are then converted to proteins in another part of the cell, such as growth and repair hormones, among other things. You can think of the DNA gene sequences as a series of centipedes all strung end to end, where each centipede is a gene. Each little body segment of each centipede is one of four different types of molecules, like square, triangle, circle, and trapezoid. When the genes (centipedes) are copied, each of the segments are also copied to make a new centipede, a messenger making its way across the cell to structures called ribosomes. These ribosomes are like the German code machines in World War II, where the centipede messengers are fed in and are translated into amino acids that are strung together to make proteins, enzymes, and so forth.

As we age, our bodily functions, including the brain, slow down. Using the language of the gasoline engine, the "RPMs" (rounds per minute; a round is one revolution of the crankshaft in a gas engine as all of the pistons fire) in the human body are not determined by the heart, the muscles, the kidneys, or the liver; the brain determines the RPMs, or our intrinsic operating speed. This operating speed, located in the brain, drives our daily activities, our thirst for knowledge, the way we process stimuli, and so forth.

A generalized decrease in speed or intrinsic operating energy level is a normal part of the aging process. Our DNA very likely governs this process, and as you now realize, one of the primary sites of activity of the hyperbaric oxygen therapy is the DNA. So, in addition to treating certain diseases that affect the brain, it makes sense to consider hyperbaric oxygen as a potential anti-aging tool.

It is believed that one mechanism involved in aging is the aging of the DNA itself, which may consist of a shortening of the ends of the chromosomes, called telomeres, as cells divide. As these telomeres become shorter and shorter, the cells eventually stop dividing. Brain cells are a little different in that they appear not to divide and multiply as we age, though we do form new neurons. However, we don't know how much the growth and generation of new neurons contributes to brain function.

When speaking about hyperbaric oxygen and aging, I've made an argument that HBOT may have a role in slowing the aging process, or at least the premature part of the aging process that is due to injury[1]. The argument is based on HBOT's repair capability, and goes like this:

1. Part of the aging process is the accumulation of tissue injury due to the many insults discussed in previous chapters. We can think of this almost as premature aging.
2. HBOT acts at the DNA level to stimulate growth and repair hormones and influence the cell receptors for these hormones.
3. These hormones, in reverse, act directly and indirectly at the DNA level to stimulate cell growth and division.
4. Growth and repair are anti-aging processes.

Therefore, HBOT acts to reverse "premature" aging processes partly through its action at the DNA level on growth and repair processes.

In addition, HBOT may have beneficial effects on aging at the level of DNA aging itself. I say this based on the fact that we already know that HBOT affects cells at the DNA level, as discussed previously. If HBOT can induce tissue repair indirectly by turning on the growth and repair hormone genes, it is not such a stretch of the imagination to think that HBOT may also have direct reparative effects at the DNA level. Essentially, HBOT might be able to override, correct, repair, accommodate, or alter damage to the genes or chromosomes and even perform these same functions on the parts of genes responsible for aging. This is all very speculative, however.

Interestingly, I've treated 30–40 or more patients with genetic disorders using HBOT—and they improved. By inference, HBOT has to be either acting on the DNA at the site of the defect, the abnormal gene's product, or the gene product's site of action. Unfortunately, at this point it is impossible to say at which site(s) HBOT is acting.

One of these patients is a little girl with a genetic seizure disorder who has had significant improvement with HBOT. Other examples include a number of children with Down syndrome treated by a colleague of mine in Montreal, Dr. Pierre Marois. Dr. Marois called me a few years ago to discuss the cognitive improvements he had seen in a number of Down syndrome children he had treated with HBOT. Last year I was fortunate enough to treat my first Down syndrome patient, and my results matched those of Dr. Marois. The patient, a young woman in her mid-twenties, was able to express herself better, experienced improved cognition and motivation, and was generally more interested in life.

We can also cite a well-known case of a child's genetic mitochondrial disorder showing dramatic improvement with HBOT: the now famous Gracie Kenitz case. The child progressed from an 11-pound three-year-old with intractable seizures to a 45-pound five-year-old who walks and talks. I recently saw her at a medical convention, and the change in her has been nothing short of life-altering. In fact, it has also had such a life-altering effect on her mother, Shannon Kenitz, that she has become the director of a hyperbaric association (the International Hyperbarics Association) and opened a hyperbaric clinic in Madison, Wisconsin.

I used to think that genetic diseases were the only disorders in which HBOT would have no effect. However, I now think differently about the possibilities of HBOT in genetic disorders. Specifically, if we can affect all of these genetic disorders, why couldn't HBOT have a positive effect on the DNA aging process and improve the length and quality of life? I think it can, but I expect that it will take time for the future to unfold on this matter.

In the last 10 years or so, I've heard various reports about well-known individuals and the use of HBOT, perhaps for anti-aging purposes, although that's not been confirmed. For example, when people I meet casually or socially learn that I'm in hyperbaric medicine, they invariably mention the late Michael Jackson. Now, I suppose that many people have seen a picture in one tabloid or another of Michael Jackson purported to be sleeping in a monoplace (single person) chamber. I'm then asked to give the reasons he might have had this treatment. Is it to preserve his youth or, of all things, did he sleep better in a chamber? The impression many people got was that he was using it as a tool to preserve his youth.

Unfortunately, I don't know the truth behind any of the reports of Michael Jackson and hyperbaric oxygen therapy. Certainly, within the medical community reports have circulated that he was treated with hyperbaric oxygen after his hair caught on fire while making a commercial for Pepsi. This would make sense, because HBOT for acute burns is one of the approved uses and typically is reimbursed. HBOT for burns results in faster healing, less skin grafting, fewer surgical procedures, and a decreased infection rate. Animal studies on hyperbaric oxygen for burns also have shown strong evidence for its value, and supports its application in humans.

Some years back, I saw Oprah Winfrey interview Michael Jackson, and she tried to get to the bottom of the hyperbaric oxygen controversy. She essentially said she would ask him what everyone wanted to know. She'd had a tour of his house, and saw every room, and wanted to know where the hyperbaric chamber was. Jackson's answer was that he didn't know where the rumor started but that he didn't have a chamber and certainly didn't sleep in one. However, it wouldn't matter to me if he had used a chamber in this way. Recall Dr. Teller: he used HBOT on a daily basis for years, and stayed mentally sharp until reaching very old age. While I don't recommend that individuals buy their own chambers and self-treat, I do respect the willingness to experiment and find ways to improve quality of life at any age.

What Accelerates the Aging Process?

Various lifestyle issues can accelerate the aging process. This is of particular concern to the Baby Boomer generation, because we weren't always wise in our youth—and our children haven't been wise either! As I said before, the post-WWII generation was famous for its widespread "experimentation" with a variety of drugs. While some stayed on that path for only a short time or refrained altogether, others became active users of all sorts of drugs. Today, I hope that hyperbaric oxygen will add to the positive side of the cultural ledger and revolutionize medicine so that we can repair the earlier damage.

As my contemporaries reach middle age, I hear their concern about declining brain capacity based on previous behavior. Put another way, these individuals confide their hope that being stupid when they were young hasn't taken too much of a toll in terms of reserve brain capacity, which will show up as they grow older. I believe that HBOT may be the singular tool that helps such people recover brain function, much like the case of Jason in Chapter 11. Unfortunately, many middle-aged men and women who did not spend their youth as part of the counterculture still may have picked up habits that can reduce reserve capacity in the brain and other organs.

The "Lecture" We Can't Repeat Enough

It's well known that cigarette smoking decreases the average life span by approximately 15 percent, so if our life expectancy is nearly 80 years, this decrease amounts to a 12-year reduction in life span for smokers. Just as important, smokers often have markedly reduced quality of life during their last years. They often suffer chronic lung disease, strokes, heart attacks, vascular disease in the legs, cancers, repetitive infections, multiple operations, and other chronic diseases. It's impossible to overstate the destructive effects of smoking. Some people in middle age now may be watching the ravages of smoking in their aging parents. For many, it's a horrible, slow march—or crawl—to an early death.

Most definitely, cigarette smoking affects the brain in pronounced ways. Each cigarette puts carbon monoxide in the blood, which injures brain cells and causes damage to the lining of blood vessels. Carbon monoxide causes delayed death of neurons, and it binds to hemoglobin and lowers the oxygen content. As you know, smoking accelerates vascular disease, too. But each injury to the body does not occur in isolation, but rather, they combine to cause a progressive, slow injury through the effect on both the large and small blood vessels leading to the brain. This is what leads to early dementia, as well as to strokes.

While I'm on the subject of substances that harm the brain, alcohol deserves a mention, too, because it is another major toxin. When used in moderation, alcohol reduces stress and actually shows some benefits to overall health (although we don't need it to promote health). On the other hand, excess amounts of alcohol kill brain cells and progressively thin out the brain.

The combination of alcohol and tobacco is particularly devastating to the brain. Sadly, most doctors, and probably most families, too, have seen this first hand. Currently, we see the effects prominently among our World War II veterans. During that war, cigarettes were part of standard issue, included with GI rations. Consequently, a huge percentage of that generation of men became addicted to cigarettes. The high incidence of alcohol abuse combined with decades of smoking has led to a high incidence—a profusion!—of strokes, heart attacks, lung diseases, vascular problems, and cancer. We began to see the consequences of smoking and/or alcohol when these veterans approached their 50s, 60s, and early 70s.

The population of men in our veterans' hospitals provides an overview of a generation and the Veterans Administration (VA) acquired significant statistics about the health of the World War II generation in this setting. In addition, cigarette smoking among that generation became prevalent among non-military men and swept through a generation of women as well. In fact, if you look at cigarette advertising, beginning in the 1940s and 1950s and continuing through the 1960s, 1970s, and beyond—you will see that cigarette companies targeted women, and they responded in droves. Even today, the most common new smoker is a teenage girl.

It goes without saying that if alcohol abuse and tobacco disappeared from our cultural scene, we would see dramatic health improvements, and a far lower total healthcare bill. While I know that won't happen soon, we have thankfully seen reduced smoking rates, even among our military personnel.

A Case in Point

I once treated a man in his early 70s, who had lived a hard life of smoking and drinking, plus general carousing and brawling. Earl had a number of episodes in which he'd lost consciousness, and also had carbon monoxide poisoning from working around gasoline and diesel engines most of his life. He got along because his wife took care of him, but that fact only masked his cognitive decline. When she died, it became obvious that he couldn't care for himself, and his grief couldn't explain his level of dysfunction. For example, he was often confused, a situation that affected him during several attempts to travel to visit his son.

During his last attempt at travel, Earl became ill, sought medical care, and was admitted to a hospital with massive intestinal bleeding. Once stabilized, a work up was done and he was discharged from the hospital. He continued on his trip. Subsequently, another hospital admitted him, again because of intestinal bleeding. After being treated, he left and started out for his son's home. Finally, though, Earl "found himself" near the state where his son lived, but was extremely confused.

At one point, Earl got on and off the interstate at the same exit, traveling in a repetitive loop. His erratic driving drew the attention of the state police and they pulled him over. When he told them that he was lost, the police asked that he stay in a parking lot and sleep for the evening. But, confused again the next day, Earl started following a car he believed belonged to his son, which then led to a confrontation on the highway when the passengers in the other car noticed his behavior.

It soon became clear to these other people that Earl was terribly confused.

For example, he had the heat on full blast in his car on an extremely hot summer day. Earl was taken to yet another emergency room, where he was diagnosed with dehydration and dementia, but then (and I know this is hard to believe) after treatment, the emergency department discharged him!

Fortunately, he finally made it to his son's home, but his episodes of confusion included bizarre behavior such as waking in the middle of the night and running naked through the house. Before this disturbing travelogue of events, some of Earl's relatives had consulted me about possible treatment for dementia. I had recommended bringing him to New Orleans, but not all the family members were in agreement. At the time of their consultation a few months before, Earl was still at home and only mildly confused. The new surroundings, both during his travels and at his son's home, especially at night (this is a well-known phenomenon called "sun-downing" in medical parlance), were enough to cause his florid deterioration. When this happened everyone agreed that something needed to be done.

I wanted to gather his medical records, summarize his condition, and obtain brain imaging. I asked that Earl's son drive his father to New Orleans, but they decided to fly him in. I strongly warned against this, and en route to Louisiana, Earl had an acute psychotic episode during the flight in which he became delusional, loud, threatening, irrational, and short of breath. So, although he was manageable when he got on the plane, during the flight when the oxygen level decreased to the 8,000 foot level upon depressurization of the cabin he "decompensated" with the psychotic episode. The flight crew had to alert air marshals, and when the plane landed, medical personnel took him off the plane and to a hospital where doctors diagnosed pneumonia. Apparently, the decrease in blood oxygen level caused by the pneumonia (and chronic lung disease) was further compromised by the decrease in oxygen level in the plane. The psychotic decompensation in flight and the underlying dementia were not noted by the hospital.

When he finally reached New Orleans, he was agitated, slightly confused, and kept talking about his breathing difficulties. He'd also lost a considerable amount of weight over the previous few months. I hospitalized Earl and we thoroughly evaluated him, but found no obvious pathology with his lungs or other organs that explained his dementia. However, on SPECT imaging his brain appeared abnormal.

After we began HBOT, Earl progressively improved in all areas, including his thought processes, mental abilities, and appropriateness. He also got his appetite back and began to gain weight. His shortness of breath was actually anxiety-related, and not a true lung condition. Repeat SPECT brain imaging showed improvement after 40 treatments. It's important to note that what showed on the imaging was consistent with the clinical improvements we measured.

Ultimately, Earl was able to live independently, with his son periodically checking on him. This is another case where I'll leave it to the patient and his family to define the "miracle," but when Earl started treatment, he was at the point where he'd likely have ended up "managed" with medications in an institutional setting. He would have required 24-hour observation, at the very least, and potentially may have lived out his remaining days in a lock-down facility.

Even putting aside the enormous improvement in Earl's quality of life, not to mention the peace of mind for his children, the cost-saving benefit of just 40 hyperbaric treatments was most impressive. Moreover, I don't consider Earl a freak case or an anecdote. In all likelihood, Earl's descent into dementia came about because previous lifestyle habits had reduced his brain's reserve capacity, which eventually converged with life events. Millions of individuals have variable degrees of reduced capacity and early dementia. Just imagine the potential benefit of HBOT for this population alone. We would spare patients and their families enormous emotional suffering, along with cost savings that would benefit our whole society.

Some Hidden Risks

The cumulative insults to the brain that occur over a lifetime contribute to premature aging and what I call the "tired brain." Among the risk factors are the chemical and toxic exposures that occur throughout our lives. Every year in the United States, between 5,000 and 7,000 new chemicals are synthesized and released for commercial use. It's not surprising that the number of environmentally related illnesses has increased over the years, just as the amount of chemical exposure in air, water, soil, and food products has increased.

Almost everyone knows that we adulterate our foodstuffs with chemicals and various processing agents. When I consider where we find ourselves in terms of environmental toxins, I'm reminded of one of my high school teachers, Solomon Guggenheim—Mr. G. He taught Latin and an advanced language course, which was very popular at Santa Ana High School. Although Mr. G. was considered a bit eccentric, he was also ahead of his time in countless ways.

Mr. G. encouraged creative, expansive thinking, and we discussed the futuristic ideas of R. Buckminster Fuller and other authors. The reason I'm mentioning Mr. G. is that he was the first person I'd known who strongly believed that we were being poisoned by our food, and he adhered to an organic diet. He had us bring in boxes and cans from home and we would review all of the chemicals that were "hidden" in the food. He'd point to the back of his hand and say, "Everything you eat ends up right here," meaning that the chemicals we ingested ended up in our cells and contributed to ill health.

Unlike the rest of us, Mr. G. bought his food from organic farmers and producers and drank only milk from dairies in which the cows grazed on grass not treated with DDT or other pesticides. Mr. G. had reason to be a true believer, in that he'd been a sickly child with chronic lung problems and frequent infections. He had also been legally blind, able to see only with thick glasses (the proverbial "Coke bottles"). At age 17, Mr. G. took his health in his own hands and began an organic diet. Eventually, his health vastly improved and his vision returned to normal. I have often thought about his vigorous health—rarely missing a day of school in spite of spending all day around young people with their numerous colds and flu.

Although I couldn't have predicted this at the time, Mr. G. made me (and others, too) conscious of what we eat and, perhaps more than that, how we live. What seemed eccentric (although fascinating) at the time is now part of mainstream conversation and "respectable" speculation. I mention this in particular because we don't know the extent to which the chemical "soup" that we inhale in the air and ingest in our food contributes to the aging of our brain.

Stress and the Aging Brain

Stress is another important, if often hidden, risk factor for brain aging. Stress causes release of stress hormones, which increase blood pressure, increase heart rate, and on a long-term basis can permanently affect our vascular system. Stress causes the "human machine" to run at a higher RPM. The most extreme example of stress, post-traumatic stress disorder (or PTSD), has affected our returning veterans by the hundreds of thousands. It has now been shown that after years of PTSD the size of the brain changes: it actually shrinks in size. The combination of stress hormones, vigilance, sleep deprivation, and other injurious components of PTSD cause brain cells to die at an alarming rate.

An extreme example of a stressor is what happens to the body when it's "hit" with substances such as methamphetamine or cocaine, both of which dramatically speed up basic functions: blood pressure rises, the heart beats faster, and the arteries constrict. We can liken chronic stress to a lesser dose of cocaine or methamphetamine.

While this isn't a stress management book, it goes without saying that we all need to examine stress as a personal health issue. Sometimes, though, events occur over which we have no control. In the fall of 2005, the whole country looked on as hundreds of thousands of people were "slammed" by the stress involved in going through a major hurricane, which, if they were lucky, only temporarily displaced them.

On the other end of the spectrum, some were subject to physical stress, along with emotional distress, as they attempted to survive with minimal water and food for many days. If you had the occasion to visit the stricken area of New Orleans even months after the hurricane you realized that the stress continues to a significant degree with all of the hardships imposed by the cleanup and rebuilding process. This situation shows us that no one is immune to the impact of stress. We can only try to cope with it so that it doesn't become a chronic situation. The long-term recovery from major events, such as war or natural disaster, should include attention to the potential for the stress to become chronic and affect the brain.

Isn't Aging Normal?

If we use the term premature brain aging, then what do we call normal aging? This is a difficult question to answer, to say the least. Normal aging of the body, including the brain, is a combination of genetics and all of the factors previously mentioned. We are born with a genetic profile, and then we intentionally or unintentionally add "insult to injury" to the brain through the process of living—stress, chemical exposure, lifestyle, illness, accidents, and so forth.

When we discuss using HBOT for diseases that occur among the elderly population or we talk about brain rejuvenation, this is not meant to deny aging or to pretend we can defy death. What we want to achieve is "good aging," which we can define as living as well as we possibly can for whatever time we spend in our older years.

Defining the Normal Brain

We only have the ability to look back at the factors that have contributed to premature aging. In other words, we see the result and then look at events in the past to try to figure out the cause. A few examples help illustrate this. In 1997, I initiated a study using SPECT brain blood flow imaging to see the range of patterns among "normal" people in the population. This boiled down to how we defined "normal."

I started with two groups of individuals who professed never to have been drinkers or smokers. These were Mormons and Baptists, and in addition to the lifestyle factors, they also said they had not abused other substances, nor had they experienced trauma to the brain. After careful screening, I ended up with a small group of individuals in whom my diagnosis of "normalcy" depended on their honesty.

What I found were some of the most beautifully clean, homogeneous normal brain blood flow "pictures" I've since imaged in 26 years of practice. I then designed a formal study in which I tried to identify a population of those with normal brains, as seen on SPECT, to compare to the individuals who had been chemically poisoned in the previously mentioned industrial accident in Bogalusa, Louisiana.

I then recruited 75 individuals from the general population (not specifically Mormons and Baptists), and had each complete a detailed neurological questionnaire documenting all previous insults or potential insults in their life. I asked about alcohol, drug use, caffeine intake, episodes of traumatic brain injury, loss of consciousness, known chemical exposures, SCUBA diving history, altitude exposures, sexual activity with the risk of HIV, and a list of all their medications. I also asked about any neurological symptoms.

The husband of a nurse that I worked with had volunteered for scans, and when we displayed his on the computer monitor, I immediately brought him over to the scanner and asked him about his questionnaire, specifically, "What information did you leave out?" This man's scan was grossly abnormal. It was actually consistent with his somewhat spacey demeanor, which I had thought was just his normal personality.

This man admitted that he'd had at least five episodes of traumatic brain injury with loss of consciousness; each incident had occurred when he was drunk. He'd passed out and hit his head after a fall. In each episode, he hadn't awakened immediately, so his friends carted him away. He'd never gone to an emergency department, and had written these episodes off as what it felt like to wake up hung over. But the brain scan showed the damage. This man was a college graduate and functioned at high levels, but it was clear that he had a significant amount of hidden injury. (By the appearance of the brain scan, his reserve capacity was probably minimal at that point.)

As another example, a relative of mine began to develop dementia in her late 50s, and a neurologist diagnosed her with Alzheimer's. She hadn't been tested, but that diagnosis matched the symptom profile and was the diagnosis just given to the neurologist's mother who had symptoms similar to my relative's.

I recommended a brain blood flow scan since Alzheimer's has a characteristic pattern we can see on this type of scan. She came to New Orleans where after a formal history and physical exam, I concluded that she didn't have Alzheimer's, but rather, she had dementia secondary to a variety of insults. In particular, she'd been a smoker and a moderate to a (possibly) heavy drinker for the better part of four decades. She'd had an incident in which she'd fallen and hit her head on a rock and had lost consciousness. She then experienced subsequent confusion and some neurological symptoms that same night and in the following days.

Like the man discussed above, she was never medically evaluated for this traumatic brain injury and her current neurologist never asked her about traumatic brain insults. Very shortly after the fall, however, her family noticed a decline in her cognitive abilities, and her symptoms increased over the next few years.

With this woman, a significant traumatic brain injury was layered on top of chronic alcohol and tobacco use. When I examined her, I found minor neurological abnormalities, but her SPECT brain imaging told more of her story. Directly underneath the right side of her forehead (which took the impact of her fall) she had a significant area of low blood flow. The rest of the brain was diffusely abnormal, consistent with chronic alcohol and tobacco use and traumatic brain injury.

A colleague of mine, a nuclear medicine radiologist specializing in SPECT brain imaging, read her scan, but I didn't supply any history other than to say she'd been diagnosed with Alzheimer's. He agreed that the scan was totally inconsistent with Alzheimer's. He called particular attention to the right front of the brain and asked me about previous trauma.

Unfortunately, the family declined to proceed with HBOT, and I learned not long ago that my relative died in a nursing home with dementia. This woman was an example of a person whose brain was prematurely aged by alcohol and tobacco; a traumatic brain injury then compromised the rest of her reserve capacity. Her sad fate was premature dementia and death.

Preventing or Reversing the Signs of Aging

In certain situations, I would not hesitate to recommend HBOT to reverse some early signs of "tired brain." We have seen that hyperbaric oxygen can repair or reverse various types of brain injury. But in terms of overall health, preventive care has never been more important, and, as you know, prevention is largely on your shoulders. This is why I mentioned the situations above in which earlier lifestyle choices and head injuries influenced aging. So, given what we know, my best advice is simple: minimize excess in all areas of one's life to maximize brain health.

Interestingly, the notion of a life in balance is reflected in what we see in the brain of a healthy normal person on SPECT brain blood flow imaging. The normal brain is a picture of balance, with all the different regions of the brain having roughly similar blood flow, thus giving us a picture of homogeneity. I have included a brain scan of a normal person so that you can see the balance and appreciate what a normal 3-dimensional surface reconstruction looks like. (See the scan on page 1 of the photo insert.)

Too often, people wait until they are older before they curb their excesses. They say they just don't have it in them to stay out late and drink a lot anymore. By the time that happens, though, they may not have it in them, quite literally, because it's already gone. So goes the line in Joni Mitchell's song, "You don't know what you've got 'til it's gone."

To the extent possible, avoid traumatic brain injury. Approximately two million known traumatic brain injury incidents occur every year in the United States. The actual figure is likely much larger, especially when we consider the number of brain injuries never mentioned to doctors, let alone treated. As you can see from these examples, fairly serious falls resulted in brain injury seen on scans years later, yet these individuals never were taken to an emergency department for evaluation. In both cases, alcohol intoxication covered up what were traumatic brain injuries.

Thanks to our Iraq and Afghanistan veterans and some retired NFL players who developed early dementia, the national spotlight is at last focused on the long-term effects of TBI as a cause of early dementia. As our experience with HBOT and chronic TBI increases we are likely going to see that HBOT will help delay or ameliorate early dementia. Today, patients experiencing premature cognitive decline make up nearly 20 percent of my practice.

What about Hair Growth and Sexual Regeneration?

These claims, going back to the 1920s and reappearing in the late 1960s and early 1970s, sounded sensational because we didn't know how hyperbaric oxygen therapy actually worked. That made it easy to discredit HBOT, and it's true that "amazing" claims are often held up to ridicule. But now we know that these side effects are just manifestations of hyperbaric oxygen therapy's effect on chronic wounds in other areas of the body, such as the brain or the pelvic blood vessels, which supply the nerves for erection, to address just one example. In fact, if some patients claimed that impotence was reversed, that made some sense, especially if there was a vascular cause of the impotence. This is frequently the case in diabetics, where small blood vessel disease affects the nerves. Most commonly seen in the feet, patients develop neuropathy and lose sensation. This damage to the blood vessels is responsible for the foot wounds, described in Chapter 9, but this damage can also occur with other nerves, and it is the likely cause for erectile dysfunction. So, once you understand that HBOT affects the entire body, it's easy to see how HBOT applied to repair a foot wound would simultaneously do the same to a wound in the pelvis, where low blood supply and oxygenation cause dysfunction in the nerves controlling erection.

Another explanation for HBOT's effects on these blood vessels and nerves has just recently been discovered. We now know from multiple scientific studies in the past few years that HBOT is intimately involved with nitric oxide function in the body. Under certain circumstances, HBOT causes an increase in nitric oxide. Nitric oxide is a chemical in the body that acts as a type of messenger that indirectly causes dilation of blood vessels. It is the messenger that is primarily involved with obtaining and sustaining erections in men during sexual arousal. Viagra, the erectile dysfunction pill, is similarly involved with the nitric oxide pathway. Knowing these facts about HBOT and Viagra, it's easy to understand how past claims of hyperbaric oxygen improving impotence could have some merit.

Renewed libido can also be explained using the chronic wound argument. With chronic brain wounds HBOT acts on areas of the brain affected by premature aging, as in the damage that occurs in stroke or dementia, for example. Again, a wound in the brain similar to one in the pelvis or the feet should respond the same way to hyperbaric oxygen. We may be growing new blood vessels in the damaged areas of brain and bringing them to life again, much like what I did in the rat traumatic brain injury experiment. Alternatively, we may be dilating blood vessels in the damaged areas.

Given what we know about HBOT's effects on nitric oxide and blood vessel dilation and its dramatic effect on blood flow in the SPECT brain imaging in this book, it's not such a stretch of the imagination to think of HBOT in dementia or brain wounds as "Viagra for the brain." I believe we will hear more reports of overall rejuvenation as HBOT is used more frequently for a wide range of conditions, especially those that frequently occur in the older population. (I encourage patients to tell their doctors about these positive side effects of treatment, and I invite you to share your story on my website.)

In the past, documented reports about hair growth were also inexplicable. I have seen evidence of it in the fathers of two of my pediatric patients. These men accompanied their children into hyperbaric chambers. One man, whose son had a near-drowning episode, brought pictures with him to show me that he grew hair where he had been bald for some time. Interestingly, this man was the only male in his entire family·on either side that had developed baldness, and his hair loss had occurred when he was in his early 30s, about 15 years prior to his exposure to HBOT.

After I asked a few more questions, I learned that this man had untreated sleep apnea for many years before he began to lose his hair. In all likelihood, sleep apnea was the cause of his baldness. The most common target organs for sleep apnea are the heart and brain. In this particular man, the scalp was likely sensitive to the nighttime reductions in oxygenation and it thus caused his hair to fall out without regrowth. The repeated exposure to hyperbaric oxygen stimulated the scalp and thus new hair growth. While I don't tout hyperbaric oxygen therapy for balding and hair growth, it's easy to see how a scalp injured by low blood flow or low oxygenation could be just another wound in the body responding while the body is under hyperbaric oxygen.

Rejuvenating As We Age

I liken the revolutionary potential of hyperbaric oxygen to the revolutionary nature of joint replacements, organ transplantation, artificial organs, and other breakthroughs in medicine. Many of these advances particularly benefit the elderly population. We need look no further than joint replacement. If I consider only what I have seen among my elderly patients, I can speculate that HBOT could be the most important medical tool we can offer to our elderly population.

Mental confusion, loss of cognitive ability, a constant feeling of fatigue, and other symptoms rob many older individuals of their quality of life. However, I have seen that HBOT has the ability to rejuvenate and energize my older patients and allow them to function at higher levels, which enriches their quality of life. This has been a reproducible finding.

I didn't discover this rejuvenating effect of HBOT. A variety of physicians and researchers in the U.S. reported this in the 1960s and early 1970s. In his book, *Hyperbaric Oxygenation: The Uncertain Miracle*, Pulitzer Prize-winning author Vance Trimble discussed the many doctors who noticed an effect on their elderly patients, some of whom were receiving hyperbaric oxygen for other conditions. Improved vitality was the most significant reproducible finding, including a reawakening of sexual interest and improved sexual vigor.

At the time, these results were kept quiet for fear of creating a tabloid sensation. Besides, the physicians couldn't explain the results, which added to the potential for sensationalism. We only recently learned about hyperbaric oxygen's effects on the DNA and brain blood flow and metabolism. We also have the animal model that shows improved cognition and vascular density. So, it makes all the sense in the world that hyperbaric oxygen therapy would invigorate sensory centers of the brain, including the centers that control libido. After all, sexual interest, performance, and erectile function are all brain-based phenomena controlled by nerves. This sexual rejuvenation could occur at any age, so younger individuals with certain brain injuries or diseases would experience this benefit, too.

A Wellness and Prevention Tool

Imagine that HBOT is a "standard" treatment for elderly men and women who show the first signs of senility. Given what we know, and have already replicated many times over, it's possible we could prevent or significantly delay loss of independence or autonomy among the elderly. In addition, HBOT could improve the quality of life for those already living in nursing care centers. If you are an in-home caregiver for an elderly parent or other person, then you can imagine how much your quality of life would improve, too.

We could go back another step, and offer periodic HBOT to ameliorate minor acute insults to the brain, caused by environmental toxins, trauma, and other agents or events. Doing so would boost and regenerate the aging brain and perhaps prevent senility. I agree with Vance Trimble, who decades ago suggested that someday we would use hyperbaric oxygen therapy as a wellness tool to keep people functioning at a high level.

The Most Important Endorsement of HBOT in Anti-Aging and Dementia

This book chronicles the powerful effects of HBOT on the lives of many people, including some patients of mine. However, HBOT has touched me on a very deep and personal level. While writing this book, I found myself in the midst of a considerable amount of personal trauma. Hurricane Katrina had just wiped out my personal residence and possessions, my former-wife was stricken with Grade IV colon cancer, and my second wife and I, along with my children, scattered out west where I tried to make a living as we rebuilt our lives.

While working in California, I had the opportunity to visit my mother, whom I had treated for early dementia using HBOT four years earlier in 2001. After a series of unfortunate events, namely severely low blood pressure from surgical anesthesia, she became intractably dizzy and developed memory problems. As it turned out, she had suffered a stroke and became demented.

Back in 2001, after ineffective therapies and a failure to diagnose my mother's stroke, I brought her to New Orleans and performed a SPECT brain scan on the same scanner I had used for hundreds and hundreds of other patients. There, in living color, was her stroke—the reason for her early dementia. I promptly began a course of HBOT and she became animated and quick-witted again, along with noticeable improvement in her energy level. I began to again see the mother I'd known for 49 years. Unfortunately, halfway through her treatment she developed a severe upper respiratory infection and I had to discontinue her treatment. She flew home and gradually began to decline again.

I had kept in touch with her frequently over the subsequent four years, but I didn't appreciate the extent of her deterioration until I visited her after Hurricane Katrina. She was now sleeping 10-12 hours a night, napping every day, was unable to drive, and had no short-term memory. She was on two dementia drugs, an anti-depressant, and pain medication for her severe arthritis, back pain, and sciatica. She'd become increasingly sedentary and because of severe arthritis, she needed an adult on each side to help her walk short distances. No longer able to follow a conversation, my mother couldn't remember the names of my children. My brother, a general surgeon, and I gave her six months to live.

I was torn and conflicted. I spend my life treating patients with HBOT and my mother was dying for lack of HBOT. We started making arrangements and were able to secure HBOT for her in California, over the extreme skepticism of my brother. Less than six months later my mother was a different person. We had weaned her from all of her dementia drugs, anti-depressant, and pain medication. She began to walk under her own steam, became animated once again, and was able to carry on a conversation. In addition, she became competitive and could even beat my brother and sister-in-law at cards.

We continued her treatment until she was no longer improving. At the same time, after approximately 250 HBOTs, she grew tired of the treatment. She enjoyed a good quality of life in her remaining years, all the more so for not being doped up on a cocktail of prescription medicines. My family visited her in the summer of 2009 and she was mobile enough to shoot a few baskets with my kids in the driveway. Not only had the HBOT helped her dementia, but her arthritis was under control, and she was less dizzy than she had been in the past 15 years.

In 2012, she celebrated her ninetieth birthday, and eight months later finally passed away, six years after we started the HBOT. Her death was not due to her dementia or a medical condition; she had tripped on a rug and fallen late one night and fractured/dislocated her shoulder. Faced with a surgical pinning, she decided that she had lived a full life and it was time to "cash in her chips." Two weeks later she died in her sleep, for no other reason than she had lost the will to live.

An Important Caveat

Because we are seeing a certain "popular" application of oxygen in spas and oxygen bars, as well as increased use as a wellness tool, we must address the potential for receiving too much oxygen. To date, we still haven't established the ideal dosing guidelines for HBOT. What we *do* have is clinical management, which means a treating doctor observes the patient's response to a given dose of hyperbaric oxygen and then adjusts the dose according to the person's condition.

Joseph Priestly, the English chemist, philosopher, and clergyman who discovered oxygen in 1774, said something that has become famous in the field and remains appropriate to this day:

> "...though pure dephlogisticated air [this was a term for pure oxygen] might be useful as a medicine, it might not be so proper for us in the usual healthy state of the body: for as a candle burns out much faster in dephlogisticated than in common air, so we might, as may be said, live out too fast and the animal powers be too soon exhausted in this pure kind of air."

Using modern language, Priestly was essentially saying that we accelerate combustion and, potentially, aging, if we take too much oxygen. In modern terms, we call this oxidative stress. Like so many things involved in human health, too much or too little of something, from medications to nutrients to sunshine, can lead to adverse reactions. There must be a happy medium at which injuries and insults to the body, including the ravages of aging, can be reversed or limited over time with HBOT. This includes our ability to maintain health and vitality as we age. As we move ahead with greater application of HBOT, I'm confident we will sort out the issue of dosing and optimal and less than optimal amounts. This process is well underway, and I have continued to explore the entire dosing range of oxygen and pressures, tailoring patients' treatment based on their individual response.

PART III

HOW YOU CAN TAKE ADVANTAGE OF HBOT

U NTIL NOW, HBOT MAY HAVE SEEMED SOMEWHAT abstract, and perhaps it still seems a bit mysterious. However, the following chapters provide essential information to prepare you or a loved one for the experience of treatment. Among other things, I discuss the types of chambers you may encounter in various treatment settings and describe the way treatment is carried out. Most people I speak with are also curious about the process of locating and obtaining treatment, as well as handling reimbursement issues, so I have included relevant information about those important topics.

In addition, because HBOT is an emerging treatment and still on its way to full acceptance, know that both opportunities and roadblocks exist. In this section, I attempt to provide a glimpse into "medical politics" as it relates to HBOT and future research. Because I know the value of this therapy, I remain very optimistic about its future. So, rather than discouraging you, this discussion is meant to empower you as patients and as citizens whose influence can and will change the course of medicine in this country.

CHAPTER 13

THE TREATMENT EXPERIENCE AND COSTS

MOST PEOPLE ARE CURIOUS ABOUT HBOT ON A basic level. They often ask questions about the hyperbaric chambers; specifically, they wonder how the treatment feels. Of course, most of us ask questions about any medical treatment, but this one arouses particular curiosity. The concept of a "chamber" has a certain fascination for people— and may even trigger some apprehension. I'm confident, however, that the information below will help clarify the nature of the treatment experience.

Prescriptions for Hyperbaric Oxygen Therapy

At physician-run free-standing facilities, patients generally do not need a prescription before they schedule an appointment for a consultation with a hyperbaric physician. However, some, but certainly not all, insurance companies require that another doctor make a referral to a hyperbaric doctor, much like they would to any other consultant, as a requisite for reimbursement. I've treated patients with neurological injuries for many years without such a referral requirement. In addition, because many of these hyperbaric applications were so new, I didn't expect another treating physician to have sufficient knowledge to refer, and many doctors hesitate to refer patients for treatments they know little about.

Generally, a referral can be simply a request for a consultation by the facility's medical director. This means that the referring doctor does not need to be quite so concerned about liability in this situation, since he or she is only asking for an opinion from the hyperbaric physician. In that case, the patient who chooses to pursue the treatment does so at his or her own risk. I explain these subtle differences, because you could encounter these situations in your own quest for treatment, especially if you have the potential for insurance reimbursement.

At facilities run by lay (non-medical) personnel and which don't have an active medical director, the owners will require a prescription. The owners of the facility often determine the prescription, but they need a physician to "sign off," so to speak. I don't recommend this method of obtaining treatment, and instead I advise you to seek care at physician-run facilities. In these facilities, doctors who deliver the hyperbaric oxygen therapy write the orders and adjust the dose to a patient's response. In general, they are also more knowledgeable, and trained to handle any complications that may arise.

Will Insurance Pay for My Treatment?

The cost of HBOT and how those costs are paid remain among the most complicated issues in our medical system. So, while I address it here, I am aware that some of what I report today may change tomorrow. However, I can make a few general statements and try to discuss the direction we're heading in terms of the business side of HBOT.

The 15 "typically reimbursed" indications are presumed to be reimbursed by insurance companies. However, each insurance company seems to have its own private list that no one understands or even has knowledge of until the provider bills that insurance company or attempts pre-approval for reimbursement.

In addition, each insurance company may have set reimbursement rates or preferred provider discount contracts and predetermined limits on the numbers of HBOT treatments they will reimburse. It is not uncommon in our hospital-based facilities to get piecemeal approval for HBOT on a given patient. For example, the insurance company may approve 10, 15, or 20 initial treatments, and then require a medical report before authorizing additional treatment. This can be problematic, because in chronic conditions we may not see substantial change in the appearance of a wound by 10 treatments; new blood vessel growth often occurs in the range of 12 to 15 treatments. This is also problematic because gaps in treatment can occur while the insurance company is in the process of authorizing treatment—and this process can take several days.

Government reimbursement lists are similar to insurance companies. Medicare and Medicaid rigidly adhere to their own list, which differs slightly from the

15 indications. However, there is no pre-approval process, no set limit on the number of HBOTs, and no piecemeal reauthorization.

The amount of reimbursement for each HBOT is another story, because hospital billing rates vary widely. Generally, the rates are rapacious, considering that the cost of oxygen is between $3–20 per HBOT, depending on whether you are breathing oxygen from a mask or hood tent or are in a pure oxygen chamber. One of our local for-profit hospitals charges $525 for 30 minutes of treatment for the "technical" portion of the fee and $400 for the physician component. That amounts to about $2,775 or $3,700 for each 90- or 120-minute standard HBOT, respectively.

If your insurance company won't pay, you can often negotiate a cash discount or payment plan with the hospital, but it is still very expensive. The identical HBOT at a free-standing HBOT facility is usually much less. At our facility in New Orleans the standard billing rate to the insurance company is $495 for the technical portion (it is the same for 90 or 120 minutes). The standard physician fee is $341. So the total charge for a 90- or 120-minute HBOT is $836. You will often find more room for negotiation at free-standing facilities. As you can see, it pays to make some phone calls as you search for treatment facilities.

Government, meaning Medicare (federal) and Medicaid (a state-managed federal program), reimbursement is markedly less. Their rates are fixed within a narrow range around the country, but differ depending on region, whether you are an inpatient or outpatient, and whether you are receiving the HBOT in a hospital-based or free-standing facility. For inpatients, the hospital cannot bill Medicare/Medicaid for HBOT; the reimbursement comes out of the global Diagnosis Related Group (DRG) reimbursement. This is a set amount reimbursed to the hospital by the government for all of the care in the patient's entire hospital stay, and is based on the patient's diagnosis. The doctor's reimbursement is a separate professional fee. In 2015, Medicare paid the physician about $93 and the patient is responsible for an additional $23 for every HBOT. Medicaid pays the doctor about $116/each HBOT and there is no patient co-pay.

In the outpatient setting, Medicare reimbursement varies according to hospital-based or free-standing status. In a hospital-based HBOT center, Medicare currently pays the hospital about $83 for every half hour of compression time. The doctor fee is, again, separate and identical to the fee quoted previously. In a free-standing center (at least in Louisiana), Medicare and Medicaid no longer pay for HBOT.

Medicaid differs from state to state, but in Louisiana, for example, outpatient Medicaid at a hospital based facility pays the hospital a set fee on a different scale than Medicare. The true figure is difficult to ascertain from hospital to hospital because it is based on the hospital's year-end "cost report." It is roughly similar to the Medicare payment rate, however. The doctor fee is the same as a Medicaid inpatient or about $116/each HBOT with no patient co-pay.

For the diagnoses covered in this book, generally referred to as "off-label" diagnoses, reimbursement is uncertain, often surprising, and always improving. Very little information on off-label reimbursement for inpatients exists, since so few patients are treated for off-label diagnoses in hospital HBOT centers. However, for the ones that I have treated, insurance company reimbursement has been surprisingly good.

For Medicare and Medicaid inpatients, again, reimbursement comes out of the DRG. Because of this fact and others, many hospitals are reluctant to treat off-label inpatient diagnoses. For outpatients, there is similarly little data since most hospital-based centers do not want to treat off-label diagnoses period. In addition, the hospital rates are usually so high that most people cannot afford the out-of-pocket expense. Occasionally, patients negotiate "arrangements" with the hospital to treat an outpatient for an off-label diagnosis. Frankly, at this point, these arrangements are often political: the patient is the grandson of a hospital board member or a doctor's child, and the charges are often not openly discussed because the "cash" rate is far less than the amount billed to insurance companies for the identical treatment with a "typically reimbursed" diagnosis.

And, now for the most important information about this issue: for outpatient free-standing "off-label" HBOT, the situation is totally different. From 1990–2000, including the five to six years under a formal experimental program, our facility obtained insurance reimbursement for about 20 percent of our patients, often at markedly reduced fees. From 2000–2007, this 20 percent frequency seemed to increase slightly. At our facility, for the remaining 80 percent of patients we subsidized the cost of HBOT and charged $150/HBOT. With inflation, the charge is now $200/hour, with nearly all treatments being one hour long. In the past eight years, patients pay this hourly rate for treatment and then submit the bill to their insurance company. Increasingly, they are receiving reimbursement, especially for treatment of chronic TBI.

In general, the insurance billing charge/hour of treatment for off-label free-standing facility HBOT is the same as it is for typically reimbursed indications/hour, but the overall charge is less because the treatments are usually only 1–1.25

hours, instead of 1.5–2.5 hours for the 15 indications. The cash rate, however, is between $125–300/HBOT at physician-attended facilities and $75–125/ HBOT at non-physician attended facilities. For a variety of reasons mentioned elsewhere in this book, I recommend obtaining HBOT from a doctor-attended facility.

After reading this, you're probably thoroughly confused, primarily because this is a very confusing situation, and reflects the mess we find in our healthcare system and healthcare reimbursement systems. I am confident that I'm not saying anything that surprises you.

To sum up, I've provided two tables I hope you will find useful. Remember, however, that every medical situation is different. Actual reimbursement depends on the facility, location in the country, diagnosis, reimbursement source, and your aggressiveness in obtaining reimbursement.

TYPICALLY REIMBURSED INDICATIONS

Reimbursement	Hospital Inpatient	Hospital Outpatient	Free-standing Inpatient-Daily transfer from hospital	Free-standing Outpatient
Insurance	Yes. ~$1,000/ HBOT for hospital and $250 for doctor.	Yes. ~$1,000/ HBOT for hospital and $250 for doctor.	Maybe. ~$1,000/HBOT total for the free-standing facility and doctor.	Yes ~$1,000/HBOT total for the free-standing facility and doctor.
Medicare	Yes. Included in DRG. Doctor paid $93/ HBOT + $23 patient co-pay.	Yes. ~$83/30 minutes of compression + ~$93/HBOT doctor fee + $23 patient co-pay.	No. Not in the seven state fiscal zone that includes Louisiana.	No. Not in the seven state fiscal zone that includes Louisiana.
Medicaid	Yes. Included in DRG. Doctor paid ~$116/ HBOT; no patient co-pay.	Variable from hospital to hospital, but similar to Medicare. Doctor paid ~$116/HBOT; no patient co-pay.	No. Not in the seven state fiscal zone that includes Louisiana.	No. Not in the seven state fiscal zone that includes Louisiana.

OFF-LABEL DIAGNOSES

Reimbursement	Hospital Inpatient	Hospital Outpatient	Free-standing Inpatient-Daily transfer from hospital	Free-standing Outpatient
Insurance	Variable frequency and rate; up to ~$1,000/HBOT for hospital and $250 for doctor.	Variable frequency and rate; up to ~$1,000/HBOT for hospital and $250 for doctor.	Variable frequency and rate; up to ~$1,000/HBOT total for facility and doctor.	Variable frequency and rate; up to ~$1,000/HBOT total for facility and doctor.
Medicare	No. Done at hospital and doctor expense or patient may be responsible for charges.	No. Done at hospital and doctor expense or patient may be responsible for charges.	No. Done at hospital and doctor expense or patient may be responsible for charges.	No. Done at hospital and doctor expense or patient may be responsible for charges.
Medicaid	Hasn't been tested to my knowledge.	Hasn't been tested to my knowledge.	Hasn't been tested to my knowledge.	Yes, in 29 states so far.

Again, this situation is changing monthly. Progressively, more states are beginning to reimburse for outpatient free-standing off-label HBOT, especially for traumatic brain injury. For the most current information on this, contact your state Medicaid program; or better yet, enroll in the Medicaid for HBOT List at www.medicaidforhbot-subscribe@yahoogroups.com.

A few final points: There is no specific breakdown on charges and costs based on the type of chamber used for HBOT. However, any charge reflects all of the costs incurred in delivering HBOT service, so a large multiplace facility with a big capital investment will likely cost more, unless they are treating a very large number of patients. Another facility with one or two hard-shell monoplace chambers that also provides other medical services, such as internal medicine, surgery, pediatrics, and so forth, can charge substantially less. Further still, if the monoplace chambers are the portable chambers, the cost may even be less.

Other Payment Options

A few options exist for patients whose insurance provider will not pay for HBOT and who cannot otherwise afford HBOT. Occasionally, patients can be entered into an existing experimental trial. The problem with these, however, depends on the design of the trial, and if it has a placebo group a chance exists that you won't get HBOT for your condition.

Not-for-profit foundations exist and are continuing to sprout that will fund HBOT for patients. I recommend that you search online for these and check their individual requirements.

Choosing a Hyperbaric Facility

1.5 Atm

People often ask about the best way to choose an HBOT center and a doctor who uses HBOT. I tell patients they need to shop for their doctors like they shop for anything else, like plumbing services, appliances, electronics, a new home, a mortgage lender, and so forth. Again, I recommend that you choose a facility attended by a doctor. In terms of safety, this is especially important when using the hard-shell chambers (the ones made of steel and acrylic, as opposed to the portable or "soft shell" chambers, which are made of soft synthetic materials) and going to at least an atmosphere and a half. Even given its potential usefulness as a wellness tool, HBOT is still a medical treatment and should be administered by medically knowledgeable practitioners.

Assuming a non-emergency situation, I often advise patients to visit the center, talk to patients who are being treated there, interact with the staff, and above all talk to the doctors on staff. Ask them about their experience. Given what you now know about the field as a result of this book, you may want to find out how they became interested in hyperbaric medicine. These questions will help you gauge their level of interest in their patients.

Best Publishing Company maintains a list of hyperbaric centers in the U.S. and some international sites (see HBOT.com for a copy of this list). Of course, I also recommend using the Internet to locate various forums and discussion groups. Nowadays, this is actually where many people start their search. When you become part of these groups you will find individuals who have been treated at various places and can exchange information on the quality of the facility and the care they received. These online forums are a great source of feedback and provide a rapid exchange of information. This is as true for HBOT as it is for virtually the entire medical marketplace. These groups can significantly help someone searching for hyperbaric oxygen therapy services.

Of course, be careful about what you take away from the Internet. As we all know, anyone with a keyboard can appear to be an expert. One of the best sites is a Yahoo site run by David Freels, the father of Jimmy Freels, a child with cerebral palsy. David is a fount of information, especially on government reimbursement and the Medicaid program.

The HBOT Chambers

In monoplace chambers (see Figure 6), which only accommodate one patient at a time, you enter the chamber and the door is closed behind you. You are in a quiet, insulated environment. When we turn the oxygen on to pressurize the chamber, you hear a whooshing sound that becomes white noise. The chamber atmosphere heats during compression because of the energy generated by forcing more oxygen in to increase the pressure.

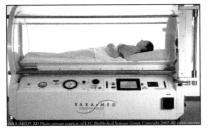

BARA-MED® XD Photo appears courtesy of ETC BioMedical Systems Group. Copyright 2007. All rights reserved.

FIGURE 6. The figure depicts a typical "hard-shell" monoplace chamber. The usual construction and configuration are steel ends, one of which opens to allow a patient to slide in on a stretcher equipped with rollers. The cylinder is usually double-hulled like a storm window and made of thick acrylic. The chambers are rated to 3 atmospheres absolute (66 feet of seawater equivalent pressure). A technician or nurse sits by the console and monitors the gauges and valves that control gas entry, exit, and pressure. The chamber rolls on wheels and weighs about 2,000–2,500 pounds. Some models can weigh as much as 5,000 pounds.

Soon your ears will start to feel a "pressure" or fullness. Actually, it is a contraction of the airspace behind the eardrums—the space in the ear canal in which some young children experience ear infections—as this space begins to decrease in size. At this point, you will need to yawn, move your jaws, swallow, or pinch your nose and send air into the Eustachian tube at the back of the throat. This tube communicates with the middle ear air pocket, which then gently moves the eardrum outward and "pops" the ears, as we say. This is a painless feeling similar to what happens during commercial airline flights. You will continue to pop your ears as you travel to the desired pressure. However, the deeper you go the less frequently you will need to pop your ears, because you have progressively smaller changes in volume to the air in the middle ear space. To modulate these pressure changes in the middle ears we sometimes use soft plastic earplugs that fit in the ear canals, much like the ones used in swimming. It seems these earplugs make it easier for patients to adjust to the pressure changes in the middle ear.

As you eventually reach the desired pressure, the chamber cools to room temperature and you lay quietly for the duration of the treatment. Once at depth you can't tell that you are in a hyperbaric environment, even though you may feel better. In other words, you don't feel the effects of the pressure itself. Patients hear only the white noise of the compressed air or oxygen blowing through the chamber. This white noise is likely why many people sleep in the chamber. They can hear nothing from the outside unless someone speaks to them through a microphone. This is particularly true for the hard-shell chambers, those made of steel and acrylic, as opposed to the less soundproof portable chambers. (Due to recent legal problems between the portable chamber manufacturers, we have not pictured any of the portable chambers here. We instead refer you to the Internet for examples of the different sizes and configurations of these chambers.) Due to their limited visibility, these hyperbaric chambers can have a cocoon-like feeling, insulated from cell phones, alarms, beepers, and all manner of ambient noise and confusion—and normal visual stimuli. However, they often have one or two small "windows" or portholes, instead of a full length see-through acrylic hull. Overall, the chamber is a relaxing and peaceful environment.

Once the prescribed amount of time at depth is over, the chamber is decompressed and more oxygen is let out of the chamber than is forced in, thereby decreasing the pressure.

Since energy is taken out of the chamber, the chamber cools. You will feel fullness in your ears again, but now the air in the middle ear space is expanding and will force its way out of the ear into the Eustachian canal without pain. You can pop your ears or just let the air go out.

The chamber will finally stop decompression at a slight pressurization above sea level pressure. The door is opened and there is a slight escape of gas. Depending on the condition being treated, you could feel refreshed, slightly fatigued, or not different at all when you leave the chamber. Those being treated for neurological conditions may experience improvement in the areas in which their symptoms manifest.

In multiplace chambers (see Figures 7 and 8), which accommodate more than one person, you would usually sit in the chamber, and you are compressed on air. You experience all of the same sensations, and because other people usually are in the chamber, too, you are free to interact with them.

Once you reach the desired pressure you don a clear plastic hood or mask, like pilots use, and breathe oxygen through the hood. We use the hood because the chamber atmosphere is

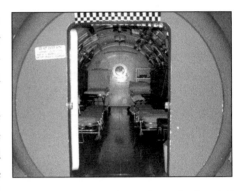

FIGURE 7. This figure depicts the inside of a typical multiplace chamber, the chamber featured in Figure 8. The main lock or treatment lock is seen with four stretchers in place. Each stretcher is sitting where three individual airline style seats are in the folded up positions. At the back of the main lock is the metal door that leads to the emergency compartment of the chamber. It is approximately 1/3 the size of the main lock. Over the head of each chair or stretcher are the gas manifolds that attach to the hood demonstrated in Figure 8.

just air; to give the patient pure oxygen, the whole chamber would need to be filled with oxygen, as is the case with a monoplace chamber. This is expensive, so we can deliver oxygen through the hood, with air breaks every 20–30 minutes, during which the hood is removed and the patient breathes pressurized chamber air. (In the monoplace chamber, air breaks can be delivered through a mask that gives air to the patient.) The ascent to surface in the multiplace chamber is done on air, with the hood off, but patients experience the same cooling as takes place in the monoplace chamber.

Patients also ask about "life inside the chamber," or what they can do while they're inside, assuming that they are not severely disabled. (And remember, given the range of applications for HBOT, many patients will not have obvious disabilities.) What they can do is somewhat determined by the chamber atmosphere. If the chamber (either multiplace or monoplace) is compressed with pure oxygen, the patient's clothing and activities are dictated by fire risk. The patients must be in all cotton or high percentage cotton garments and

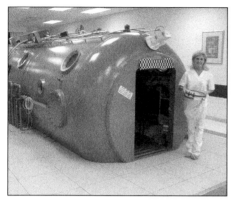

FIGURE 8. Depicted is a typical multiplace chamber, with Nurse Juliette Lucarini Harch demonstrating the clear plastic hood worn by patients while in the chamber. The hood consists of a small ring with a rubber neck dam that fits around the patient's neck creating a seal, and a clear plastic bonnet which covers the patient's head and attaches to the ring. Plastic oxygen intake and exhaust hoses attach to the hood from inside the chamber and inflate the hood (they are coiled in the hood in this picture). This is a 32′x8′ diameter "dual-lock" chamber, meaning it has a main compartment (that seats 12 patients) and a secondary compartment (for emergency entrance and exit). The chamber doors are on hinges and seal from the inside. If there is an emergency in the main lock, personnel can enter the secondary lock, compress it to the depth of the main lock, and enter the main lock through the connecting door. Multiplace chambers are custom-made to any size and thickness of steel in order to fit the desired use, with portholes made of acrylic. This chamber is rated for over 300 feet of seawater of pressure and has a hull thickness of about 5/8 inches.

must not have any fire accelerants with them, such as oil-based liquids, makeup, lotions, hairspray, matches, paper, or metal that can be a source of sparks. If the chamber is compressed on air, then fire hazard is much less and the restrictions are similarly less.

So, in the monoplace chambers which are typically compressed with pure oxygen, patients can watch television or videos through the acrylic shell or portholes, or they can sleep. In the multiplace chambers, which are typically compressed with air, they can similarly watch television or videos through the acrylic shell or portholes, but they can also take certain reading material inside, since the chamber atmosphere is not pure oxygen and hence not a significant fire risk. In addition, they can talk to other people during the compression, decompression, and air break phases since they don't have their hoods on during these times. They usually can't sleep, however, since the hood is removed and replaced on their heads multiple times during the treatment.

The great majority of HBOT in the United States is done on an outpatient basis, while a smaller percentage of patients receive HBOT while they are hospital inpatients. Obviously, patients given HBOT for medical emergencies may need medical transport to a hospital with a hyperbaric facility.

What about Side Effects?

By now, you realize that HBOT is a very safe medical procedure—one of the safest procedures we have. However, like all medical procedures it is not without risk. Fortunately, the most common are relatively minor. Equally fortunate, the most severe risks are also the rarest. But because of these risks, I strongly recommend that HBOT is delivered by and under the supervision of physicians who are knowledgeable about HBOT.

The most common problem encountered in a chamber is difficulty clearing the ears, and less commonly, the sinuses. Active asthma, as previously mentioned, is a theoretical problem because it could result in "air trapping" in poorly ventilated small segments of the lungs that can burst and send air into the bloodstream on ascent. However, this is extremely rare, and we can make accommodations for most asthmatics (see Chapter 11 for a discussion of HBOT and asthma.) Individuals with other lung problems, such as emphysema, can also have problems with air trapping during HBOT, but this is equally rare.

Patients with severe congestive heart failure must be screened carefully before treatment is undertaken. The slight increase in arterial resistance caused by HBOT could worsen the heart failure condition. We can still offer these patients HBOT, but using markedly reduced pressures.

Patients often ask if they will be sleepy before or after treatment. The best answer is, "It depends." Those with chronic fatigue may be sleepy before treatment, but then feel improved energy after treatment. This is variable, however, so only individual experience will tell.

Many normal individuals experience a little fatigue after a treatment, especially at higher pressures, since we are stimulating the metabolism a bit with the excess oxygen. In other words, we are oxidizing patients, or burning fuel. It's a little like stepping on the gas and increasing engine RPMs. Many people with brain injuries, however, experience an improvement in neurological activity or energy level after a single treatment or a group of treatments, as the HBOT treats the brain injury.

Patients often ask me about the risk for seizure during HBOT, but as it turns out, we treat many patients with seizure disorders (see Chapter 2) with hyperbaric oxygen therapy. (We have documented this since the early 1990s, when we treated a series of near-drowning patients and individuals with seizure disorders and found that seizures are responsive to hyperbaric oxygen.) A number of Chinese authors have actually presented research on this topic. However, we must be extremely careful with dosing, since the brain that seizes has a lower threshold to oxygen sensitivity and oxygen toxicity. Therefore, in these cases, I start with much lower pressures and observe the patients carefully. I adjust the dose based on the patient's response to the HBOT.

The Ventilator Question

I'm often asked if it's possible to receive HBOT while on a ventilator, and yes, it is possible, but must be approached with great care and caution. This type of treatment is considered a critical care dive and the vast majority of free-standing facilities are not equipped to handle such a technical dive. They can be dangerous because of problems with ventilators and the lungs and the changes in pressure as the chamber is compressed and decompressed.

The ventilator for multiplace chambers also cannot achieve high ventilatory rates, which means that if babies need to undergo critical care dives, they often have to be hand-bagged in the chamber (see Chapter 5). This is a less than optimal condition, but in life and death situations it may be the only option.

I often advise waiting until patients can be weaned off the ventilator before receiving HBOT at a free-standing clinic. Otherwise, the costs are prohibitive, as more medical personnel and intensive doctor supervision are necessary for every dive.

Are There Reasons Treatment Must Stop?

Yes, and some of these involve symptoms of oxygen toxicity. These can occur in any patient undergoing HBOT, and we also look for the timing of the symptoms to reveal the cause. For example, if neurological symptoms appear early in a treatment course, this often is a sign that too great a dose of oxygen is being used. I have a theory that shifts in brain blood flow are responsible for some of these symptoms. For example, I once performed a SPECT imaging test on a diver after he had hyperbaric oxygen therapy while on a face mask of supplemental oxygen. What we saw in that image was a reduction in blood flow to the normal brain as the blood flow improved to the damaged brain. This illustrates the shift in brain blood flow, and if it happens that the blood flow to the damaged area is reduced, then that alone could lead to deterioration in neurological function.

When it happens later on in the course of therapy, neurological deterioration can be a sign of too much cumulative oxygen and so is true oxygen toxicity. However, we have ways to remedy this situation. We can take a break in treatment, decrease the pressure, shorten the length of exposure, or reduce the frequency of treatments. As I have mentioned many times in this book, the key principle is to properly dose HBOT for individual patients, and adjust the dose based on their response to HBOT. As the years have passed, I have become extremely sensitive to the signs of plateau, overdosing, oxygen sensitivity, and the need to change course. Make sure the HBOT facility you choose has a physician who is watching your progress closely.

The Other Side of the Issue

If you talk with your family doctor, he or she might talk about a downside of this treatment. It is possible that hyperbaric oxygen therapy could worsen some conditions, and it is certainly true that I have seen situations in which patients became worse. Because I was puzzled, I collected data on a series of patients whose conditions worsened.

In general, what I found and documented were cases involving patients in which too much oxygen resulted in deterioration in their condition. Sometimes we saw this at the outset of treatment. Half of the cases I documented were mine and occurred during the early years of my investigation of hyperbaric oxygen therapy; the others were patients from elsewhere in the United States and in other countries. In these cases, the treating facilities (most of them had no physicians involved) were operating under the precept that hyperbaric oxygen therapy could only improve patients, so the negative effects were inexplicable, puzzling, and often ignored. (I reported these results at the 2001 Symposium on Hyperbaric Oxygenation and the Brain Injured Child. The Proceedings are published by Best Publishing Company).

Based on what we saw, almost all of these negative outcomes resulted from dosing problems; most often, too much oxygen was used. Other times it was caused by blood flow shifts in the brain from constriction of blood vessels. Hyperbaric oxygen constricts blood vessels, and in certain situations, too much constriction could shunt blood flow away from damaged areas and increase symptoms.

We know that adjusting the dose can ameliorate this. What I documented suggested that the patients we looked at had not been given the right dose, which means a combination of pressure along with duration and frequency of treatments. It's significant that many of these patients had experienced neurological improvement either before the dose was adjusted (usually increased), or after adjustments (usually decreased) were made to reverse the negative effects. The patients usually got into trouble because the people administering the HBOT were unaware of these side effects and continued treatment, even when the patients began to deteriorate. Their presumption was that everyone gets better with HBOT and the neurological deterioration was just something that would get better with more HBOT. The important point here is that with careful monitoring of the dose by knowledgeable physicians there is little risk of permanent negative effects.

When HBOT Is Not Appropriate

Knowing when *not* to use HBOT is as important as knowing when it may be beneficial. Unfortunately, this can be a difficult task. In acute injury, HBOT acts upon basic disease processes common to a variety of different injuries. In chronic pathology, the processes are also very similar, almost irrespective of the different initial causes. Because of this, it's conceivable that hyperbaric oxygen therapy may be appropriate for the great majority of medical conditions. Since we haven't yet defined the range of conditions, it's difficult to know when it would be inappropriate.

However, I would say that in true brain death, hyperbaric oxygen therapy is not useful. By brain death, I mean absence of any neurological activity by clinical and laboratory parameters, including no signs of meaningful awareness, a flat electric brain recording (electroencephalogram or EEG), and a SPECT brain scan that shows no brain blood flow. In these circumstances, performing hyperbaric oxygen therapy to try to recover neurological function is almost certainly futile.

While this may seem obvious, it is surprising the number of phone calls I have received asking if HBOT would be helpful in cases that appear to involve brain death. Much more often, however, the phone calls are about patients in coma with various degrees of neurological activity and the family is being encouraged by physicians to discontinue life support. In many of these cases adequate testing has not been performed to substantiate brain death. My answer to these families is that HBOT may be appropriate and I encourage them to first obtain the testing to exclude brain death and then try to get HBOT for their loved one.

As a final caveat I would like to discuss a topic that often embroils the medical question of whether HBOT can be helpful in comatose patients. That topic is respect for a patient's self-determination and autonomy. Sometimes medical decision-making at the end of life devolves into squabbling amongst family members about the true wishes of the comatose person. Some family members argue that their loved one would want any and all measures regardless of the quality of life that resulted from aggressive medical interventions. Others will cite conversations where they heard the patient say that they never wanted to be kept alive by tubes and machines. We have seen this played out in the media in a number of sensational cases over the years. This is why it is so important that you make your end-of-life wishes known while you are of sound mind, so that there will be little question of your intentions when the time arises. It's best to do so in writing, on tape, CD, or some permanent recording so that you end your life the way you want to end it, with dignity.

The Special Exception

Organ transplantation is a special case in which HBOT could be useful even when brain death is involved. HBOT delivered to the brain dead donor and recipient immediately before transplantation could possibly suppress some of the reperfusion-inflammatory injury that occurs to the transplanted organ immediately after the procedure. This may be particularly important if the transplanted organ has to be transported significant distances, thereby increasing the time before the transplant procedure can begin. The longer the organ is without oxygen the greater this reperfusion injury can be.

Beyond situations involving brain death, it's difficult to delineate other conditions where hyperbaric oxygen therapy is inappropriate. Often, the mantra of hyperbaric critics that "there is no evidence" for HBOT in a given condition is limited by language barriers, or better put, our cultural habit to speak only a single language in the United States. Let me explain. In the mid-1990s, I got my hands on the abstracts from the 7th International Congress on Hyperbaric Medicine, held in Moscow. I was amazed at the breadth of over 300 papers presented. For at least a decade before the conference, the Russians had been applying HBOT to everything under the sun and finding positive results in many situations. For example, they have treated asthma, peptic ulcer disease, chest pain due to heart disease, and a variety of chronic disease conditions that reinforced my research and belief that the boundaries for hyperbaric oxygen therapy were near limitless.

This is also true for contraindications, or risks, of the treatment. Even conditions listed as "absolute" contraindications for hyperbaric oxygen, including pneumothorax (the abnormal presence of air in the chest between the lung and chest wall), are essentially relative contraindications. Nearly every single contraindication including the worst pulmonary conditions can be successfully accommodated. In fact, over the last 30 years my group has treated patients with nearly every pulmonary contraindication in a hyperbaric chamber without harm. But of course, in these situations, the doctor has to carefully and skillfully accommodate the patient's condition.

The other reason that precludes making broad statements about what conditions we should exclude from HBOT is that brain injuries are idiosyncratic. They are like a fingerprint of that individual and a combination of the person's normal brain, plus the genetically determined blood supply pattern in the brain, along with the individual peculiarities of the brain injury.

To add further complication, every person has a different response and tolerance to increased levels of oxygen, which is one major reason that research results have varied widely. Susceptibility or individual tolerance to oxygen is best understood when considering experiments and information involving oxygen toxicity.

A given patient can respond to the same dose of oxygen in a different way on any given day or hour. A previous oxygen toxicity reaction caused by exposure to three atmospheres of oxygen for two hours on one day might be precipitated by a mere one-hour exposure another day or a three-hour exposure on a third day. This remains an unpredictable factor; we can't characterize a person's response beforehand.

CHAPTER 14

ROADBLOCKS AND GATEWAYS
TO THE FUTURE

D ESPITE SOME OF THE SETBACKS AND ROADBLOCKS
involved in moving HBOT into mainstream medicine once and for
all, I remain optimistic about its future for you and your loved ones.
However, as it currently stands, finding HBOT in the United States is not a
straightforward process; in fact, it involves some twists and turns, and raises the
issues ever present in the story of this treatment. HBOT's journey into wide
acceptance also sheds light on the intricacies of medical economics and politics,
and because availability and reimbursement for HBOT may be complicated
at times, research issues also become involved. However, I urge you to use the
information in this book to guide discussions of treatment with your healthcare
providers, as well as to spread the word about the treatment. I have always
believed that medical consumers have far more power than they know.

Thus far, I have discussed the historical context in which HBOT developed,
the way in which it works in the body, and the scientific arguments for its
effectiveness as a treatment for numerous diseases. As I've said before, I believe
the misperceptions about hyperbaric oxygen therapy are rooted in the inability
of earlier pioneers to adequately define HBOT and explain how—and therefore
why—the treatment works. This is why the argument that HBOT is a brain
repair drug and acts on the DNA and other cellular structures is so important
to its future. This understanding allows us to see the magnitude of potential for
hyperbaric oxygen therapy, particularly in the treatment of the neurological
diseases discussed in this book. It's also important to understand that HBOT

is very effective for many diseases that are not yet on the list of approved applications.

What Does "Off-Label Use" Mean?

This is a critical term for those seeking treatment because it represents an issue that could stand in the way of obtaining reimbursement from your health insurance provider. But let's start at the beginning. As you probably know, doctors still take the Hippocratic Oath, which over the history of medicine dictates that a physician will attempt to treat patients and prescribe therapies with possible benefit while doing a minimum of harm. Hence, we hear the phrase, "First, do no harm."

In the United States, with the advent of the Food and Drug Administration (FDA), this traditional Hippocratic practice of medicine took on a new term: off-label, used with respect to an FDA-approved drug or device. Briefly, FDA approval means the FDA has approved marketing of the drug or device by the manufacturer for certain indications, which is known as "labeling." For instance, an antibiotic may be approved and labeled by the FDA for use in treating infections in various organs or organ systems of the body that are caused by specific organisms sensitive to that antibiotic. Once any drug or device is approved by the FDA, all doctors licensed to practice in the United States are allowed to use that drug or device in any way they choose to treat their patients. In other words, a doctor may know that a particular FDA-approved drug is effective to treat a condition for which the FDA has not yet labeled it. Using a treatment in this way is compatible with the Hippocratic practice of medicine, but in today's medical context it is now called an "off-label" use of an FDA-approved drug or device.

It usually surprises people to learn how much medical treatment is composed of off-label use of FDA-approved drugs and devices. Take the drug Zyban, first approved by the FDA as the drug Wellbutrin—an antidepressant. A psychiatrist noted that patients who were smokers and also depressed lost their craving for cigarettes once they began taking Wellbutrin. As this phenomenon became known, physicians all across the country began prescribing Wellbutrin to help patients quit smoking. So, doctors wrote millions and millions of prescriptions for this off-label use of Wellbutrin.

It's important to understand that this off-label prescription is entirely legal.

The FDA does not regulate the practice of medicine, but only prohibits the manufacturer from advertising a use for a drug or device for which the FDA has not labeled it. The drug company that made Wellbutrin performed studies on its use in smoking cessation, and when they found evidence to support this use, they reapplied to the FDA to approve Wellbutrin for smoking cessation. The FDA complied; Wellbutrin used for depression was still called Wellbutrin, but Wellbutrin for smoking cessation was named Zyban.

In pediatrics, scarcely any of the routine medications given to children have actually been tested on children. Almost all were tested and approved for use in adults and then used off-label in pediatrics. I have to chuckle when I hear critics of HBOT for pediatric neurological diseases attempting to disparage HBOT because it is an "off-label" use.

Except for chambers introduced before 1977 and a few models since then, all chambers in the United States are FDA-approved, therefore "labeled," for the original 13 uses for HBOT. They are not labeled for the two newest indications. However, in an earlier meeting with the FDA group that approves hyperbaric chambers in the United States, members of this group admitted that as they more thoroughly examined the evidence they realized that a considerable number of the approved uses did not have sufficient scientific proof to warrant labeling. Nevertheless, those remained the approved uses of hyperbaric chambers in the United States, and anything beyond this is considered off-label. Astounding as it may seem, nearly all of the neurological indications described in this book are considered off-label. (As you'll recall, we listed the approved uses in Chapter 3.) Keep in mind, however, that this situation exists only in the United States. In many other countries, the neurological conditions discussed in this book are considered standard accepted indications for hyperbaric oxygen therapy.

In addition, the unlabeled chambers mentioned above have no restrictions on them and hence there is no true label or off-label use. Those chambers can be used to treat any disease as long as a doctor prescribes it (just like all the other chambers), but the term off-label is not applied to them.

In the early 2000s, Environmental Tectonics Corporation, through the urging and assistance of the IHMA, submitted an application to the FDA to have one of their new chambers labeled for treatment under a doctor's prescription, without tying the labeling to any particular diagnosis. Essentially, there was no such thing as using the chamber "off-label." I have to admit the practice of medicine seems crazy at times, but this distinction is actually critical. When a doctor or an insurance company wants to discourage or prohibit the use of something, they say it is "off-label," hence, "bad" or "useless." This is often the way HBOT is dismissed. And if the indication the patient asks about is not on the approved list, then many doctors are quick to point that out. Hospital hyperbaric departments have also used this as an excuse not to treat.

As a patient, you should know that the FDA has *not* prohibited use of HBOT beyond the accepted indications list. So, no matter how the chamber in a facility is labeled, you should be able to receive hyperbaric treatment for an off-label indication.

It is likely that most of the neurological applications will remain off-label for some years into the future. FDA approval will not come until a substantial amount of research money is devoted to generating large clinical trials. As we all know, this can take years and years—even decades. But your medical care should not depend on political infighting, which can delay approval and availability even more. More importantly, whether something is label or off-label has nothing to do with whether it works or whether it can be offered to a given patient. And it should not unduly influence your decision to try the treatment, especially when evidence shows the possibility that it will help your condition.

The importance of FDA labeling, however, is that labeling makes it easier to obtain HBOT for a given condition in the hospital setting. Many hospital hyperbaric units will use the lack of FDA labeling as an excuse to deny a patient HBOT unless the patient has inside connections. The other important factor is that FDA labeling can facilitate reimbursement from an insurance carrier since FDA approval implies that substantial research has proven the effectiveness and safety of the drug or device for a labeled condition. However, as previously mentioned the FDA approved a good number of the thirteen indications for HBOT without adequate scientific proof.

Why Research Challenges May Affect You

As you've read in this book, hyperbaric physicians use treatment protocols for a variety of applications. However, HBOT tends to be an individualized therapy and responses to it are varied. Today, with our improved SPECT brain blood flow imaging, we now have a way to assess early on if a particular individual can respond to hyperbaric oxygen. However, we still don't know whether that dose is the best dose unless we look at a SPECT image after every different dose of HBOT. While this is certainly possible, it is prohibitively expensive, and therefore impractical.

This individual susceptibility causes difficulties in research, especially when the studies include only a small number of cases. If we all have a different susceptibility to a different dose of oxygen, giving a single dose or a narrow dose range will render a response in only a certain percentage of patients. This may not be large enough to provide the statistical significance generally desired in scientific studies.

Sometimes medical research is described in a generalized way and may leave the impression that virtually anything can be studied using one standard methodology. For example, individual responses to drug doses exist, too, but major studies funded by pharmaceutical companies are able to overcome this with massive amounts of capital. They may also enroll many thousands of patients in a study; such large numbers allow investigators to overcome individual idiosyncrasies. In addition, many drugs, particularly antibiotics, do not rely so much on an individual susceptibility to the antibiotic. Instead, it's dependent on a bacterium's response. If it's been shown in tissue culture or a test tube, for example, that the known offending bacterium is killed 99 percent of the time by a given drug, we know that when we give it to patients they have a 99 percent chance that if the antibiotic reaches the bacterium it will be killed. In other words, it's not as dependent on each individual patient as it is with an exposure to hyperbaric oxygen.

Research Data and Reimbursement Issues

These research issues may come up not only when you and your doctor consider undergoing HBOT, but also when insurance companies or public health agencies are involved in approving and reimbursing care. For example, at this point we can't accurately predict the cost benefit return for HBOT, especially in certain cases such as years after a stroke or when Alzheimer's is advanced, or in severe birth injuries. Cost benefit analysis is usually done for a patient on an individual basis, in a retroactive fashion. It is my hope, however, that eventually, as HBOT is used more widely over the next few years, we'll have large numbers of patients we can compare—especially those who received HBOT compared to those with similar diagnoses who did not. Collecting and analyzing data to reach meaningful conclusions often requires investments in adequate funds to hire skilled researchers. I'm sure I don't need to tell you that funding for a host of worthy projects is always scarce.

The situation is somewhat different when considering individual benefits as compared to cost. For example, if you or your loved one undergoes HBOT, you can assemble medical bills before and after treatment, and use this evidence to justify HBOT and its reimbursement. In terms of overall future acceptance with severe birth injury it likely wouldn't take many cases to prove cost benefit, but at present we still have, relatively speaking, few cases involving birth injury in the United States. If we include the Chinese studies we have nearly 1,000 cases from which to make our argument. Those of us who treat these children do so after the fact, and frankly, the cost of medical care for a child born in extremis usually results in months of care in a neonatal ICU. Hospital costs are in the hundreds of thousands of dollars and sometimes exceed one million dollars. Because of this, we could see a turn of the tide in the treatment of these children if as few as five or ten children known to have severe birth injury received HBOT and subsequently had far fewer ongoing problems that required a lifetime of various treatments. Unfortunately, we haven't been able to generate data on this in the United States as yet.

What You Should Know in Emergency Situations

Although I wish I could reassure you about the availability of treatment in emergency settings, I can't do so at this time. But I can offer a reason why research can both help and hinder your quest for treatment, particularly if you are seeking HBOT for acute severe traumatic brain injury. Multiple studies in animals and humans, including metabolic studies (which look at various blood markers that measure metabolism, such as the way the body uses glucose) and studies that measured intracranial pressure or swelling have now shown that HBOT in acute severe traumatic brain injury can significantly reduce mortality. Yet, HBOT is not routinely or frequently used in these cases, in part because the reviews have been inadequate and in some cases, suppressed.

In 1992, results of the Rockswold study of acute severe traumatic brain injury were released[1]. These results showed that the group of patients who did not receive HBOT had a 150 percent increased chance of dying compared to those who received HBOT. Put another way, the HBOT patients had a reduction in death rate of 60 percent. These are astounding figures, and one would have thought the cable news shows would have been filled with stories about this great advance in emergency medicine. However, the study results were cast in a negative light that generated a non-scientific moral judgment. Specifically, the results were dismissed essentially because researchers had not found a greater percentage of patients in the hyperbaric group in the "good outcome" category, even though there was a highly significant reduction in death if you received HBOT.

Sadly, the "good outcome" category was defined as the highest functioning group, those patients who at least potentially could return to work or to a nearly normal lifestyle. But remember, these patients suffered severe brain injury; many were close to death. It was ludicrous to expect these patients to fully recover from these significant brain injuries and once again function at their pre-injury level. The fact that so many more within the control group died speaks to the severity of their injuries.

What should have been shouted from the rooftops is that so many were saved—it was a monumental scientific achievement that had great implications on a human level. In almost no other area of medicine is saving life and reducing mortality disparaged or discounted, as I recounted in the earlier discussion of TBI. Frankly, the way the article was interpreted, hyperbaric oxygen saved a bunch of severely brain damaged individuals who would become a drag on the medical system. Hence, we saw a moral judgment that we should not apply a therapy that saves a group of non-productive, non-functional, high expense individuals.

We can take this kind of twisted reasoning one step further. If we apply the same dysfunctional reasoning, why do we give any therapy to a severely brain injured individual if we know it will result in a severely disabled individual? For example, individuals with a gunshot wound to the head or a head injury from a high-speed motor vehicle accident in which the patient stops breathing at the scene are in a high mortality group. Even if they survive, they have a poor outcome. Emergency procedures at the scene, such as securing the patient's airway, breathing for the patient, and obtaining ambulance transport are going to result in lessening the mortality of the patient. However, we don't stop our efforts at the scene. We don't say that since this patient is going to be a drag on the medical system, let him or her die at the scene. Rather, we do everything we can to save these injured individuals. Why wouldn't we add HBOT to save even more?

In December 2009, I asked this same question to a group of the top brain injury specialists from the U.S. military and civilian medical communities at the Department of Defense Consensus Conference on HBOT and Traumatic Brain Injury, held in Arlington, Virginia. The conference was convened as a result of the HBOT treatments I delivered to brain injured servicemen, along with the pressure Bill Duncan and Martin Hoffmann had brought to bear in Washington, D. C.

After Dr. Rockswold presented a review of HBOT in acute severe traumatic brain injury, I asked him and the audience why we weren't using HBOT to save more of our brain injured soldiers. I cited the example of the soldier who is shot in the head on the battlefield and whom we know is going to have a severe brain injury and long-term disability. Given that he is going to be "a drag on the medical system" why don't we just stand there, say a prayer, and let him die? There was stunned silence as all realized that we are applying the rules unevenly when it comes to HBOT in acute severe traumatic brain injury. I was told that we would take it up at another conference.

Let's remember that it's not up to the medical profession to make this kind of a moral and financial judgment. It's simply not our place to decide what degree of recovery is "worth it" or "acceptable." Families make these decisions, and ultimately, society in general is involved. And, speaking as a doctor, it is not up to me to define your good outcome; or, as I've said in this book, your miracle. My job is to offer the best treatment options I'm aware of and supply scientific evidence to make informed decisions.

The families of those who were given hyperbaric oxygen therapy and survived at least had the possibility of a continued relationship with their loved one on some level. In addition, these surviving patients also had the opportunity to receive other therapies that could help them improve—advance them to higher levels of functioning. They are also candidates for new therapies that may be developed or discovered some years into the future from which they may benefit at that time. Death precludes all of these options.

Based on what we currently know, we can't measure outcomes from traumatic brain injury and stroke at one year. The brain continues to develop, remodel, and improve for years and years after the injury. Had they been followed over a period of years, the group receiving HBOT may have gone on to function at higher levels than the control group. Since I have seen this long-term improvement in patients myself and treated hundreds of them years after their injury, I know this is possible.

I mention the Rockswold study because it is an example that tells us of the monumental effort involved in reversing worn out attitudes and inadequate reviews about HBOT for acute severe traumatic brain injury. These attitudes have developed over the last 40–50 years and are entrenched in much of the neurological medical community, but among some in hyperbaric medicine, too.

What's important here is that the Rockswold study was not a single isolated study. In the 1970s, the Germans[2] had shown that the pressure of HBOT subsequently adopted by Rockswold had a beneficial effect on brain metabolism in 30 patients with either severe traumatic brain injury or severe stroke. They followed this article with a randomized prospective controlled trial, the "holy grail" of medical research[3], like the Rockswold study on patients with the traumatic mid-brain syndrome. A similar study was done in France with positive results in the younger group who received HBOT[4].

A mid-brain syndrome patient is someone whose mid-brain and lower structures are the only working portions of their brain. These patients are in a coma on a ventilator with no response to any stimulation. Essentially, this is the identical type of group in Rockswold's study that had such a good response to HBOT.

The Holbach study also showed the same 60 percent reduction in mortality in the HBOT group, or 150 percent increased chance of death in those who did not receive HBOT. Moreover, the ones who lived had better outcomes than the non-HBOT group. Dr. Rockswold (a neurosurgeon, not a hyperbaric physician) couldn't believe Holbach's results were true, so he wanted to do the definitive study to confirm Holbach's findings—and that's exactly what he did.

Let's belabor the point just a bit more. Subsequent to Holbach and Rockswold, Dr. H. Ren in China duplicated both of these studies and found, you guessed it, the same 60 percent reduction in mortality in the HBOT group and 150 percent increased chance of death in the non-HBOT group[5]. Four countries, four studies, four nearly identical outcomes.

As if that wasn't enough, in 2001 Dr. Rockswold and his daughter went back and did some more fine-tuning and found that a single HBOT in acute severe traumatic brain injury had a profoundly positive effect on the damaged brain's metabolism that had never been recorded in the history of science and medicine[6]. The Rockswolds concluded that HBOT should be delivered as soon as possible after severe traumatic brain injury. Sadly, this has not happened. So, why aren't we using HBOT in acute severe TBI?

In 2001, Bill Duncan, Dr. Neubauer, and I met with Dr. John Eisenberg, the director at Medicare's Agency for Healthcare Research and Quality, the evidence arm of Medicare that makes recommendations on reimbursement for new therapies. Dr. Eisenberg commissioned a study of the scientific literature on HBOT in neurology. I was invited to be a peer reviewer and consultant to the project and sent the study investigators at the Oregon Health and Science University's Evidence Based Practice Center fourteen FedEx boxes with literature from my files.

Unfortunately, the conclusion reached, now known as the AHRQ Report[7], was based on misinterpretation and misunderstanding of all of the literature I just cited above. Furthermore, the main authors of the commissioned study didn't have the credentials or scientific backgrounds in hyperbaric medicine and brain injury neurology to properly interpret the literature based on its science. In August 2004, the traumatic brain injury component of the AHRQ report was published in the *Archives of Physical Medicine and Rehabilitation*. In a Letter to the Editor finally published in April, 2006, titled "Medicine That Overlooks the Evidence[8]," I pointed out how the authors of the AHRQ study ignored the science and came to their inaccurate conclusions.

Meanwhile, the Hyperbaric Oxygen Committee of the Undersea and Hyperbaric Medical Society rejected my application in 2001 to have acute severe traumatic brain injury added to the vaunted 13 "accepted indications" list, citing the need—initiated that day, mind you—to change the manner in which they score and approve new indications. Acute severe traumatic brain injury just happened to have one of the highest scores of any of the 13 accepted indications in terms of scientific evidence. Curiously, these "new rules" were conveniently rescinded in 2006 to allow the inclusion of the newest "accepted indication," central retinal artery occlusion.

To belabor this even further, the Drs. Rockswold just published yet another proof of effect of HBOT in acute severe traumatic brain injury. In a 2010 issue of *Journal of Neurosurgery*[9], Drs. Rockswold showed that HBOT had a markedly beneficial effect on brain function that was significantly greater than oxygen at normal atmospheric pressure and room air. An editorial accompanied the article; for the first time, HBOT was lauded as a potential significant therapy for acute traumatic brain injury. But the Rockswolds weren't done yet. They published yet *another* study, this time about a protocol of once-daily HBOT, plus three hours of oxygen for three days in a row. As in all the previous studies, they found a major reduction in mortality. In addition, they demonstrated an improvement in favorable outcomes, thus negating the main complaint lodged against their first study.

How many studies does it take? I don't know; but the evidence of effectiveness of just a few HBOTs delivered soon after severe traumatic brain injury is overwhelming and far exceeds the evidence for the standard of care.

The point of all of this discussion, which is rather boring—until your loved one has acute severe traumatic brain injury and is in danger of dying—is that the scientific evidence supports the use of HBOT in acute severe traumatic brain injury to save lives. Period. However, a badly flawed "evidence-based medicine" review by primary authors with pharmacy and bioinformatics degrees enters the picture, along with a rejection based on "rules changes" and politics by a committee whose decisions affect reimbursement. These flaws are no minor matter. At this point, they mean that you cannot obtain HBOT for your acute severe traumatic brain injury, even when it decreases your chance of dying by 60 percent. This comedy, or rather "tragedy" of errors and misinterpretation and misunderstanding of the science—and its implications—leads me to one very important conclusion: The medical profession at the institutional level cannot be trusted to act in the public's best interest medically when it comes to making scientific decisions that determine reimbursement for medical care. It is time for the lay public to be brought into the medical reimbursement decision-making process.

At this point you have the scientific evidence to demand the application of HBOT to save the life of your loved one with acute severe traumatic brain injury, and I strongly encourage you to do so.

The other reason why the lay public needs to have a deciding voice in medical reimbursement has to do with the hyperbaric medicine specialty itself. I've talked about the boom-bust cycles of HBOT, in large part due to over-optimism and "amazing" claims, coupled with inadequate definition and understanding of

HBOT. It also has been a medical orphan at times, lacking adequate protection and defense, so to speak, even by its practitioners. For example, the Hyperbaric Oxygen Therapy Committee of the Undersea and Hyperbaric Medical Society has no current neurologist or neurosurgeon member, and has had neither since 1986. How can you defend, let alone promote, HBOT for neurological applications if you have no one with special knowledge or experience in this field? You can't. Furthermore, the curious political climate in the hyperbaric medicine field has held back the therapy and kept it from advancing into neurorehabilitation.

While I won't go into this in detail, personal, non-medical issues within the hyperbaric medicine field itself have been at the root of the lack of advancement of HBOT in neurology for the past 30 years. Unfortunately, these influences continue to this day, although they are slowly waning as a result of—for lack of a better term—"the natural order of things." Once again, I'll quote quantum physicist Max Planck: when he was dismayed by the lack of acceptance of his and Einstein's mathematical proofs, he said: "Science progresses funeral by funeral." While I'm no Einstein or Planck, and this is not rocket science, my problem is that you, your brain-injured loved one, and I cannot and should not have to wait for the doctors to die in order for the science to advance! We need it yesterday.

Finally, I believe the lay public is at least vaguely aware of the "culture of medicine," meaning that doctors allow long-held assumptions within their fields, and personality issues, too, to influence attitudes toward treatment. Until recently, medical information and the profession itself existed as a relatively insular world. However, all of this has changed. The Internet alone, not to mention cable news networks and a plethora of science and health channels, have made it possible for everyone to access scientific literature.

No longer is vital medical information sequestered or made inaccessible even to those in another medical specialty. The entire public can read and review articles. This will help move HBOT, and other therapies, into the mainstream.

An Additional Factor

Another impediment to receiving immediate care is the growing trend for corporate hyperbaric medicine. By this I mean that all over the country, companies install hyperbaric wound care departments in hospitals. However, these are limited care operations—open Monday through Friday, "business hours" only, and many of them lack on-call or weekend service. Unfortunately, babies are not always born during banker's hours. Right now, we need these hospital facilities to be available 24 hours a day to treat emergencies as well as the elective outpatients.

In 1999, this type of artificial restriction hit home when a neighboring hospital emergency department wanted to transfer two severely carbon monoxide–poisoned patients to our facility. (As it happens, Hurricane Katrina subsequently destroyed this hospital.) However, a hyperbaric chamber was in a professional building just across the parking lot from that hospital. Both patients could have been in hyperbaric chambers long before they reached my facility. To my surprise and shock, that facility didn't treat carbon monoxide poisoning, which as you recall, is one of the conditions for which HBOT is approved.

This situation makes no sense at all. That facility had chambers and a hyperbaric physician. "Time was brain" (to quote the famous stroke treatment catchphrase in the past tense) as the carbon monoxide continued to destroy and damage these patients' brain cells, They could have easily treated both of these patients, whose lives, after all, were held in the balance. But the facility claimed they didn't have a doctor on call; thus, they didn't offer emergency services.

In a series of questions that turned into demands, I was finally able to speak with the hyperbaric physician who in fact was available, but he held fast to the policy—no night and weekend services. And these patients had the bad luck to be injured on a Saturday at 10 o'clock in the morning! The two patients came to our facility, which was run 24 hours a day, 7 days a week. The decision against maintaining this type of availability is likely due to the bottom line. It's expensive to pay doctors and staff to be available 24 hours a day. Moreover, it is expensive to treat these emergencies. More importantly, many carbon monoxide poisoned patients are in the lower socioeconomic groups that are least likely to have medical insurance, a fact that is not lost on the corporate providers of hyperbaric services.

This situation points to a couple of issues that relate to birth injuries. Obviously, if a hyperbaric chamber is in every obstetrics department we would not have to worry about the immediate availability of treatment for newborns. However, if a chamber is available in emergency departments, then it could treat patients of all ages. What we *don't* need, however, is greater proliferation of "half services," that is, HBOT available only in offsite professional buildings whose medical staff can't or won't respond to true emergencies.

My ideal labor and delivery rooms would be equipped with a hyperbaric oxygen chamber. A simple 32- to 40-inch diameter chamber would be able to accommodate a neonate and an inside attendant. Although a multiplace chamber would be ideal, a smaller chamber may be adequate. With a small chamber in place, infants born in distress, perhaps because of ruptured placenta or other conditions in which they are deprived of both blood and oxygen, could immediately be placed in a hyperbaric chamber, thereby treating the reperfusion injury and low oxygen components of the injury without delay.

Case Study Research

Although we've engaged in ongoing attempts to obtain funding from the National Institutes of Health to investigate using HBOT in a rigorous fashion, we've encountered tremendous resistance. The details of the controversy are not important here, but they involve differences in ideas about some specific treatment methodologies. In addition, as you now understand, some in medicine generally oppose HBOT for all but a few narrowly defined applications.

However, when you are educating yourself about the multiple applications of HBOT, the importance of case studies can never be understated or minimized. Case studies are the seeds that generate most research and help lay the foundation for plausibility of effectiveness when there is no knowledge of the underlying mechanisms of disease or treatment. Unfortunately, within medicine, a bad habit persists with respect to case studies, and that's to pejoratively refer to them as "anecdotes," which as I previously said, is "an amusing narrative or hearsay account." When we have a series of case studies with the same results they are referred to as "a series of anecdotes." But, as I point out, it's insulting to patients to have their medical history referred to as "anecdotal." To the patient and their family there is nothing amusing about the devastating nature of their injury and their plight. I've often quipped to colleagues that in medical school we should submit to psychosurgery to have this word removed from our brains.

In addition, each case study is not just another case study; they aren't all the same. Some are very powerful, and the most telling are the chronic cases, the patients who have suffered from some affliction for years and exhausted literally every therapy in the process, often to no avail. Then, and often through a series of events, they try a new treatment and experience a change for the better.

To what do we attribute the positive change? A miracle? Divine intervention? I suppose, but we don't like to talk about that in "science." How about the "placebo effect?" But this means that during the previous years (and treatments) patients didn't really want to get better, but they suddenly decided to believe in this therapy and, voila! It worked. We end up with explanations that the patient liked the doctor or trusted the big orange pill. Or, in some cases, it was apparently just time for the person to get better—it's explained as the natural history of the disease. We even address the problem of "malingering," that is, the patient grows weary of their "con game," and decides to "act normal."

I thought I had heard it all—until I heard the latest creative explanation of the placebo effect offered by the Department of Defense doctors in their HBOT concussion study. They explained that the "ritual" of going in a hyperbaric chamber, namely resting, watching a movie, or taking a snooze daily was responsible for the significant improvement in cognition and symptoms.

In all of these years, the vast majority of my patients with neurological problems just want their brain back—their lives back—by whatever means, regardless of whether they are on Workers' Comp Insurance, disability, or are involved in litigation. And many have tried myriad therapies unsuccessfully until they found HBOT.

The acute case, one in which a therapy is delivered close to the time of the injury that causes a remarkable unexpected clinical outcome, also makes a powerful argument. What often happens is that the patient improves, the therapy is then withdrawn, and the patient languishes. We reinstitute the therapy after a period of time and the patient makes a quantum leap in improvement, temporally related to reintroduction of the therapy. This also provides a strong argument for effectiveness of the therapy. This type of study is called a "single case causality study" or "n of 1 proof." (Causality means the therapy caused the improvement and "n of 1" refers to the number of patients in the study, 1.)

Overcoming the Dilemma of Finding Emergency Treatment

Part of the treatment dilemma involves the existence of some hyperbaric medical societies that threaten their members with disciplinary action if they treat conditions that do not appear on a very narrow list of indications (listed in

Chapter 3). The clever way this is stated is "treating for profit." The demand is that any physician in these medical societies who treats conditions outside this narrow list should only do so under a research protocol or for free. What has resulted is a "speak-easy" situation at hospitals. For example, doctors increasingly call me from hospitals around the county to ask about treatment of children or adults with acute neurological emergencies. These doctors may ask not to be identified, but they go on to treat the patient and hope word doesn't get back to their professional associations. (I know that situation sounds hard to believe, given what you're learned about HBOT. Likewise, with chronic brain injury, some doctors in hospital-based hyperbaric departments override the "Big Brother" effect of these medical societies.)

Knowing that obtaining emergency treatment isn't always easy, what you can do right now is locate the nearest hospital with a hyperbaric chamber. Then, in an emergency the family can ask that the person be taken to that hospital. Obviously, there is a trade-off if significant extra transport time is involved, that is, if the HBOT hospital is not the nearest facility. Certainly, if the person is at risk of dying unless he or she received immediate care, then life-saving is the priority and the patient must be transported to the nearest hospital.

At a hospital equipped with HBOT, you will at least have a chance to obtain treatment for an acute emergency, even if it is not on the current narrow list of indications. If you have a working vocabulary of HBOT (and this book should give you that), you can talk about the evidence of the benefits with the treating doctor. In these cases, the physician may look at the evidence you cite and then treat your loved one. (The Resources includes websites with information and the chapter notes provide a convenient list of references that you can use.)

I won't pretend that at this time it is easy to obtain HBOT on an emergency basis. Even physicians sometimes must resort to more drastic measures. For example, Dr. Jeffrey Weiss is a doctor living and working in southern Florida. His child was involved in a near-drowning episode and rushed to the hospital. He gathered information from me and others about HBOT for his son, but he was unable to get the hospital to allow him to provide HBOT, and had to get a court order before he could go forward.

At the time, I spoke with the hospital administrator and a neurologist in my attempt to get them to treat Jeff's son. In fact, they called me to see if there was any science behind Dr. Weiss's desire to obtain HBOT for his child. Even with all the medical professionals involved and the science I placed in front of them, the major sticking point was the same old thing—misinformation and negative bias against HBOT that had been generated against a notable hyperbaric physician in their community. Despite the many obstacles put in front of him, Dr. Weiss was eventually able to have a hyperbaric chamber brought to the hospital, and he continued HBOT for his son long after hospital discharge. At the time of the near-drowning, the uniform prediction among the doctors was that his son would not survive or if he did he would be in a vegetative coma. Jeff's son is far from that today; he is alert, awake, and has some cognition and ability to communicate.

I realize this situation sounds bleak. But I suspect that as the general public reads about this treatment and sees reports of its use on television (as happened in late 2005 and early 2006 in the Sago mine accident), then individuals will push hard for HBOT in acute situations. With increasing frequency, families are willing to seek court orders, as Dr. Weiss did. In particular, I expect this to happen when evidence exists to show that hyperbaric oxygen can have a significant impact in acute brain injury. As I have mentioned above, the evidence is strongly in favor of treating acute severe traumatic brain injury. Your best tool to pressure for HBOT is knowledge of the treatment.

Beyond the Emergency

The great majority of neurological cases I have treated in the past 26 years and some of those described in this book have been chronic cases, often three to five or more years old. (The oldest injury occurred 44 years prior to treatment.)

You've read about some of these individuals in this book, and in a few cases, you've seen the imaging done that documented their injuries and improvement. This process will help you decide for yourself whether or not these adults and children are just a "series of anecdotes."

I believe that we can treat an astounding range of neurological diseases with hyperbaric oxygen. This makes sense, if you accept my premise that the initial exposure or insult is not so important since different injuries stimulate the inflammatory reaction, thus generating common residual pathology. For this reason, HBOT likely can repair the damage done in a vast number of different neurological diseases.

I came to this conclusion after five and a half years of investigating many patients with brain-based abnormalities using hyperbaric oxygen and SPECT brain imaging. (This was the Perfusion/Metabolism Encephalopathies Study referred to earlier.) At international meetings on HBOT, we see the range of diagnoses for which the Japanese, Chinese, and Russians have used HBOT. As I pointed out before, in 1981, Russian researchers reported over 300 different HBOT studies on everything from peptic ulcer disease to chronic bronchitis, heart disease, neurological disorders, and so forth.

The Chinese and Japanese also report HBOT use for cancer in combination with radiation or chemotherapy, childhood cerebritis (inflammation and infections of the brain), seizure disorders, cortical blindness in children, and other diseases. As a generic drug for brain injury repair, hyperbaric oxygen is potentially limitless.

The free-standing outpatient hyperbaric facilities cropping up in many cities across the United States are often unable to treat the acute conditions because they are not equipped for medical emergencies. However, they are capable of treating more chronic forms of brain injury, so you may be able to find this help closer to home than ever before. So, if you can't get HBOT in an emergency setting, you can get it as soon as you are out of the hospital in the post-acute setting.

I hope that obtaining hyperbaric oxygen therapy for sub-acute and chronic neurological conditions will soon no longer be a problem. In fact, much of the increased availability is going to be driven by patient demand. This has already occurred in Canada and in the United States with respect to the treatment of cerebral palsy. I have every reason to believe that this trend will continue as patients seek doctors willing to ignore the threats of restrictive medical societies.

In reality, until HBOT is widely available and accepted for stroke or any other condition you must become the patient-pioneer or care-finder-pioneer. And this is as true of HBOT as it is for many therapies, especially those that your doctor may not be aware of. This is essentially what has occurred with chiropractic, acupuncture, chelation therapy, and even the judicious use of nutritional supplements. Virtually everyone acknowledges that the patients who get the best medical care and have the best health outcomes are aggressively involved in their care. In other words, being proactive usually brings the best results.

The Financial/Reimbursement Issue

For acute severe brain injury resulting from such things as near-drowning, stroke, or cardiac arrest, hyperbaric oxygen therapy has been delivered in hospitals when patients' families have presented evidence to their primary physicians, who in turn asked the hyperbaric medicine physician to deliver the therapy. These situations are becoming increasingly common. It means that the hyperbaric physician doesn't have the responsibility of suggesting or initiating the therapy, but is acting at the request of other physicians. In these situations, the hyperbaric doctor feels protected, and as such, is more willing to administer the treatment, especially when some published data can be presented to them.

In contrast to HBOT for acute brain injuries, it is easier to both receive HBOT for chronic brain injuries and receive reimbursement authorization for it. An increasing number of facilities throughout the United States, primarily free-standing facilities, are evaluating and treating patients with chronic brain injury. Much of this use of HBOT was fueled by the mothers of children with brain injuries (see information about MUMS in Chapter 7 and Resources.) These facilities do not require detailed "proof," such as randomized controlled studies, beyond already existing published information in order to undertake a trial of hyperbaric oxygen therapy. In addition, in increasing numbers, patients are successfully obtaining reimbursement from insurance companies, especially when they're able to document the improvements. In a number of my current cases, I have even been able to obtain reimbursement from Workers' Comp insurance.

Patient Documentation

Documenting a patient's response to treatment can be done through video exams taken before and after treatment, medical reports by practitioners who have examined the patients before and after, and reports by other care-givers. I've mentioned doing video exams, and I believe they are important for many reasons, not the least of which is the contribution they make to the big picture. While many of my patients are not part of a formal study, their improvements are there for all to see, regardless of insurance reimbursement. These video exams become part of a body of information that supports at least trying HBOT under certain circumstances, and have value beyond what they accomplish for an individual patient. Of course, where possible, SPECT brain blood flow imaging also provides documentation. I believe patients should ask for this imaging, even though it is expensive.

An "improved bottom line" is perhaps the most important form of documentation to any insurance company or third-party payer. It's sad that medical care has been reduced to a dollars and cents issue in the United States, but if patients can show a reduction in healthcare cost, this is a critical factor. By this I mean that the costs to the payer after HBOT are less than they were before treatment, and are likely to continue to be less over the long-term. The insurance company then sees HBOT as a current investment that may bring them the return of reduced costs for that patient down the road. In that case, the investment looks sound, so they're more likely to authorize reimbursement.

As an aside, medical savings accounts or health savings accounts may help some individuals pay for HBOT should a future need arise. These accounts allow reduced insurance premiums while the owner puts the balance of the premium into a medical IRA. A contribution to a medical savings account is tax deductible, but separate from normal IRA contributions. The owner of the funds that accrue in the medical IRA can use the money for medical therapies with minimum restrictions. In other words, if the insurance company will not pay for hyperbaric oxygen therapy, a medical savings account often will.

Looking for Help to Pay for Treatment

Currently, no single funding source is available for patients who cannot afford the treatment. Some organizations have started to generate the funds to treat patients in need. An organization based in Nevada, Miracle Flights for Kids (www.miracleflights.org), as well as a number of the major airlines are now providing markedly discounted flights to families with brain-injured children who must leave their home area to obtain HBOT. In order to make use of these programs, you must ask the airlines about them or call Miracle Flight for Kids. A number of other volunteer air flight organizations have announced similar programs.

These days, it's unlikely that you'd need to travel outside the country to receive HBOT. Many facilities exist in the United States that treat patients with chronic problems. Although in the past, some patients went abroad for treatment, for the average person travel and lodging costs are prohibitive. Fortunately, we are far enough along in making the treatment widespread that we've lessened the need to travel long distances to find treatment. However, when travel is required, some hotels near hyperbaric facilities offer special rates because the patient and a family member move into the hotel for several weeks at a time.

The network of Ronald McDonald House facilities are another national provider. Until it was damaged by Hurricane Katrina, many of my patients stayed in the New Orleans Ronald McDonald House. However, thanks to generous donations, it was reopened in August 2006. These facilities are the largest providers of housing for the brain-injured children who come to my clinic. We are indebted to them, and continue to support their annual fundraiser, The Hugs and Kisses Chocolate Ball.

Educating Yourself—and Your Doctors

The publications of the International Congresses on Hyperbaric Medicine are good sources of information for patients, and also for doctors. These books (available through Best Publishing Company; see www.bestpub.com) contain multiple studies done in the Far East, Russia, and other countries on hyperbaric oxygen therapy in neurological and other conditions.

While it's true that some doctors don't consider this type of publication (those coming from symposia, workshops, and so forth) reliable information, when we look at the mosaic of scientific evidence available, these publications have a place. In fact, any written material published in a proceeding of the International Congress on Hyperbaric Medicine may influence your doctors, at least to the extent that they become educated about treatment taking place in another part of the world. To reiterate, when oxygen is elevated to pressure it acts like a drug and has many drug effects, such as DNA signaling capability. When your doctor understands this, it can have a positive effect on your medical care. Remember, many doctors only want to see that someone has done it before them so they don't have to be the pioneer.

The Internet has become the premier source of information for many patients. Many hyperbaric centers have websites, and you will find a surprising array of facilities, doctors, and organizations providing information on hyperbaric oxygen. The Internet is also a way to find treatment sites in your locale. Currently, various organizations are looking into providing training, protocols, and oversight of hyperbaric facilities and also fostering additional applications of HBOT.

While this book is not a scientific compendium, you may want to give a copy to your doctors, or short of that, a copy of some of the references provided. This exposure will enable them to better understand HBOT; plus, it opens a dialogue between you and your doctors about new treatments.

Long-Term Optimism: You Have Great Power

Despite my obvious strong feelings about some of the "messier" problems in the way medical care is delivered, I remain optimistic about the future of HBOT. The reason I'm optimistic is essentially because we are in an information age, and you have the power to present your doctor with research data about HBOT for a variety of conditions. Earlier I mentioned a doctor in Florida who was forced to take legal action to have his son (who had nearly drowned) obtain HBOT. This is an extreme measure, and not something I'm advocating in a general way, although in some situations it may indeed become the only avenue of recourse.

Many doctors and others who are part of the matrix of decision-makers in medicine often tell patients who ask questions about various treatments that more studies are needed. True, more studies are needed in many areas of medicine, including HBOT. But, in the area of brain injury, more studies are needed only to refine the dosage for the lesser levels of brain injury.

In terms of research, I would like to see long-term follow-up studies on those who survived acute severe traumatic brain injury. If we embarked on a large study, we might be able to refine the way these patients respond to HBOT both in the acute and chronic stages of their condition. This would be possible, because at least some of these surviving patients could then go on to blocks of treatments at a later date when the injury is chronic.

On the optimistic side, we're seeing an increasing awareness of HBOT and reappraisal of it as a viable medical treatment. I believe this positive perception is now achieving critical mass, which is good news for patients. It means that you or your loved one will be more likely to gain access to some of the off-label uses of HBOT. Of course, it also assumes that you're willing to look for doctors and hospitals whose administrators and medical committees and boards are not afraid to try this treatment.

The New Patient and the Old Paternalism

Lay public involvement with insurance companies' medical review panels and with the Centers for Medicare and Medicaid Services is one of the more important ways to influence the future application of HBOT. That sounds daunting, and it is, but the process to bring greater freedom of choice into healthcare has to begin somewhere. It's also needed, as cost often drives reimbursement decisions, not necessarily what is best for patients' health.

I'm suggesting this new avenue of influence based on the assumption that the lay public is capable of becoming medically well-informed and sophisticated enough to make decisions for themselves and their families. It has taken some time to reverse the old paternalism in medicine, the "doctor knows best and will take care of you" attitude that dominated healthcare in our society and elsewhere. The paternalistic model of medicine would still prevail across the board were it not for patients chipping away at it.

While the dissemination of information over the Internet and the availability of medical knowledge is certainly part of this trend, we can't forget that medical paternalism has been challenged for decades. Just as an example, hospitals have modern birthing rooms because women fought for them, and men no longer are sent off to waiting rooms while their wives are surrounded by medical staff. (I recall hearing about one father's waiting room being called "The Stork Club.") That one change came about from the bottom-up, so to speak, primarily from women demanding better and educating themselves and their doctors. I mention the above changes because patients, not the medical establishment, brought them about. They grew out of the larger women's movement, and today, we need new and already existing groups of health consumers to bring about equally revolutionary changes.

"We're Dancing as Fast as We Can"

Doctors who believe that HBOT is beneficial for a vast number of diseases are working hard to educate patients and other doctors. It has been an uphill battle, but we're seeing the top of the mountain. Ultimately, however, we will complete the climb to the top when patients join with us. In fact, we must have the lay public with us to achieve the critical awareness necessary to move HBOT into the mainstream—and become a household term.

Fortunately, many organizations have formed to help foster awareness of HBOT. In addition, patients' families, often overjoyed by the medical results of hyperbaric oxygen therapy in their loved one, are compelled to pursue reimbursement through Medicaid or other bodies. This has been particularly prominent among parents, especially mothers and one well-known father, who have publicized the results of treatment for their children. Likewise, those whose dysfunction continues because they have not been able to get this treatment also have advocates. These advocating organizations are bringing pressure (pun intended) to bear on the medical establishment and on the medical societies that continue to work against wide application of HBOT.

All of these factors contribute to the rising critical mass of awareness. I believe this is ultimately what will catapult hyperbaric oxygen therapy into the future. This has been a difficult road, but overall, I'm extremely optimistic and upbeat about the possibilities.

CONCLUSION

WHEN IS HBOT RIGHT FOR ME OR MY LOVED ONE?

As I've often said in this book, HBOT was discredited in the past because it was used for so many different and seemingly unrelated diseases. Some of its detractors thought the therapy was indiscriminately touted as a cure-all for every human ill. In 1987, this point was "infamously" made in an article, "Hyperbaric Oxygen: A Therapy in Search of Diseases," by Genevieve Gabb and Dr. Eugene Robin[1].

In short, the Gabb and Robin article offered a scathing criticism of the therapy, including a list of approximately 132 diagnoses for which HBOT had been used. The list includes many of the typically reimbursed indications we have today, a good number of the diagnoses I have written about in this book, and many others that I haven't.

For instance, Gabb and Robin mention radiation necrosis, decompression sickness, and carbon monoxide poisoning, which are reimbursed indications. They also mention retinal artery insufficiency, chronic brain ischemia (low blood flow), multi-infarct (stroke), and dementia, diagnoses I've discussed in this book. Gabb and Robin also listed many diverse conditions I haven't mentioned here. Just a tiny sample includes: scleroderma (an autoimmune disorder in the rheumatoid arthritis family), frostbite, brain cyst, tetanus, cerebral vasospasm (constriction of the arteries in the brain), and liver failure.

While I agree with Gabb and Robin that there was a paucity of solid clinical studies supporting HBOT at that time, the tenor of their discussion showed their bias, which was generally unscientific and even inaccurate, not to mention negative. Hyperbaric experts were enraged and quickly pointed out some of the animal and human studies supporting hyperbaric medicine. However, both they and Gabb and Robin lacked a fundamental understanding of HBOT's action on the basic disease processes characterizing such a huge number of diseases. Or, put another way, since these authors couldn't connect the dots between various diagnoses, they were unable to show how the web of dots beautifully illustrates the vast potential of this treatment.

Like others before them, those who criticized HBOT didn't realize that the therapy doesn't treat specific diseases as such, and should not be defined by the diseases it treats, but rather, HBOT treats the processes that cause and perpetuate the diseases, and it does so through gene modulation. Those who are confused about this basic premise, the foundation of HBOT, would naturally conclude that HBOT was much like a ship without a destination, haphazardly sailing into one port after another as it searched for its true home.

It's ironic, but this infamous list of diseases Gabb and Robin provided to make their "unflattering" point may in fact be a list we'd find quite useful today. When I scrutinize the long list of diagnoses in their article, I can group them into acute vs. chronic diseases, and further divide them along the lines of basic underlying disease processes at work. Then I can identify documented HBOT effects on these disease processes. By the time I'm finished analyzing this list, bringing with me an up-to-date understanding of HBOT, then I understand that HBOT may be an effective treatment for many of these diagnoses. I can at least understand why and how HBOT was used in the great majority of them. So, in effect, I connect the same dots that only confused Gabb and Robin, and "sew" common threads throughout this once seemingly jumbled maze of diseases.

With the treatment understood, it then follows that the discussions in this book illustrate why considering HBOT as a generic drug useful for basic disease processes is perhaps its greatest strength; it's most certainly not a weakness of the treatment. Imagine the world of medicine now. What could be more exciting or useful than discovering that one treatment has benefits for diagnoses numbering not just in the single or double digits, but perhaps in the hundreds? It's only the proper dose of HBOT that separates the treatment of all of them. Beyond that, as you've seen in this book, some common disease processes for which HBOT has been useful are among those that the medical community has considered untreatable.

The basic facts of the way HBOT works are critical, not just for your understanding, but for expanding your thinking, too. Rather than providing a single list of diseases and conditions, I want you to use the principles of HBOT to consider the possibility that HBOT may help you or a loved one, even if the specific disease was not mentioned in this book.

The Beauty of the "Sensible Notion"

In some cases, such as acute severe traumatic brain injury, substantial scientific proof exists in the form of clinical studies that argue for the application of HBOT. In other situations, we haven't accumulated as much data, and if we don't think expansively, we shut a door on a treatment too soon. For example, in Chapter 1 I talked about Orval Cunningham, a pioneer in HBOT, who argued for what he called a "Sensible Notion." If, for example, HBOT is effective for the basic disease processes in disease X, then would it not be a "Sensible Notion" to think that it would be effective in disease Y, where the underlying disease processes are the same or similar?

For a variety of reasons, Cunningham's "Sensible Notion" about HBOT didn't catch on in the conventional medical community. The inability to explain the way the treatment worked, as I've done in this book, led to HBOT descending into the proverbial basement of medical thinking and out of public view.

Fortunately, what stood in the way of Cunningham's progress no longer blocks our way today. In just the last 10 years we have witnessed an explosion in the number of credible basic science experiments (in many countries) that continue to add proof of the powerful effects of HBOT on basic disease processes. The best example of this is HBOT's effect on the secondary inflammatory response (reperfusion injury, see Chapter 2) where more than twenty studies using HBOT document its benefits. The even more impressive studies are those showing that HBOT is simply gene therapy at its finest.

This is an area about which I have written and spoken extensively, and have asked the critical question: Can HBOT be viewed as a generic drug for reperfusion injury? Having read this book, it won't surprise you to learn that after carefully examining many animal and human studies, I found that it doesn't matter whether it was a rat, pig, dog, or rabbit, the brain, heart, or intestines, and heart attack, cardiac arrest, or carbon monoxide poisoning, applying HBOT before, during, or immediately after the event had an overwhelmingly positive effect.

I made this argument at the 5th World Federation of Neurological Societies Meeting in Copenhagen in 1999[2]. Since that time, at least a dozen additional irrefutable scientific articles show the same findings. Essentially, a single, well-timed dose of HBOT is the most powerful drug for reperfusion injury. At this time, we only have a few studies of this conducted on human beings, but we are accumulating the human studies. Similarly, in chronic wound states the positive studies are mounting, and because of their results, we are picking off the diagnoses on Gabb and Robin's extensive list. More importantly, we're applying Cunningham's "Sensible Notion."

While we don't yet have a consensus or definitive studies on HBOT in human stroke, for example, the Hyperbaric Oxygen Therapy Committee of the UHMS has now approved the use of HBOT for acute Central Retinal Artery Occlusion (CRAO), a stroke of the eye (see Chapter 11 for a discussion of a case of CRAO successfully treated acutely with HBOT). In Chapter 11, I also recounted the case of a woman who had "compartment syndrome" of the eye, where high pressure in the eye shut off blood flow to her retina causing total blindness in that eye. She was successfully treated hours after waking up and discovering her blindness. You may recall that her ophthalmologist described this as "just another hyperbaric miracle for the eye."

As mentioned in Chapter 11, Dr. Heather Murphy-Lavoie reviewed all of the CRAO cases that she, Dr. Keith Van Meter, and I had treated over the years. She compared our cases to a group of patients with the same diagnosis who had received only standard treatment, but no HBOT. She found that the HBOT group showed markedly better results. In other words, the HBOT group had better return of vision. She presented her results to the HBOT Committee in June 2006, and now CRAO has been added to the "accepted indications" list— the first new indication in 10 years.

What is remarkable about this decision? No randomized "double-blind" controlled studies were done for CRAO, yet a substantial amount of data for what is usually considered an untreatable disease show HBOT is effective. For me, what is most important about this decision, however, is the realization that CRAO is a "stroke of the eye."

Further, if we apply Cunningham's "Sensible Notion," what is the difference between a stroke of the eye and a stroke of the brain? In fact, both involve brain tissue. (The aphorism, "The eye is the window of the soul" also means that it's a window to the brain.) Both conditions are characterized by the same disease processes, a blood clot in an artery.

HBOT's effect on the disease processes in CRAO should be identical to its effects in the disease processes in stroke of the brain. Additionally, HBOT is approved for use in a condition known as acute peripheral arterial insufficiency, which is a stroke in an artery of the arm or leg. To buttress this argument further, HBOT has been successfully used in acute strokes of transplanted livers. Again, what's the difference between the eye, an arm, a leg, the liver, or any other organ in the body deprived of blood flow? This is the question I invite you to ask; when you do, the only answer you can come to is that HBOT is potentially effective for a list at least as large as what Gabb and Robin presented!

As seen in many cases discussed in earlier chapters, this same thinking can also be applied to chronic wound states. For decades, both Dr. Neubauer and I recommended and used HBOT for a wide range of chronic neurological conditions with a range of success. By and large, we found that the greater the amount of damaged tissue, and the greater the proportion of dead to living tissue, the greater the number of HBOTs are necessary and the more modest the results, particularly in the short term.

Therefore, in very large chronic strokes where there is a substantial amount of dead brain tissue improvements with HBOT are more modest. The main benefit in these cases is to the rest of the "normal" aged brain, particularly if the brain has been abused by alcohol and tobacco throughout adulthood.

To give an example, to date, I've treated over 35 patients with chronic near-drowning. This is the most devastating of neurological injuries because the amount of affected brain tissue is substantial. With these children, improvements are more modest than nearly every other condition I have treated. Nevertheless, HBOT has the ability to improve symptoms, such as reducing seizures and improving cognition. However, with the extensive neurological damage we see in these situations, I would never tell parents that their children will be restored to what we call a normal condition or that they will get up and walk and talk.

Returning to stroke, based on my experience and the scientific arguments, HBOT has its greatest effect in treating chronic stroke when the event was a small vessel stroke, particularly the strokes that occur in the small vessels to the white matter of the brain. In each of these little strokes, the proportion of injured non-functional living brain tissue to dead tissue is large. This means that HBOT helps to "reclaim" function in a substantial proportion of the tissue affected in each little stroke. In 2005, Dr. J. F. Vila presented a study reaffirming this exact finding[3]: improvement in motor and cognitive impairment after hyperbaric oxygen therapy in a selected group of patients with cerebrovascular disease in a prospective single-blind controlled trial.

The International Results

To give you an idea about the scope of the work in HBOT, I cited papers coming out of Turkey, for example, on the usefulness of HBOT in Reflex Sympathetic Dystrophy[4] (mentioned by Gabb and Robin above), the disease of chronic severe pain in arms or legs of patients who have experienced trauma, infection, or surgery. In some cases, patients can't tolerate even the weight of a piece of tissue paper on their hand or leg without excruciating pain. HBOT was applied to these patients and they experienced a significant reduction in pain. Italian scientists had released a similar study some years before. You saw the proof of this in the video cited earlier that documents the treatment of my patient Vickie Harrison.

In 2006, a study conducted by doctors in Turkey showed that HBOT was useful to treat pain in fibromyalgia. That same year, an animal study by Texas doctors showed that HBOT can reduce inflammatory pain, further buttressing the Turkish study on fibromyalgia.

And, so it goes...one study after another continues to slowly pick off diagnoses on the Gabb and Robin list, and this body of research continues to affirm the argument made in this book, that HBOT has generic effects on basic disease processes in both acute and chronic diseases.

A fair number of the applications for HBOT I've suggested in this book are diagnoses that have been treated in foreign countries for years. Japan, China, Russia, Italy, and other countries have lists of applications much longer than what we have been restricted to in the United States. While one can criticize any single study, we continue to see the replication of findings, or put another way, study after study in many countries produce similar results.

The obvious conclusion is that HBOT's effects on a variety of disease processes are the same in human beings everywhere. So, to determine if HBOT may benefit you or a loved one, let's turn to the Gabb and Robin article and flip the argument to identify diseases in search of a therapy for their underlying processes. This makes sense, because when all the facts are presented, HBOT may be effective for the vast majority of the conditions listed in their article.

So, where is *my* list? There isn't one, and I won't list every possible diagnosis, because if I did, the list would mislead you. A list, no matter how long, would imply that you can pick out certain diagnoses and conditions, and in failing to see your condition on the list, you might exclude the treatment from your own list of possibilities. And that is not the line of thinking I intend to encourage.

When you make treatment decisions, I want you to ask questions about the basic underlying processes of the disease in question and then find out if HBOT has been shown to have beneficial effects on those disease processes. If so, then I invite you to apply Cunningham's "Sensible Notion" and try HBOT for your condition. Then, you can add *your* condition to the list.

Appendix A

Making—and Changing—Health Care Policy

A S I'VE SAID BEFORE, MEN AND WOMEN WHO SEEK
HBOT for themselves or their loved ones are medical pioneers, every
bit as much as the scientists and healthcare professionals who are always
looking for innovative, safe, and effective treatments for their patients. To medical
consumers, it may be difficult to understand how acceptance of new treatments
can take so long, and when it happens, they ask what tips the scale. I added
this section, describing the way in which Medicare finally approved HBOT
for diabetic foot wound healing, because it illustrates the journey that a new
treatment may take to find its way into the mainstream. Because I was involved
in this process myself, I, too, became even more aware of the way healthcare
policy evolves at this particular time.

Back to 1990

In 1990, President George H. W. Bush's administration launched the Healthy
People 2000 initiative, with one of its goals being reducing healthcare costs by
the year 2000. As one of its primary targets, it named preventing amputations,
particularly among the diabetic population. This represents a significant health
issue with great personal and financial consequences. In 2003, the Agency for
Healthcare Research and Quality (a federal agency), reported that that year,
70 percent of lower limb amputations were performed on diabetics. In strictly
economic terms, this means that these men and women became dependent on
tax dollars rather than generating revenue through taxes paid on earned income.
That sounds cold, but the government was and is primarily focused on and

concerned with costly disease, due to the rising healthcare costs and their far-reaching effects.

As I described in Chapter 9, the human cost of major amputations is serious, too, and often includes significant disability and premature death. In the early 1990s, the Bush administration saw that preventing amputations would have a significant impact on the healthcare budget, plus the overall health of this significant group in the population would improve. However, they still weren't looking at all the most effective ways to bring about this result.

Then, in 2001, as president of the new International Hyperbaric Medical Association (IHMA), I was able to secure a meeting with the deputy director of Medicare, Dr. John Whyte. This occurred through Bill Duncan (who wrote the introduction to this book), a contact of mine in one of the congressional offices. Bill Duncan's personal crusade to help get approval for HBOT to treat other conditions began because one of his family members (currently, four of his family members) had been helped dramatically by HBOT received at my clinic. Through his efforts, we were able to have this meeting with Dr. Whyte.

To simplify what was a complex conversation, I asked what we needed to do to get Medicare to approve HBOT for certain conditions, and Dr. Whyte explained the evidence they required to establish new indications. At that time, I realized that we had the evidence to satisfy the requirements for approval of two new indications, one of them diabetic foot wounds. After the meeting, I began to prepare the scientific argument for the effectiveness of HBOT for diabetic foot wounds. (The second indication was acute severe traumatic brain injury, discussed in Chapters 4 and 14.)

The Complexity of the Process

Remember that the amputation prevention mandate in the Healthy People 2000 initiative began in 1990, and it was already 2001 before a meeting took place to discuss the role HBOT could have in treating diabetic foot wounds. When my senior partner heard that I was assembling evidence for HBOT for the two indications, he encouraged me to contact members of the Undersea and Hyperbaric Medical Society (UHMS) and American College of Hyperbaric Medicine (ACHM), who were petitioning Medicare for approval of hypoxic wounds, which are characterized by low oxygen levels in the wound. (We attempt to surmise the oxygen level in the wound by measuring the oxygen level through the skin immediately around the wound.) The UHMS was arguing to Medicare that individuals with these wounds are candidates for HBOT. However, while treating such wounds was common practice in hyperbaric medicine, no new evidence on this matter had been put forth in some time, and I thought the existing evidence would not meet the scientific muster demanded by Dr. Whyte.

I then asked the individuals who had the most knowledge and had done the most research about HBOT in hypoxic wounds for additional evidence and proof of this application of HBOT. The authorities in the field of hyperbaric medicine each confirmed my belief that no new data had been produced, which left us with nothing more than the existing data. Because of this, I decided that the UHMS petition to Medicare to cover additional indications would be a fruitless pursuit. Therefore, I declined to join them in their application on hypoxic wounds.

By November 1, 2001, on behalf of the IHMA I submitted the scientific argument for the application of hyperbaric oxygen to diabetic foot wounds for reimbursement from Medicare. My argument was based solely on the data showing that hyperbaric oxygen therapy could prevent major amputations.

In late December of 2001, following Medicare's rejection of the UHMS petition on hypoxic wounds, my scientific argument proceeded to evaluation. The following year, all the interested parties of the various medical societies assembled in Baltimore at the Center for Medicare/Medicaid Services (CMS) headquarters. Everyone was allowed to discuss and argue the data. However, the decision boiled down to whether or not the evidence supported the ability of HBOT to prevent major amputations.

Since I was the last to give a summary statement, I asked the evaluators from CMS if they could find any reason to deny that the data showed that hyperbaric oxygen could reduce major amputations. They began to indicate their agreement, but of course they held back a decision—these regulating bodies don't render decisions on the spot. However, later that year they issued a memo that supported the application of HBOT to reduce the number of major amputations[1].

When a common condition is approved by a major regulatory body, it has implications that take us into new territory. One important implication is that further research and clinical experience will likely refine our application of HBOT to the aforementioned hypoxic wounds. We will then be able to accumulate adequate evidence to convince Medicare that the treatment of these wounds should be reimbursed. In addition, it provides another brick in the foundation of credibility from which HBOT medical specialists can argue to our skeptical medical colleagues. Our colleagues know that therapies usually are not approved by Medicare unless there is substantial evidence of their effectiveness. We can talk about government waste, and there is plenty of it, but Medicare treatments come from tight budgets that all taxpayers fund.

It may be difficult for the lay person to understand why this approval by Medicare was such a major milestone. However, as many have noted throughout the history of hyperbaric medicine, progress has been inhibited because we haven't been able to spread the word, so to speak, about the evidence we've accumulated. The reasons are many, and certainly include, as I've said before, the political stumbling blocks that exist within medicine itself.

So far, you might wonder why this discussion has focused on who pays for the treatment and how HBOT would save the taxpayers money in the coming decades. However, dismal or not, financial considerations are part of what patients and their doctors face when they make treatment decisions. But when we get back to the basic issues, benefits for patients are the best part of this recent development within a giant medical bureaucracy.

I directed the Louisiana State University School of Medicine, New Orleans, Fellowship in Hyperbaric Medicine from 1991–2009. In that capacity, I taught my fellows always to answer one question first when they evaluate a new patient with a wound problem: is it good medicine to apply HBOT to this patient's problem or not? If it is, we then ask what the reimbursement status of the patient is to see if our decision to deliver HBOT fits reimbursement guidelines. Essentially, we have to do what is known as a "wallet biopsy." If we discover that the medical need for HBOT is not going to be reimbursed, we try to find a way to offer the patient HBOT. We did this through January 2007 by privately funding a clinic that treated patients who did not have any financial resources. (This is the same clinic at which I treated most of the brain injured patients that have shaped my career in the past 26 years.) By 2007, however, we were bankrupt. As it turns out, nearly 50 percent of our hyperbaric patients prior to that time had been treated for free. Since then, we've had to manage our budget better, but we still treat some patients at our own expense. To get back to the point, our top priority is to deliver good medicine and then we figure out how to do it. Our final task is to see if we can get treatment funded. Sometimes we can't and we treat anyway.

I'm aware of the brewing controversy over drug companies advertising their new drugs. Many doctors have made it clear that they don't like it when the ads urge viewers to ask their doctors about a particular drug. Frankly, though, healthcare is a complicated maze to negotiate and no one can claim perfect knowledge. The best doctors can't possibly know about every new development. This is why informed patients are ultimately such a great asset.

For example, right now anyone with a concern about a foot wound complication of diabetes can go to the Medicare website, arm themselves with the scientific evidence I originally assembled, and then take the information to their doctors (they can take this book, too). Ultimately, patients that have the greatest motivation to become involved in their healthcare decisions will achieve the best possible outcomes.

It's true that many insurance companies approved HBOT reimbursement for diabetic foot wounds prior to this Medicare ruling. However, since many diabetics are disabled and thus have Medicare as their medical benefits provider, they could not get the treatment for their foot wounds. With Medicare approval, more of these diabetic patients would be able to obtain HBOT. In addition, because of Medicare approval, more insurance companies that previously didn't reimburse for diabetic foot wounds will subsequently follow suit. That means that Medicare's decision will benefit healthcare consumers affected by these foot wounds, regardless of their age or disability status.

Using Consumer Power

The journey to obtain approval of HBOT for that one condition alone is instructive because it isn't an isolated event. However, consumers have more power to influence the world of healthcare than ever before. I see this every day; for many years, I've often been put in touch with potential patients because they have done the research that led them to seek HBOT. Expanded, easy-to-use resources represent a revolutionary development, and in certain situations change the direction of healthcare.

Since medical information is no longer cloistered in private medical libraries, patients are often sophisticated to the point where they serve as an important source of information for their doctors. Much of what is advertised to doctors frankly enriches drug companies or the manufacturers of expensive medical equipment. But consumers are often more interested in therapies that fall outside of the control of these powerful groups—and as I've said, consumers have more power than they know.

Just think about what happened to chiropractic medicine, a field that traditional or "conventional" medicine disparaged for decades; both as individuals and through their powerful medical societies, many physicians openly tried to discredit chiropractic. Meanwhile, patients with back pain and other orthopedic problems kept right on seeing chiropractors and complaining that they had to pay out-of-pocket for a treatment that helped them.

In the 1980s and 1990s, nonpartisan sources in other countries, including Canada, New Zealand, and Australia, conducted independent studies and reviews. When these individuals and groups returned favorable opinions to their government-run healthcare boards, this paved the way to greater acceptance for chiropractic. In the United States, chiropractic associations won a lawsuit that essentially stopped their work from being automatically disparaged by allopathic physicians. Now, thanks to consumers and chiropractors, chiropractic is on the reimbursement list of the vast majority of insurance companies and government payers.

A similar process can and should be started with hyperbaric oxygen therapy, and the International Hyperbaric Medical Association is devoted to educating both the lay and medical communities.

I hope you take away from this book the very real sense that your experiences as a patient and a patient advocate are critical to the course of medical treatment. No longer will all the policy changes come from the "top"—the doctors, insurance companies, and politicians. You have power, too, and educating yourself through books like this one is an important step on the way to fulfilling your role in changing—and creating—healthcare policy.

APPENDIX B

MORE ABOUT SPECT

S PECT IMAGING HAS HAD A ROLLERCOASTER RIDE OF its own on the way to expanded use. Over the years, reproducibility and quality control have been the biggest issues surrounding SPECT. So, while nearly all hospitals in the United States have SPECT brain scan capability, the great majority of departments rarely use it for brain imaging.

The problems involved with SPECT use include: the conditions under which the radiopharmaceutical is injected in the patient, such as the amount of noise, lighting, talking, movement, and so forth; proper positioning of the patient and minimizing movement; and finally, computer processing of the imaging. All these factors are highly dependent on the operator of the scanner, the nuclear technologist.

As a result, I recommend that you find a place that frequently does SPECT brain imaging, preferably one that has a dedicated nuclear technologist performing all the scans. I was lucky to have this luxury for many years in the form of Phillip Tranchina, whom I mentioned in the Acknowledgements of this book. This minimizes the variability in technique among operators, which I have found can make a big difference, much the way specializing in any area of knowledge or work makes a difference in skill levels.

Ideally, you want the brain scan done under the identical conditions with the identical dose with the same acquisition (the actual acquiring of the radioactive counts by the scanner as the patient lies on the scanning couch) and processing every time the patient is scanned.

What the radiologist who reads the SPECT brings to the table, so to speak, is equally important to the value of the imaging. SPECT brain imaging is a small part of nuclear medicine and 99 percent or more of all nuclear medicine departments do not recruit their own "normals." ("Normals" are individuals who have no obvious neurological condition and so are neurologically "normal." On rare occasions, these individuals are recruited by a radiology department to undergo a free SPECT scan so the radiologist has a good appreciation of what a normal brain and hence, brain scan, looks like on that scanner.) Therefore, the great majority of radiologists do not have experience reading "normal" SPECT brain scans. This can lead to a normal reading of a very abnormal brain, and this has implications when it is placed in a patient's chart and becomes part of that person's permanent medical history.

In 1990, when I first started performing this imaging, I began to encounter this problem. For example, the first scan was determined to be "normal," and after repeating the scan following the first HBOT or a series of HBOTs, the radiologist had to go back and reinterpret the first scan because the second scan was much improved and "more normal." Finally, the radiologists stopped interpreting the first scan until I had performed a scan after the first treatment. Then, they could see what truly was "more normal." In fact, at the end of the first year the chief radiologist reading the SPECT scans thanked me for the "after HBOT" scans to show him what they were missing on the first scan.

The Future of SPECT

I expect the problems with the uneven quality of SPECT will improve in the near future. As time of writing, a number of companies are now offering high-quality, high resolution reproducible SPECT brain imaging. Some of them have databased their imaging and compared their database to those done of normal individuals. This is key: over the years, I've recruited 85 people we would classify as "normals," and have a detailed neurological questionnaire from each of them. I also interviewed each of these individuals to review their questionnaire. I was able to document their smoking history, drug use, caffeine intake, brain injury, medication, and so forth, and their neurological history in detail so I knew what was being registered on the scan. This has helped immensely in interpreting the patient scans I have seen over the years. A sampling of these normals is included in the book and on the website.

GLOSSARY

As you read this book, you will encounter various terms, some associated with specific medical conditions, others related to HBOT. Because I want you to gain a depth of understanding about this therapy, I have included definitions and explanations to provide a working knowledge of the language you will hear when hyperbaric oxygen is discussed. I've arranged them in alphabetical order, but you will see that when taken together they represent a coherent terminology you're likely to hear and use when discussing this treatment.

ACUTE: This refers to an injury at the onset of a disease or condition that has just happened; in medicine, it implies the immediate time at which an injury or accident occurs, essentially, a fresh injury or sudden change in condition. It also includes the period after the injury during the first few days. Sub-acute refers to the period of time after an injury or event between the first few days or so and the chronic period. Of course, a large overlay and gray zone exists between the sub-acute and chronic periods.

AT DEPTH: This refers to being in the chamber under pressure, usually at the final treatment pressure. When we pressurize the chamber, we go from surrounding ambient pressure (one atmosphere absolute if we are at sea level) to the treatment pressure. When patients are under pressure greater than atmospheric pressure they are said to be in the chamber "at depth."

ATMOSPHERES OF PRESSURE: The earth's atmosphere consists of nothing more than "air" that is about 21 percent oxygen, 79 percent nitrogen, and a tiny percentage of other gases, such as carbon dioxide. Yet despite the seeming "nothingness" of air, it has weight. That weight of all of the air from the surface to the edges of the earth's stratosphere is measured at the earth's surface as atmospheric pressure. It is about 14.7 pounds per square inch (psi), or about one third of the pressure in a typical car tire. This 14.7 psi is called one atmosphere absolute.

Imagine digging a hole in the earth. As we descend deeper, we have an increasing amount and density of air from the top of the hole (which includes all of the air above it to the stratosphere), at surface level, to the bottom. This increased amount of air in the hole exerts greater pressure as we descend deeper into the hole. Similarly, when we dive underwater, rather than the weight of air, the weight of the water exerts pressure and is added to the weight of the air on top of the water, extending to the stratosphere. Every 33 feet of seawater below the surface is equivalent to another atmosphere of pressure or equivalent to the entire weight of the atmosphere of air extending up to the stratosphere.

With HBOT for acute conditions, we usually treat at the equivalent pressure of 33–66 feet of seawater of pure oxygen. For chronic neurological conditions it is usually less, the equivalent of 16.5 feet of seawater or less. (Remember, in both cases we add the weight of air, or one atmosphere at sea level, to each of these pressures).

CHRONIC: This term implies the passage of time. In medicine, we say a condition or situation is chronic when it has reached a clinical plateau and is no longer changing. In neurology this typically refers to at least six months to one year after an event. We now know that improvements from rehabilitation of an injury can have a much longer time course, but are still in the chronic phase.

DIVE: A slang term for a hyperbaric treatment, it has its roots in diving medicine. When receiving a hyperbaric treatment, you're subjected to increased pressure and you breathe air or oxygen at increased pressure. It is identical to taking a SCUBA dive, meaning that in both cases you breathe air or oxygen under pressure. The only difference in HBOT is the lack of water to cause the increased pressure. Instead of having to descend underwater, we increase pressure with an air compressor or oxygen tank that forces increased air or oxygen into the hyperbaric chamber. Essentially, it is a "dry" dive.

DOSE: Since HBOT is a drug, doctors use the term dose to describe the amount of the drug delivered to the patient. In the case of HBOT, we believe it is the increased amount of oxygen and pressure. As with all drugs, we can think of the dose in terms of the childhood story of the three bears: a mama bear dose, a papa bear dose, and a baby bear dose that's just right. We're trying to find the baby bear dose that's right for any given patient and his or her disease.

In HBOT, the right dose is a combination of the absolute pressure of the treatment, the pressure of increased oxygen, the duration of each exposure, frequency of treatments, and the total number of treatments delivered at the particular time in the course of the patient's disease. The tricky part of HBOT dosing is that no one has the ability to discern the ideal dose for each patient and the condition. Instead, we use approximations based on experience, research, and medical reports. Further compounding the problem is the fact that we don't yet know the minimum amount of increased oxygen and pressure it takes to get the job done. SPECT brain imaging has helped us gather data, and I am currently working on a more individualized dosing technique.

The early HBOT pioneer, Dr. Orval Cunningham, found that the small amount of increased oxygen that could be obtained by pressurizing air to 1.3 times sea level atmospheric pressure and beyond (just 30 percent additional oxygen) was enough to save the lives of patients dying of the flu. This is the same amount of additional oxygen used in some portable air chambers to treat children with cerebral palsy. So it appears that even small increases in oxygen and pressure can have beneficial effects. This means that the dose of oxygen necessary to ameliorate a patient's condition can range from the slight increases used by Cunningham, up to the six atmospheres of 100 percent oxygen used by my partner for cardiac resuscitation—and every combination of pressure and percentage of oxygen in between.

EVIDENCE-BASED MEDICINE: For many in the medical field, evidence-based medicine includes only those treatments that have been shown to be effective through a narrow lens, especially double-blind studies. Lack of those studies (which may be completely impractical and not particularly wise in many cases) sometimes leads to dismissing some of the most effective therapies, including HBOT. However, a better definition of evidence-based medicine is more inclusive. The best statement I know comes from researcher David Sackett, (paraphrased earlier in the book.)

This is how Sackett defines evidence-based medicine: *The conscientious, explicit, and judicious use of current best evidence in making decisions about the care of individual patients. The practice of evidence based medicine means integrating individual clinical expertise with the best available external clinical evidence from systematic research*[1]. More recently, this has been described as the "integration of best research evidence with clinical expertise and patient values[2]."

HERNIATION: Disks are the rubber–like cushions that sit between each vertebra in our spine. They absorb shock and help our spine bend. Each disk is similar to round pieces of gum that have a soft center. The outer rim of the disk is firm and tough and the inner core is softer material. When someone herniates a disk, the soft center portion ruptures through the tough outer "tire" and presses on the spinal cord or nerves, causing extreme pain.

HYPOXIA: This term refers to a decreased level of oxygen relative to a certain norm. Commonly, the normal level of oxygen is the amount in air at sea level, which is about 160 mm mercury pressure, or 21 percent of atmospheric pressure at sea level. In normal, healthy people this translates to a level in the blood of about 90 mm mercury pressure. While there is a range of normal for oxygen levels in the blood at sea level, any measurement considerably less than these numbers is considered hypoxia. At altitude, however, the atmosphere is less than 21 percent and blood levels are less than 90 mm mercury pressure. The atmosphere and people are hypoxic relative to sea level, but because human beings can adapt to altitude, we can tolerate the hypoxia. In order to cause a hypoxic insult, a significant reduction in oxygen must exist, and, of course, a much less reduction in oxygen level at altitude than at sea level.

HBOT ATTENDANT OR INSIDE OBSERVERS: These individuals accompany patients inside multiplace chambers. They can be hyperbaric technicians or more highly trained or skilled medical personnel.

HBOT TECHNICIANS: In the context of HBOT, these individuals are trained to operate hyperbaric chambers. They can have a variety of different basic degrees, but most are EMTs (emergency medical technicians) who traditionally staff ambulances.

INSULT: Used in a generic fashion, it describes injury processes that affect the brain. We use it to refer to anything that has a negative impact on the brain, such as a traumatic blow or force, a loss or decrease of oxygen, a loss or decrease of blood flow, a toxin, a toxic drug, and so forth.

PRESCRIPTION: The actual order given by your hyperbaric physician for HBOT, for example, 1.5 ATA/60 minutes, twice/day, five days/week consecutively, for 4 weeks; total number of treatments = 40.

SURFACE AIR: This term refers to the ambient room air that is present at the "surface," which in HBOT is the room where the hyperbaric chamber is sitting. Surface air is not all the same, however. If you are at an altitude of 5,000 feet, the surface air is not the same as surface air at sea level; at altitude there is quite a bit less oxygen. So, pressurizing someone with surface air in Denver is not the same as pressurizing someone with surface air at sea level; you get different doses of oxygen.

TREATMENT BLOCKS: In hyperbaric medicine, you will hear treatments spoken of in "blocks." These are the concentrated number of treatments needed to effect change in an acute or chronic condition. In acute conditions, we inhibit the acute inflammatory and destructive processes that cause much of the long term damage. In this acute stage, we have found that we need only a few treatments delivered early on to quench the inflammatory process.

However, once the chronic pathology is established, we are then treating a different clinical situation; we are trying to grow new tissue, among other things. This process requires many more treatments, which usually start with a block of 40. This number can taper as we deliver more treatments, and in some cases, patients have more than one block of treatment; however, in all cases, the dosing must be individualized.

Treatments generally last one to two hours, with blocks of treatments are administered over successive days. Ideally, when treating chronic conditions, no more than a day or two should elapse between treatments, but this is not written in stone. Again, we must adjust the dose to the patient. Depending on the dose of HBOT and the severity or acuity of the illness, treatments can be delivered repetitively up to four or more times per day or for prolonged periods of time (6, 12, 24 hours or more).

Resources

T HE FOLLOWING REPRESENTS A SAMPLE OF THE KINDS of resources currently available as you seek more information about HBOT, or perhaps search for treatment facilities close to your home.

Pass these resources on to family and friends, so they, too, can find the help they need for their individual health issues.

You will find links to all of these resources at HBOT.com

Paul G. Harch, M. D. (and the website for *The Oxygen Revolution*)

IMPORTANT NOTE: One of the critical features of this book is the series of Internet links to videos, articles, newspaper pieces, patient testimonials, and so forth, all of which powerfully illustrate the healing power of hyperbaric oxygen therapy. These have been noted throughout the text, and are meant to augment the information in this book, leading you to resources that will expand your knowledge of this important treatment.

To view these news articles and patient testimonials, go to www.HBOT.com and click on the "Oxygen Revolution" tab on the home page, which will take you to all of the videos mentioned in this book.

The website has become massive over the years, and is an important complement to this book. There is a wide range of information, from the most basic facts about HBOT, to studies, discussions of SPECT, FDA labeling, case reports, references to a variety of publications, videos of patients, press releases, and more.

Information on HBOT

American College of Hyperbaric Medicine:

www.hyperbaricmedicine.org

This was the original hyperbaric medical society founded by the late Dr. Richard Neubauer and colleagues in 1983. It has changed quite a bit over the years and is now primarily focused on wound care, the typically reimbursed hyperbaric indications, certification, regulatory issues, practice protocols, quality assurance, and establishing relationships with Medicare.

Best Publishing Company

A company which specializes in hyperbaric medicine and diving texts, books, and science. They maintain a map of hyperbaric centers: www.bestpub.com/periodicals-and-subscriptions/find-a-hyperbaric-chamber.html

American College for Advancement in Medicine (ACAM):

www.acam.org

The members (primarily physicians) of this professional organization are interested in the latest in integrative/complementary medicine, and take an open-minded approach to several therapies, including HBOT. Their website includes a "doctor locator" service, which may help you choose a provider in your area.

Decision Memo for HBOT for Hypoxic Wounds and Diabetic Wounds of the Lower Extremities:

This is the Decision Memo and discussion of the medical literature and argument that I submitted on behalf of the International Hyperbaric Medical Association to obtain reimbursement for HBOT in the treatment of diabetic foot wounds. The approval was subsequently granted by Medicare based on this argument.

The 129 reference scientific argument was the basis for the decision (viewable on HBOT.com).

HBOT for Health:

http://health.groups.yahoo.com/group/hbotforhealth/join
HBOT for Health is a support group for people who are currently undergoing HBOT, or who are considering giving HBOT a try. It's a place where people can share their HBOT success stories, discuss the protocols they are utilizing, and give encouragement to people who are interested in starting HBOT. Unlike many of the yahoo HBOT groups, this group is open to people of all ages with a wide variety of medical conditions.

International Hyperbaric Medical Association (IHMA):

www.hyperbaricmedicalassociation.org
I'm one of the founders of this association, which was designed to advance hyperbaric oxygen therapy across the entire spectrum of medicine. The principles of the organization are essentially those espoused in this book. The site presents the latest information about hyperbaric medicine, a wealth of resources for patients and medical professionals, and links to other information to assist you in finding treatment for yourself or a loved one. The IHMA also has a sister organization, the IHMA Foundation (www.hyperbaricmedicalfoundation. org), which is a nonprofit corporation that accepts tax deductible donations for research, education, and treatment.

Textbook of Hyperbaric Medicine, K. K. Jain, editor, Hogrefe & Huber Publishing (January, 2009), www.hhpub.com

I've mentioned this book within the chapters, and if you're interested in the scientific side of this topic, then I invite you to look at this textbook. While technical, it compiles chapters from numerous contributors and offers another look at the kind of future in healthcare for HBOT that I presented here and offer to you. The distinguishing features of this book are the open-minded editor and publisher and the review of the international literature of HBOT for any disease not on the typically reimbursed list.

For MS patients:

www.hyperbaricoxygentherapy.org.uk
This is the United Kingdom site about the patient-organized network of treatment centers for multiple sclerosis.

The Undersea and Hyperbaric Medical Society:
www.uhms.org
The oldest and largest of the hyperbaric medical societies. Holds regular national and regional meetings. Responsible for the current list of typically reimbursed indications.

Special Needs Resources

Exceptional Parent:

www.eparent.com

This magazine addresses the parents of special needs children. It is one of the most comprehensive resources of its type and the owner, medical director, and editors are not afraid to investigate and report on controversial topics and treatment. The magazine is a highly respected publication that appeals to both parents and healthcare professionals. Their website is full of information and features tutorials and other educational resources. The site also provides links to other resources and posts research updates.

Honest Medicine:

www.honestmedicine.com

Julia Schopick, a patient advocate and writer, hosts this site, which contains a variety of helpful articles and resources. Julia is working with others to make significant changes in the way individuals interact with the medical system. She includes information about many different treatments and has interviewed me about hyperbaric medicine. Her book *Honest Medicine*, published in 2011, includes an extensive discussion of the ketogenic diet (used for pediatric seizure disorders), which I mention in my discussion of HBOT and cancer treatment.

Medicaid for HBOT:

www.medicaidforhbot-subscribe@yahoogroups.com

This is a subscriber list with thousands of members that helps parents navigate through the state-run Medicaid programs to find treatment for their children. It is run by David Freels, who has become a parent-advocate after his experience obtaining HBOT for his child, Jimmy Freels. The site is heavily weighted toward HBOT, Medicaid law, and Medicaid reimbursement for HBOT in pediatric neurology. It chronicles the multiple legal decisions/triumphs in favor of Medicaid reimbursement of HBOT for Jimmy Freels.

Miracle Flights for Kids:
www.miracleflights.org
This organization arranges transport for children and families who must leave their homes to find appropriate medical treatment.

MUMS (Mothers United for Moral Support):
www.netnet.net/mums
Based in Green Bay, Wisconsin, Founder and Director, Julie Gordon established this group to assist parents of special needs children. The organization was dedicated to its network of parents with similar concerns and provided both support and information about medical resources of all kinds. It was a pioneer organization in the use of HBOT for cerebral palsy, for example, and it was devoted to helping parents obtain appropriate treatment for their children, including HBOT. It no longer does parent-to-parent matching, but is still a resource for parents.

Ronald McDonald House Charities (RMHC):
www.rmhc.com
These charities help families who need housing while their seriously ill children are receiving medical treatment away from home. This website will help you locate a facility in the U.S. and abroad. I have experience with this organization through the New Orleans Ronald McDonald House, and I highly recommend consulting the website for more information.

REFERENCES

Chapter 1

1. In his book, *Hyperbaric Oxygenation: The Uncertain Miracle* (published by Doubleday in 1974 and now out of print, but available from the International Hyperbaric Medical Association website) Pulitzer Prize–winning author, Vance Trimble, discussed the rich history of hyperbaric medicine.
2. *NOAA Diving Manual: Diving for Science and Technology, 4th Edition*. National Oceanographic and Atmospheric Administration, U.S. Department of Commerce. Editor, James T. Joiner. Best Publishing Company, Flagstaff, AZ, 2001.

Chapter 2

1. Harch PG., Late treatment of decompression illness and use of SPECT brain imaging. In Treatment of Decompression Illness, 45th Workshop of the Undersea and Hyperbaric Medical Society (eds. RE Moon, PJ Sheffield). UHMS, Kensington, MD, 1996, 203-242.

Chapter 3

1. The Hyperbaric Oxygen Therapy Committee Report, Chairman, Hampson NB, Undersea and Hyperbaric Medical Society, Kensington, MD, 2003.

Chapter 4

1. (Ewing, R., McCarthy, D., Gronwall, D. and Wrightson, P.(1980) 'Persisting effects of minor head injury observable during hypoxic stress', Journal of Clinical and Experimental Neuropsychology,2:2,147 — 155. http://www.tandfonline.com/doi/abs/10.1080/01688638008403789).
2. Harch PG, Neubauer RA.," Hyperbaric Oxygen Therapy in Global Cerebral Ischemia/Anoxia and Coma," Chapter 18. In: Jain KK (ed). Textbook of

Hyperbaric Medicine, 4th Revised Edition. Hogrefe & Huber Publishers, Seattle WA, 2004.

3. Heckerling, PS, "Occult carbon monoxide poisoning: a cause of winter headache," American Journal of Emergency Medicine, 5 (3) 1987: 201-4. 43.

4. Dolan MC, Haltom TM., Barrows GH, Short CS, and Ferriell KM,"Carboxyhemoglobin levels in patients with flu-like symptoms," Annals of Emergency Medicine, 16(7) 1987:782-6.

5. Stoller KP, "Quantification of neurocognitive changes before, during, and after hyperbaric oxygen therapy in a case of fetal alcohol syndrome," Pediatrics, 116(4) 2005: e586-91.

Chapter 5

1. Cowan F, Rutherford M, Groenendaal F, et al., "Origin and timing of brain lesions in term infants with neonatal encephalopathy." Lancet, 361(9359), March 1, 2003: 713-4.

2. Hutchison JH, Kerr MM, William KG, Hopkinson WI, "Hyperbaric oxygen in the resuscitation of the newborn," Lancet, November 16, 1963; 13:1019-22.

3. Hutchison JH, Kerr MM, Inall JA, Shanks RA, "Controlled Trials of Hyperbaric Oxygen and Tracheal Intubation in Asphyxia Neonatorum," Lancet, April 30, 1966 1(7444): 935-9).

4. Liu A, Xiong T, Meads C. Clinical effectiveness of treatment with hyperb aricoxygenforneonatalhypoxic-ischemicencephalopathy:systematic review of Chinese literature. British Medical Journal: BMJ, doi:10. 1136/ bmj. 38776. 731655. 2F (published 11 May 2006).

5. Harch P, Kriedt, C, Van Meter, K, Sutherland, R, "Hyperbaric oxygen therapy improves spatial learning and memory in a rat model of chronic traumatic brain injury," Brain Research, 2007; 1174:120-29).

6. Senechal C, Larivee S, Richard E, Marois P., "Hyperbaric Oxygenation Therapy in the Treatment of Cerebral Palsy: A Review and Comparison to Currently Accepted Therapies," Journal of American Physicians and Surgeons, 2007; 12(4):109113.

Chapter 6

1. http://circ.ahajournals.org/content/131/4/e29.full.pdf#page=151
2. Hossman KA, Chapter 11: "Disturbances of cerebral protein synthesis and ischemic cell death," In: Progress in Brain Research, Vol. 96, editors. K. Kogure, K. A. Hossmann, and B. K. Siesjo, Elsevier Science Publishers, 1993, 161-177
3. Neubauer RA, Gottlieb SF, Kagan RL, "Enhancing 'idling' neurons," Lancet, March 3, 1990; 335 (8688):542.
4. http://journals.plos.org/plosone/article?id=10.1371/journal.pone.0053716

Chapter 7

1. A detailed discussion of this can be found in the AutismOne Radio Interview I did on June 28, 2005. The entire transcript is published: P. G. Harch and T. Small, Interview with P. Harch: The application of hyperbaric oxygen therapy in chronic neurological conditions by Paul Harch and Teri Small, Medical Veritas: The Journal of Medical Truth, 2 (2) 2005: 637-Ref. 00084

Chapter 8

1. Plassman BL, Havlik RJ, Steffens DC, et al., "Documented head injury in early adulthood and risk of Alzheimer's disease and other dementias," Neurology, 55(8) 2000: 1158-66.)
2. Information on the Congressional testimony about the Alzheimer's patients appears on the IHMA website, www.hyperbaricmedicalassociation.org
3. Neubauer RA., "Treatment of multiple sclerosis with monoplace hyperbaric oxygenation," J Florida Medical Association, 1978; 65:101-104.
4. Neubauer RA. "Exposure of multiple sclerosis patients to hyperbaric oxygen at 1. 5-2 ATA: a preliminary report," J Florida Medical Association, 1980; 67: 498-
5. Fischer BH, Marks M, Reich T, "Hyperbaric-oxygen treatment of multiple sclerosis. A randomized, placebo-controlled, double-blind study," New England Journal of Medicine, 308(4) 1983:181-6.
6. Steele J, Matos LA, Lopez EA, et al, "A Phase I study of hyperbaric oxygen therapy for amyotrophic lateral sclerosis, Amyotroph Lateral Scler Other Motor Neuron Disord, 5(4) 2004:250-4.

7. Neretin Via, Lobov MA, Kiselev SO, LagutinaTS, Kir'iakov VA, "Effect of hyperbaric oxygenation on the recovery of motor functions in vertebrogenic myelopathies, [Article in Russian], Zh Nevropatol Psikhiatr Im S S Korsakova, 85 (12) 1985:1774-8.

Chapter 9

1. Summary of Evidence: Diabetic wounds of the Lower Extremities, http:// www.cms.hhs.gov/mcd/viewdecisionmemo.asp?id=37
2. Abidia A, Kuhan G, Laden G, et al., "Hyperbaric Oxygen Therapy for diabetic leg ulcers—a double blind randomized controlled trial," Undersea & Hyperbaric Medicine, 2001;28 (Suppl):64.
3. Alex J, Laden G, Cale AR, et al., "Pretreatment with hyperbaric oxygen and its effect on neuropsychometric dysfunction and systemic inflammatory response after cardiopulmonary bypass: a prospective randomized doubleblind trial," Journal of Thoracic and Cardiovascular Surgery, 130(6) 2005:1623-30.

Chapter 10

1. http://www.ncbi.nlm.nih.gov/pubmed/20637561
2. This was trade named P-gel and was the subject of a nationally syndicated news program called "Medical Breakthroughs."
3. McAlindon TE, Formica MK, Fletcher J, Schmid C, "Barometric Pressure and Ambient Temperature Influence Osteoarthritis (OA) Pain, Results of a National Web-Based Prospective Study," American College of Rheumatology Meeting, San Antonio, TX, Oct. 18, 2004. Presentation Number 596.
4. Verges J, Montell E, Tomas E, et al., "Weather conditions can influence rheumatic diseases," Proc West Pharmacol Soc, 2004;47: 134-6.

Chapter 11

1. Reillo MR, "Hyperbaric oxygen therapy for the treatment of debilitating fatigue associated with HIV/AIDS," Journal of the Association of Nursing in AIDS Care 4(3) 1993:33-8).
2. http://journals.plos.org/plosone/article?id=10.1371/journal.pone.0065522.
3. http://emedicine.medscape.com/article/310834-overview#a6
4. http://www.ncbi.nlm.nih.gov/pubmed/16539861

5. http://www.ncbi.nlm.nih.gov/pubmed/25988526

6. Richard O'Brien, "Scorecard: Chamber Mates," Sports Illustrated, June 13, 1994, p. 10.

Chapter 12

1. This was the argument I presented to the American Academy of Anti-Aging Medicine in Las Vegas in December 2004. (This can be viewed on my website.)

Chapter 14

1. Rockswold GL, Ford SE, Anderson DC, et al. Results of a prospective randomized trial for treatment of severely brain-injured patients with hyperbaric oxygen. J Neurosurg 1992; 76(6):929-934.

2. Holbach KH, Caroli A, Wassmann H. Cerebral energy metabolism in patients with brain lesions of normo- and hyperbaric oxygen pressures. J Neurol 1977; 217(1):17-30.

3. Holbach KH, Wassmann H, Kolberg T. [German]. Verbesserte Reversibilitat des traumatischen Mittelhirnsyndroms bei Anwendung der hyperbaren Oxygenierung (Reversibility of the Traumatic Mid-Brain Syndrome with Hyperbaric Oxygen. Acta Neurochir (Wien) 1974;30:247-56

4. Artru F, Chacornac R, Deleuze R. Hyperbaric Oxygenation for Severe Head Injuries. Eur Neurol, 1976;14:310-318.

5. Ren H, Wang W, Zhaoming GE, et al. Clinical, brain electric earth map, endothelin and transcranial ultrasonic Doppler findings after hyperbaric oxygen treatment for severe brain injury. Chi Med J 2001; 114(4):387-390.

6. Rockswold SB, Rockswold GL, Vargo JM, et al., "Effects of hyperbaric oxygenation therapy on cerebral metabolism and intracranial pressure in severely brain injured patients," J Neurosurg 2001; 94(3):403-411.

7. McDonagh M, Carson S, Ash J, et al., "Hyperbaric Oxygen Therapy for Brain Injury, Cerebral Palsy, and Stroke. Evidence Report/Technology Assessment," No. 85 (Prepared by the Oregon Health & Science University Evidence-based Practice Center under Contract No 290-97-0018). AHRQ Publication No. 04-E003. Rockville, MD: Agency for Healthcare Research and Quality. September 2003.

8. Harch PG. "Medicine that Overlooks the Evidence," Arch Phys Med Rehabil, April 2006; 87(4):597-3.
9. Rockswold SB, Rockswold GL, Zaun DA, Zhang X, Cerra CE, Bergman TA, Liu J. A prospective, randomized clinical trial to compare the effect of hyperbaric to normobaric hyperoxia on cerebral metabolism, intracranial pressure, and oxygen toxicity in severe traumatic brain injury.

Conclusion

1. Gabb G, Robin ED. "Hyperbaric Oxygen: A Therapy in Search of Diseases," Chest. December 1987; 92(6):1074-82. Review
2. Harch PG. "Generic Inhibitory Drug Effect of Hyperbaric Oxygen Therapy (HBOT) on Reperfusion Injury (RI)", Eur J Neural, 2000; 7 (Suppll 3):150
3. Vila JF, Balcarce PE, Abiusi GR, Dominguez RO, Pisarello JB. "Improvement in Motor and Cognitive Impairment After Hyperbaric Oxygen Therapy in a Selected Group of Patients with Cerebrovascular Disease: A Prospective Single-Blind Controlled Trial Undersea," Hyperb Med. Sep-Oct 2005; 32(5):341-9.
4. Kiralp MZ, Yildiz S, Vural D, Keskin I, Ay H, Dursun H. "Effectiveness of hyperbaric oxygen therapy in the treatment of complex regional pain syndrome." J Int Med Res. 2004 May-Jun; 32(3):258-62.

Appendix

1. Summary of Evidence: Diabetic wounds of the Lower Extremities, http://www.cms.hhs.gov/mcd/viewdecisionmemo.asp?id=37

Glossary

1. Sackett D, et al. "Evidence Based Medicine: What It Is and What It Isn't," BMJ 312, no. 7023 (1996).
2. Sackett D, et al. Evidence-Based Medicine: How to Practice and Teach EBM (New York: Churchill Livingstone, 2000), 1.

Index

Abidia, A., 165
abscesses, brain tissue, 56
acute injuries or situations, 33–34, 38–40, 90–91
acute peripheral arterial insufficiency, 267
addictions, drug and alcohol, 191–193
Agency for Healthcare Research and Quality, 248, 271
aging
    acceleration of, 203
    caveat on HBOT for, 218
    cumulative brain insults and, 207–208
    DNA and, 199–200
    Earl's case, 205–207
    HBOT endorsement for, 216–218
    normal, 209–212
    preventing or reversing signs of, 212–213
    rejuvenating during, 215
    smoking and, 203–205
    stress and, 208–209
    tissue injury and, 201–202
    wellness and prevention, 216
AIDS (Autoimmune Deficiency Syndrome), 183–184
air baths, 18
air embolism
    Greathouse case, 49
    HBOT approved for, 55
    Tom's case, 45, 46
airplanes, oxygen pressure in, 206
alcohol. *See also* fetal alcohol syndrome
    abuse of, 191–193

aging and, 204, 210–212
detoxification, HBOT and, 8
oxygen bars and, 196–197
traumatic brain injury and, 212–213
in utero brain damage and, 115
Allen, Curt, Jr., 62, 63, 77, 95–97
ALS (amyotrophic lateral sclerosis), 157–159
Alzheimer's disease, 8, 145, 147–148, 211–212
American College for Advancement in Medicine (ACAM), 286
American College of Hyperbaric Medicine (ACHM), 272–273, 286
American Diabetes Association, 162
amputations, 274. *See also* diabetic foot wounds
anecdotes, definition of, 72
anemia, severe, 56
animal studies
    on acute stroke, 121
    on acute toxic overdose or poisoning, 90–91
    on brain injuries, 113–114
    on burns, 202
    on carbon monoxide poisoning, 38
    on chemotherapy and heart damage, 188–189
    on chronic brain injuries, 113–115
    on cognition and vascular density, 215

on decompression sickness, 36
on HBOT dose, 75
on inflammatory pain, 268
positive effects of HBOT in, 264, 265
on reserve capacity, 143
on stroke, 121
on TBI, 42–43, 54, 244
on trauma and bone growth, 169
anterior cruciate ligament (ACL) repair, 170–171
APGAR scores, 103
approved indications, HBOT, 55–57
    acute severe TBI and, 248
    disciplinary action for treating outside of, 253–255
    off-label uses and, 240–241, 242
Archives of Physical Medicine and Rehabilitation, 248
Argentina, Type II diabetes study in, 165
arthritis, 174–175
ascending paralysis, 105
asthma, 189–191, 232
athletes, 195–196, 197
atmospheric pressure, 4–5
autism
    birth injuries and, 133–134
    Brian's case, 135, 136–138
    as epidemic, 131–132
    HBOT for, 7, 132–133, 138–139
    HBOT studies, 51, 113

avascular necrosis (AVN), 170
axons, 143

babies, 106–108, 131–132, 233.
    See also birth injuries
Baby Boomers, 150, 173, 203
back surgery, 176–177
Bal, Sean, 96
Baptists, SPECT imaging of, 210
barometric pressure,
    osteoarthritic pain and, 175
Battles, Chad, 72
Beall, Jeff, 49
Best Publishing Company,
    227–228, 286
Biden, Jill, 73
birth injuries. See also babies;
    cerebral palsy
    augmenting standard care for,
        111–112
    compressions in birth canal
        and, 102–103
    data on, reimbursement and,
        244
    epidural anesthetic and,
        105–106
    global view of, 116
    HBOT impact on, 7,
        110–111
    hidden, 103–104
    induced labor and, 100–101
    "miracle" child, 109–110
    overview of, 99–100
    research on, 113
Black Hearts (Frederick), 72
bleeding strokes, 117, 120
blindness from herpes
    encephalitis, 62
blood clots. See also central
    retinal artery occlusion; TPA
    brain reserve capacity loss
        and, 145, 149
    inflammatory reaction and,
        31–32
    post-op depression and, 167
    stroke and, 117, 120, 266–267
blood flow
    chronic wounds and, 41

damage, as later HBOT
    target, 40–41
low oxygen injuries and level
    of, 30–31
blood pressure, elevated, 118,
    120–121
blood–brain barrier, multiple
    sclerosis and, 151–152,
    154–155
Bogalusa chemical spill, 92
bones, 169, 194
    necrosis, 56
borrelia burgdorferi, 181
Boyle's Law, 22–23
brain
    plasticity, remodeling, and
        development of, 246–247
    redundancy and reserve
        capacity of, 143–144
brain death, 235–236
brain decompression illness
    Greathouse case, 49–50
    heart surgery and, 166
    MS lesions and, 152
    Tom's case, 45–48
brain injuries. See also birth
    injuries; traumatic brain injury
    chronic, treatment for, 257
    HBOT for, 8
    idiosyncracies, 237
    Reagan's, 144–145
    research on, 112–115
    reserve capacity loss and,
        143–144
    types, 141–142
Brain Storm, Oxygen Under
    Pressure (video), 72
Breaux, O'Neal, 155–156
bucking, 80
bulbar ALS, 158–159
burns, 41–42, 57, 202
Bush, George H.W.,
    administration of, 271–272
bypass patients. See heart surgery

CADASIL Syndrome, 128–129
Camporesi, Dr., 170
cancer, 8, 186–189, 256

carbon monoxide poisoning
    arthritis and, 175
    as brain insult, 141
    characteristics, 88–90
    HBOT approved for, 55
    HBOT for, 8, 38
    hospital emergency rooms
        and, 251
    premature dementia and,
        146–147
    repetitive daily HBOT study
        and, 51
    smoking and, 204
cardiac arrest, 8
Carlucci, Chloe, 62
case studies, importance of,
    252–253
Cassidy, John, 133
Centers for Medicare and
    Medicaid Services (CMS), 261.
    See also Medicare
central retinal artery occlusion
    (CRAO), 56, 129–130, 185,
    266–267. See also stroke, in eye
Cerebral Autosomal
    Dominant Arteriopathy
    with Subcortical Infarcts
    and Leukoencephalopathy
    Syndrome, 128–129
cerebral palsy
    autism and, 137–138
    HBOT for, 7
    repetitive daily HBOT study
        and, 51
    research on, 114–115
    seizures and HBOT for, 42
    Tim's case, 100–102, 109–110
    use of term, 110
chambers, HBOT
    at commercial dive sites, 36
    emergency room, 108–109,
        250–251, 254
    FDA approved uses of, 241
    off-label uses for, 241–242
    types and characteristics,
        228–231
chelation therapy, 139

chemical toxins, 93–94, 141, 191–193, 207–208
chemotherapy, 188–189
Cherry, Kim, 158–159
childbed fever, 99–100
children. *See also* autism; cerebral palsy
    on HBOT experience, 138–139
    routine medications for, as off-label, 241
China
    HBOT for birth injuries in, 109, 244
    HBOT for brain injuries in, 247
    HBOT for epilepsy in, 42
    HBOT for seizures in, 232–233
    HBOT treatable diagnoses in, 55, 116, 256, 268
    repetitive HBOT in, 88
chiropractic care, 177–179, 276
cholesterol, elevated, 118
chronic conditions
    acute injuries vs., 38–40
    other disease processes and, 41–43
chronic fatigue syndrome, 183
chronic pain syndrome, 193–194
chronic traumatic encephalopathy (CTE)
    multiple concussions and, 77
cigarettes. *See* smoking
Clostridial myonecrosis, 55
clothing types, for HBOT chambers, 230–231
clotting. *See* blood clots
cocaine, 115, 209
cochlea, traumatic rupture of, 184
colon cancer, 188–189, 216
comatose patients, 236
combination drug, HBOT as, 5
compartment syndrome, 55
complex regional pain syndrome, 193–194

concussions, 46, 69, 75–76, 195. *See also* post-concussion syndrome; traumatic brain injury
    multiple, 77, 148
congestive heart failure, 232
consumers, medical, 14
    power of, 275–276
contraindications, HBOT, 237
cosmetic surgery, 167
cost benefit analysis issues, 243–244
court orders for HBOT, 254, 255
crush injuries, 55, 194
culture of medicine, HBOT and, 10, 250
Cunningham, Orval, 19–21, 41
    Sensible Notion of, 265, 266, 268
cyanide poisoning, 55, 93–94

D'Agostino, Dominic, 189
Danna, Mary, 185
decompression illness (sickness)
    HBOT approved for, 56
    HBOT for, 10, 11, 21, 25–26
    Navy vs. commercial HBOT and, 36–38
    organic brain injury and, 45–47
    Parrish case of, 34–35
delayed treatment, 94–95
dementia. *See also* Alzheimer's disease
    brain tissue loss and, 61
    carbon monoxide poisoning and, 146–147
    diagnosing, 211–212
    anoxic, 190
    reserve capacity loss and, 145–146
dementia pugilistica, 77
Department of Defense Consensus Conference on HBOT and Traumatic Brain Injury (2009), 246
    on HBOT and placebo effect, 253

HBOT studies, 74–75
    post-concussion studies, 5
depression, 167
developmental delays, 134
diabetes, 118, 161–162, 166–168
diabetic foot wounds
    bone infections and, 169
    Decision Memo on HBOT for, 286
    40-treatment protocol and, 53–54
    HBOT and, 162–163
    HBOT approved for, 56, 273
    informed patients on, 164–165
Diagnosis Related Group (DRG) reimbursement, 223, 224
diapedesis, 32
diet, in multi-modal ALS therapy, 158
diving. *See* decompression illness
diving medicine, 21–27, 36–38. *See also* Navy, U.S.
DNA, aging and, 199–200
DNA stimulation, 6–7
Doc, I Want my Brain Back (Greathouse and McCullough), 50
domicilium, 18
dopamine, 149
dosing. *See also* overdosing
    negative effects of HBOT and, 234–235
Down syndrome, 201–202
drowning. *See* near drowning
drugs
    abuse of, 191–193
    brain insult from, 141
    detoxification, HBOT and, 8
    for neurological disorders, 150, 151
    prescription, bone tissue damage and, 170
    recreational, brain reserve capacity and, 150, 203
Duncan, William A., xvii–xx
    brother's brain injury, 94–95

DoD Consensus Conference and, 246
HBOT for diabetic foot wounding and, 163
HBOT for veterans and, 4, 246
IHMA and, 188
Medicare and, 248, 272
N-BIRR Study and, 73
dysphoria, 51

ear issues, HBOT and, 228–229, 232
Efrati (Israeli researcher), 75
80-treatment protocol, 51–52
Eisenberg, John, 248
embolic strokes, 117
emergency room hyperbaric chambers, 109, 250–251, 254
emotional distress, brain aging and, 209
emphysema, 189–191, 232
End, Edgar, 25
end-of-life intentions, 236
endothelial cells, 31
England. *See also* United Kingdom
HBOT for heart bypass patients in, 166
Environmental Tectonics Corporation, 241–242
epidural anesthetics, 105
evidence-based medicine, 67–68, 69, 156, 249
Ewing, R., 70, 143–144
Exceptional Parent, 289
eye. *See also* central retinal artery occlusion
acute conditions of, 185–186

falls, TBI and, 75, 211–213
Farris, Meg, 128–129
fatigue, HBOT and, 232
FDA (Food and Drug Administration), 4, 240, 241–242
fetal alcohol syndrome (FAS), 93, 115

fever, high, 141
fibromyalgia syndrome, 193–194
Fife, Bill, 181
first responders, poisoning situations and, 91–92
Fischer, B. H., 152
food additives, organic foods without, 208
football, 70, 77, 195–196, 197, 213
40-treatment protocol, 53–54
France
air baths in, 18
HBOT for TBI studies in, 247
Frederick, Jim, 72
free radicals, 32, 33–34
Freels, David, 228, 289–290
free-standing HBOT facilities
chronic brain injuries and, 257
HBOT billing rates of, 223
off-label diagnoses and, 224–225
physician-run, prescriptions for, 221–222
treatment beyond emergency and, 256

Gabb, Genevieve, 263–264, 266, 267, 268–269
gangrene, 163
gas embolism. *See* air embolism
gas gangrene, 55
gateways to the future
education for patients and doctors, 259–260
financial/reimbursement issue, 257
informed patients as, 260
lay public involvement as, 261–262
organizations funding treatment, 258–259
patient documentation, 257–258
Geller, Nate, 76
genetic disorders, 201–202

Germans
HBOT for hearing loss, vertigo, and tinnitus by, 184
HBOT for stroke studies by, 121–122
HBOT for TBI studies in, 247
low pressure HBOT studies by, 40
Gordon, Julie, 111, 290
Gottlieb, Sheldon, 51, 101, 153
Greathouse, Dan, 49
growth factors, ACL repair and, 171
Guggenheim, Solomon ("Mr. G."), 207–208
gunshot wounds, 245–246

hair growth, 214–215
Hane, Tyler, 76–77
hanging, near, 8
hangovers, 191, 197
Harch, Juliette, 156–157, 171–172
hard-shell monoplace chambers, 228–230
Harrison, Vickie, 62, 268
HBOT for Health (Yahoo group), 287
head trauma. *See* brain injuries
headaches
carbon monoxide poisoning and, 89, 90
cluster, 193–194
migraine, 182–183, 193–194
health savings accounts, 258
Healthy People 2000, 271
hearing loss, 57, 184
heart attacks, 42
heart disease, diabetes and, 162
heart surgery, 166–168
Hecker, Tim, 71–72
heliox, 21
hemorrhagic shock, 145–146
hemorrhagic strokes, 117
Henry's Law, 24–25
Henshaw, N., 18

hepatitis vaccines, 131–132
herniated disks, 178
herpes encephalitis, 62
hip replacement, 170
Hippocratic Oath, 240
Hoffmann, Martin, 74, 246
Holbach study, 247
homeless people, brain injuries
    and, 69
Honest Medicine website and
    book, 289
hood, oxygen, in multiplace
    chambers, 230, 231
hospitals. *See also* emergency
    room hyperbaric chambers
    FDA labeling of HBOT
        chambers and, 242
    HBOT billing rates of, 223
    with hyperbaric chambers,
        emergencies and, 254
    limited care HBOT
        operations in, 250–252
    off-label diagnoses and, 224
    supplemental oxygen in, 196
Hossman, K. A., 124
Hurricane Katrina, 89–90, 209
Hutchison, J. H., 108
hydrocephalus, obstructive, 82
hydrostatic pressure, 4–5
hyperbaric centers, choosing,
    227–228
Hyperbaric Oxygen Therapy
    Committee of the Undersea
    and Hyperbaric Medical
    Society, 129–130, 248, 250
hyperbaric oxygen therapy
    (HBOT). *See also* animal
    studies; chambers, HBOT;
    research
    brain death and, 236–237
    as brain repair drug, 239
    conditions helped by, 7–9
    conditions worsening with,
        234–235
    critics of, 263–264
    definition, 12
    diving medicine and, 21–27
    dosage studies, 51–53

expectations vs. realistic
    possibilities for, 27–28
familiar uses of, 54–57
as generic drug for basic
    disease processes, 264–265
history of, 18–21
lack of information about,
    9–14
measuring response to, 61–63
other therapies and, 17–18
for Parkinson's disease, 149
patient response to, 60–61
power of oxygen and pressure
    and, 3–7
scope of uses for, 14–15,
    239–240
single vs. multiple therapies,
    63–64
SPECT imaging prior to,
    58, 59
stopping, reasons for,
    233–234
when not to use, 235–236
as whole body treatment,
    16–17
Hyperbaric Oxygenation: The
    Uncertain Miracle (Trimble),
    215
hyperglycemia, 162
hypertension, 118
hypoglycemia, 162
hypoxic wounds, 272–274, 286

ice hockey, 195
idling neurons, 41, 124–126
immune system, Type I diabetes
    and, 161
infections
    bone, 169–170
    Lyme disease, 181–182
    necrotizing soft tissue, 56
inflammatory reaction. *See also*
    reperfusion injuries
    acute injuries and, 33–34
    acute vs. chronic conditions
        and, 38–40
    in calf muscle, 173

chronic wounding and,
    41–43
diving medicine studies of,
    36–38
as early HBOT target, 40–41
heart surgery and, 166–167
overview of, 29–30
oxygen paradox and, 34–35
process of, 31–33
as secondary injury, 15
influenza epidemic (1918), 19,
    20
insulin, 161, 162
insulin resistance, 161–162
insurance companies
    chiropractic care and, 178
    HBOT for diabetic foot
        wounding and, 164
    lay public involvement with
        medical review panels of,
        261
    patient documentation for,
        257–258
    on referrals for HBOT,
        221–222
    reimbursement for HBOT
        by, 11–12, 54, 98, 222–226,
        243–244
International Congresses
    on Hyperbaric Medicine
    publications, 259
International Hyperbaric
    Medical Association (IHMA)
    diabetic foot wound care
        and, 273
    education for patients and
        doctors, 259–260
    education for patients and
        doctors by, 276
    Foundation, 287
    Medicare and, 272
    off-label chamber and, 241
    SPECT imaging and cases on
        website of, 94, 133
    website, 287
International Hyperbaric
    Medical Foundation, 73
Internet

forums, finding HBOT
  facilities using, 228
  HBOT information on,
    259–260
  literature searches using, 250
intracranial abscesses, 56
ischemic freeze, 124–126, 129
ischemic penumbra, of strokes,
  118
Israeli studies, 75, 127–128, 170
Italy
  HBOT applications in, 268
  HBOT study in, 170

Jackson, Michael, 10, 202–203
Jain, K. K., 106
James, Philip, 153–154, 155
Japan
  hangover treatment in, 191,
    197
  HBOT for brain cancer in,
    187–188
  HBOT for neurological
    diseases in, 116
  HBOT for spinal cord
    injuries in, 176, 177
  HBOT treatable diagnoses in,
    55, 256, 268
  repetitive HBOT in, 88
Joiner, LeRoy, 190
Joining Forces Initiative,
  Michelle Obama/Jill Biden, 73
Journal of Neurotrauma, 71
judgment, carbon monoxide
  poisoning and, 89
Junod, V. T., 18

Kenitz, Gracie, 202
Kenitz, Shannon, 202
King, Larry, 10
Knight, "Bubba," 170–171

Lake Powell, AZ, carbon
  monoxide poisoning at, 89
The Lancet, 106–108
learning disabilities/disorders,
  134, 135

"less is more" principle, 40–41,
  153
lipid per oxidation, 33
literature searches, 113–114, 250
Liu, Dr., 109
liver, transplanted, acute stroke
  of, 267
Locklear, Ken, 188–189
Lou Gehrig's disease, 157–159
Louisiana State University
  School of Medicine, 274
low oxygen
  blood flow level and, 30–31
  chronic wounds and, 41
  as later HBOT target, 40–41
LSU Pilot Trial, 71–73, 74
lung diseases, 20
Lyme disease, 181–182

Machado, J., 42
macular degeneration, 185–186
Maney, Patt, 74
Marois, Pierre, 201–202
Mathers, Jake, 72
Maury Povich television show,
  92
Maxfield, William, 190
McAlindon, T. E., 175
McCloy, Randal, Jr., 88
McClure, Jessica, 174
Medicaid, 98, 222–224, 226, 289
medical community, HBOT
  rejection by, 12–14
medical savings accounts, 258
medical travel for HBOT,
  258–259
Medicare
  Agency for Healthcare
    Research and Quality,
    248, 273
  applying for approval by,
    272–274
  on HBOT for diabetic foot
    wounding, 54, 163, 164,
    165
  reimbursement for HBOT
    by, 222–224, 226
Meijne, Nicolaas G., 19

mercury poisoning, 139
metastatic cancer, 189
methamphetamines, 209
middle ear pressure changes,
  HBOT chambers and, 228–
    229, 232
migraine headaches, 182–183,
  193–194
Miracle Flight for Kids, 258, 290
monoplace chambers, 228–230,
  231
"more is more" principle, 40–41
Mormons, SPECT imaging of,
  210
motor vehicle accidents, 75,
  78–79, 245–246
MRI (magnetic resonance
  imaging), 61
multiplace HBOT chambers,
  230, 231
multiple sclerosis
  blood–brain barrier damage
    and, 151–152
  controversy over HBOT for,
    152–153
  HBOT for, 8
  HBOT in United Kingdom
    for, 153–154
  Juliette's case, 156–157
  patient longevity with
    HBOT for, 155–156
  patient response to HBOT
    for, 61
  patient status in research on,
    154–155
  UK website for patients with,
    287
Multiple Sclerosis Society, 153
MUMS (Mothers United for
  Moral Support), 111–112, 290
Murphy-Lavoie, Heather, 185,
  266
musculoskeletal injuries
  arthritis, 174–175
  back surgery and spinal cord
    injuries, 176–177
  broken kneecap, 171–172
  calf muscle, 173

causes of, 169–170
chiropractic care for, 177–179
joint replacements and,
173–174
torn ACL, 170–171
myofascial pain syndrome,
193–194

n of 1 proofs, 253
naltrexone, 149
Namath, Joe, 77
National Brain Injury Rescue
and Rehabilitation Study
(N-BIRR), 73
National Institutes of Health,
251
Navy, U.S.
brain decompression illness
and, 47
on HBOT pressures, 152
HBOT research by, 10, 11,
25–26
hyperbaric chambers at dive
sites, 36
LSU Pilot Trial and, 74
near drowning
chronic, treatment for, 267
HBOT for, 8
patient response to HBOT
for, 60–61
repetitive daily HBOT and,
42, 51
Weiss case, 254–255
near hanging, 8
necrotizing soft tissue infections,
56
Nelson, Steve, 73
Netherlands studies, 11, 19
Neubauer, Richard
emphysema treatment and,
190–191
on 40-treatment protocol, 53
on HBOT dosages, 52
HBOT for MS and, 152–153
HBOT for neurological
diseases and, 11–12, 267
HBOT for stroke and,
127–128

on idling neurons, 41,
124–125
Medicare and, 248
Teller and, 122, 123
Tom's case and, 48
neurological deficits, post-
surgical, 166
neurological diseases, 256. *See
also* multiple sclerosis; reserve
capacity
ALS (amyotrophic lateral
sclerosis), 157–159
HBOT for, 11, 150–151
lifespan and, 149–150
overview of, 141–142
research on HBOT and, 113
treatment beyond emergency
for, 255–256
treatment delays and, 39
treatment guidelines for, 159
neurological throwaways, 113
neurons, idling, 41, 124–126
neurotoxins, 8
Neville, Charmaine, 128–129
New England Journal of Medicine,
153
New York Times, 78
nitric oxide, sexual function and,
213–214
nitrogen tetroxide, 190
poisoning, 91–92
Nitrox, 21
"normal individuals,"
neurologically, 277–278

Obama, Michelle, 73
O'Brien, Richard, 195
off-label diagnoses, 186, 224–226
off-label uses, 240–241
Oklahoma Veteran Traumatic
Brain Injury Treatment and
Recovery Act, 73
organ transplantation, 236
osteoarthritis, 175
osteocranioencephalopathy,
syndesmotic, 137
osteomyelitis, 56
outpatient HBOT, 231

government reimbursement
for, 223–224, 225–226
overdose, drug, 191–193
overdosing, HBOT, 52, 234
Owens, Terrell, 196
oxygen
decreased, in airplanes, 206
potential for receiving too
much, 218
susceptibility or individual
tolerance to, 237
*Oxygen and the Brain, the Journey
of our Lifetime* (James), 153–154
oxygen bars, 196–198
oxygen paradox, 34–35
oxygen toxicity, 233–234
oxytocin, 101
ozone therapy, 158

Page, Michael Duncan, 94–95
pain, 193–194
Parkinson's disease, 8, 148–149
Parrish, Ray, 34–35
paternalism in medicine, 261
patient advocacy, 111–112,
164–165, 260, 261, 275–276.
See also resources
Patriot Clinics, 73–74
payment for HBOT, 227, 233.
See also insurance companies;
Medicaid; Medicare
Perfusion/Metabolism
Encephalopathy Study, 51, 53,
112–115, 152, 255–256
peroxidation, 33
Perrin, D. J., 154
PET (positron-emission
tomography), 57–58
pharmaceutical companies, 148,
241, 275
physician-run HBOT facilities,
222. *See also* free-standing
HBOT facilities
Pitocin, 101
placebo effect, 58, 253
Planck, Max, 13, 250
plateaus, in repetitive daily
HBOT, 51–52, 234

PMNs (polymorphonuclear
  neutrophils), 31
pneumothorax, 237
poisoning. *See also* carbon
  monoxide poisoning
  HBOT to minimize, 90–91
  mercury, 139
  nitrogen tetroxide, 91–92
portable HBOT chambers, 229
post-concussion syndrome, 5,
  13, 69, 76
post-traumatic stress disorder
  (PTSD), 71, 208
power of oxygen, 3–4
pregnancy, 115
prescription narcotic addiction,
  TBI and, 70
prescriptions, HBOT, 221–222
pressure
  atmospheric or hydrostatic,
    4–5
  barometric, osteoarthritic
    pain and, 175
  hearing loss treatments and,
    184
  of oxygen, 3–4
  principles of, 40–41
Priestly, Joseph, 218
Provenza, Lou, 81
puerperal fever, 99–100
pulmonary contraindications,
  237
punch drunk syndrome, 77

radiation
  bone tissue damage and, 169
  for cancer therapy, 187–188
  delayed injury from, 56
  injuries, 40-treatment HBOT
    and, 53–54
  repetitive daily HBOT and,
    41–42
radiologists, SPECT imaging
  routines for, 277–278
reactive airways disease, 189–191
Reagan, Ronald, 144–145
recognition of HBOT, 9–10
referrals for HBOT, 221–222

Reflex Sympathetic Dystrophy,
  268
reimbursement issues
  chiropractic care and, 276
  insurance companies and,
    11–12, 54, 98
  Medicare, insurance
    companies and, 222–226
  as research roadblocks,
    243–244
  treatment and, 274–275
Ren, H., 247
reperfusion injuries, 32, 106–109,
  265
repetitive daily HBOT, 41–42,
  48
research. *See also* animal studies;
  Perfusion/Metabolism
  Encephalopathy Study
  on avascular necrosis of bone,
    170
  on brain injuries and HBOT,
    112–115
  case studies, 252–253
  challenges, individual
    responses and, 242–243
  on chronic concussion, 75
  diving medicine, on
    inflammatory reaction,
    36–38
  emergency situations and,
    244–250
  on HBOT, 68–69
  on HBOT dosages, 51–53
  on HBOT in veterans, 74–75
  on multiple sclerosis,
    154–155
  reimbursement issues and,
    243–244
  on secondary inflammatory
    response, 265–266
  on stroke, 127–128
  on Type II diabetes, 165
  by U.S. Navy, 10, 11, 25–26
reserve capacity
  of brain, 143–144
  carbon monoxide poisoning
    and, 88, 146–147

characteristics, 142
  manifestations of loss of,
    148–149
  Reagan's, 144–145
resources, 285–288
  special needs, 289–290
retinitis pigmentosa, 186
rheumatoid arthritis, 175
Richards, Ben, 72
roadblocks
  case study research
    acceptance as, 252–253
  corporate HBOT and,
    250–252
  disciplinary action for
    treating outside of
    approved indications,
    253–255
  emergencies and, 244–250
  off-label use meaning as,
    240–242
  overview of, 239–240
  reimbursement issues as,
    243–244, 274–275
  research challenges as,
    242–243
  sub-acute and chronic
    neurological conditions
    and, 255–256
Robin, Eugene, 263–264, 266,
  267, 268–269
Rockswold study (1992), 244–
  245, 247
Rockswolds study (2001),
  247–248
Rockswolds study (2010),
  248–249
Romanowski, Bill, 195
Ronald McDonald House
  Charities, 259, 290
Rossignol, Dan and Lanier, 133
Rotenberry, Charles, 72
Rovira, Chad
  HBOT for TBI in, 62, 77,
    80–81
  immune system in, 85–86
  motor vehicle accident,
    78–80

multiple therapies for, 63
negative effects of HBOT in, 83–84
returns to college, 84–85
sub-arachnoid hemorrhage in, 82
Rovira, Charlene, 78
Rovira, Marlon, 78, 80, 81–82, 83
Russia
  ALS study in, 158
  chronic lung disease in, 20
  HBOT for drug or alcohol injuries, 191
  HBOT for neurological diseases in, 116, 259
  HBOT for Parkinson's, 149
  HBOT for pulmonary problems, 190, 191
  HBOT for rheumatoid arthritis in, 175
  HBOT for spinal surgery in, 176, 177
  HBOT treatable diagnoses in, 55, 236–237, 256, 268
  pregnancy and fetal development problems in, 115

Sago mine survivor, 54, 88, 255
Sanchez, Cuau, 108
Schneider, Dietmar, 121
Schopick, Julia, 289
SCUBA diving, HBOT and, 21–27
secondary inflammatory response, 32, 265–266
secondary injury processes, treating, 15
seizure disorders, 42, 51, 70, 232–233, 256
semicircular canals, traumatic rupture of, 184
Semmelweis, Ignaz, 99–100
senility, non-Alzheimer's, 8
Sensible Notion, 265
Sept. 11 disaster, NY, 92

sexual regeneration, 213–214, 215
Siddiqui, Dr., 6
side effects, 232–233, 234–235
single case causality studies, 253
Single Photon Emission Computed Tomography. *See* SPECT imaging
sinuses, HBOT and, 232
skin grafts or flaps, 41–42, 57
sleep apnea, baldness and, 214–215
sleepiness, HBOT and, 232
small vessel stroke, 128
smoking, 118, 141, 175, 187, 203–205. *See also* carbon monoxide poisoning
Smotherman, Matt, 73–74
soft tissue necrosis, 56
SPECT imaging
  of AIDS patients, 184
  of autistic children, 133–134, 139
  in chronic fatigue syndrome, 183
  HBOT for TBI in veterans video with, 78
  of "normal" people, 210
  as patient documentation, 258
  predicting patient response to HBOT with, 61
  quality problems, 277–278
  repetitive daily HBOT and, 51
  of Rovira, 81, 82–83
  scientific studies of, 68
  significance of, 57–58
  use of, 58–60
spinal cord injuries, 176–177
sports concussions. *See also* concussions
  TBI and, 75–76
stem cells, 165
steroids, 169–170
Stoller, Ken, 77, 93
stress, aging and, 208–209
stroke

acute, HBOT and, 121–122
acute severe, "less is more" principle and, 40
of brain vs. of eye, 266–267
causes and characteristics of, 117–118
chronic, reclaiming function in, 267–268
current thinking and critical points on, 126–128
diabetes and, 162
in eye, 197–198, 266
first signs and early treatment, 119–121
HBOT for, 8–9, 124–126
neurorehabilitation goals for, 129–130
repetitive daily HBOT study and, 51
risk factors, 118–119
seeking HBOT treatment for, 122–124
sub-arachnoid hemorrhage, 82
sun-downing, 206
surgery, HBOT for, 167–168
synapses, 143
syphilis, 41

television, HBOT use reports on, 255
Teller, Edward, 122–124, 203
Teller, Mici, 190–191
Textbook of Hyperbaric Medicine (Jain), 106, 124, 287
Thomas, Zack, 195
tinnitus, 184
tired brain. *See* aging
tourniquets during surgery, 32, 173–174
toxins exposure, 93–94. *See also* poisoning
TPA (tissue plasminogen activator), 120
Tranchina, Phillip, 277
trauma, bone tissue damage and, 169–170
traumatic brain injury (TBI), 13. *See also* concussions

aging and, 210–212
in animals, 42–43
causes of, 75–76
conclusion on, 97–98
delayed treatment benefits,
    95–97
HBOT for veterans with,
    71–74
HBOT in emergency
    medicine and, 87–88
incidence in U.S., 67
"less is more" principle and,
    40
mild, long-term effects of,
    70–71
mild vs. severe, 76
mortality, HBOT and, 68–70
repetitive daily HBOT study
    and, 51
research on HBOT for,
    244–245, 247–249
Rovira case, 78–86
vascular headaches and,
    182–183
videos on HBOT for
    veterans with, 77–78
YouTube before-and-after
    videos of, 62, 77
traumatic mid-brain syndrome,
247
treatment experience. *See also*
    hyperbaric oxygen therapy
    choosing facilities, 227–228
    downside of, 234–235
    HBOT chambers, 228–231
    insurance coverage, 222–226
    other payment options, 227
    prescriptions, 221–222
    side effects, 232–233
    stopping reasons, 233–234

ventilators and, 233
Trimble, Vance, 215
Turkey, HBOT in, 193–194, 268

ulcers, on heels, 125, 186
Undersea and Hyperbaric
    Medical Society (UHMS),
    272–273
    Hyperbaric Oxygen Therapy
        Committee of, 129–130,
        248, 250
    website, 288
United Kingdom. *See also*
    England
    HBOT for MS in, 153–154
Universal Gas Laws, 22–24

vaccines, autism and, 131
Vair, Margaux, 72
Van Meter, Keith, 8, 35, 45–46,
    51
Vancouver Canucks, 195
ventilators, HBOT while on, 233
Verges, J., 175
vertigo, 184
veterans
    Afghanistan and Iraq, TBI
        and dementia in, 213
    brain injuries and, 69, 70
    DoD's HBOT studies for,
        74–75
    HBOT for brain injuries in,
        71–73
    videos of HBOT for TBI in,
        77–78
    World War II, alcohol and
        tobacco use by, 204–205
Viagra, 213–214
videos, 62, 71–72, 77–78, 128–
    129, 257–258

Vila, J. F., 268
Visger, George, 77
vision impairment, 185–186

wallet biopsies, 274
The War Within (video), 72
website, 285
Weil, Andrew, 10
Weiss, Jeffrey, 254–255
Wellbutrin, 240–241
white blood cells, 31–33, 37
white matter injuries, 128, 151–
    152, 154, 184
Whyte, John, 272, 273
Winfrey, Oprah, 202–203
Workers' Compensation
    insurance, 253, 257
wound healing. *See also* diabetic
    foot wounds
    80-treatment protocol for,
        52–53
    40-treatment protocol for,
        53–54
    HBOT for, 5–6, 9
    inflammatory reaction and,
        30
    selected problem, HBOT
        approved for, 56
wounds, chronic, 41–43, 267,
    272–274. *See also* diabetic foot
    wounds; stroke
Wright, Jim, 76

Yahoo group (HBOT for
    Health), 287
YouTube, before-and-after
    videos on, 62

Zyban, 240–241